Cardiothoracic Surgery

Editor

JOHN H. BRAXTON

SURGICAL CLINICS
OF NORTH AMERICA

www.surgical.theclinics.com

Consulting Editor
RONALD F. MARTIN

August 2017 • Volume 97 • Number 4

ELSEVIER

1600 John F. Kennedy Boulevard • Suite 1800 • Philadelphia, Pennsylvania, 19103-2899

http://www.surgical.theclinics.com

SURGICAL CLINICS OF NORTH AMERICA Volume 97, Number 4

August 2017 ISSN 0039–6109, ISBN-13: 978-0-323-53257-0

Editor: John Vassallo, j.vassallo@elsevier.com

Developmental Editor: Colleen Dietzler

Surgical Clinics of North America (ISSN 0039–6109) is published bimonthly by Elsevier Inc., 360 Park Avenue South, New York, NY 10010-1710. Months of publication are February, April, June, August, October, and December. Business and Editorial Offices: 1600 John F. Kennedy Blvd., Suite 1800, Philadelphia, PA 19103-2899. Periodicals postage paid at New York, NY and additional mailing offices. Subscription prices are $386.00 per year for US individuals, $756.00 per year for US institutions, $100.00 per year for US students and residents, $469.00 per year for Canadian individuals, $958.00 per year for Canadian institutions, $525.00 for international individuals, $958.00 per year for international institutions and $250.00 per year for Canadian and foreign students/residents. To receive student/resident rate, orders must be accompanied by name of affiliated institution, date of term, and the *signature* of program/residency coordinator on institution letterhead. Orders will be billed at individual rate until proof of status is received. Foreign air speed delivery is included in all *Clinics* subscription prices. All prices are subject to change without notice. POSTMASTER: Send address changes to *Surgical Clinics*, Elsevier Health Sciences Division, Subscription Customer Service, 3251 Riverport Lane, Maryland Heights, MO 63043. **Customer Service (orders, claims, online, change of address): Telephone: 1-800-654-2452 (U.S. and Canada); 314-447-8871 (outside U.S. and Canada). Fax: 314-447-8029. E-mail: journalscustomerservice-usa@elsevier.com (for print support); journalsonline support-usa@elsevier.com (for online support).**

Reprints. For copies of 100 or more, of articles in this publication, please contact the Commercial Reprints Department, Elsevier Inc., 360 Park Avenue South, New York, New York 10010-1710. Tel. 212-633-3874, Fax: 212-633-3820, E-mail: reprints@elsevier.com.

The Surgical Clinics of North America is also published in Spanish by McGraw-Hill Interamericana Editores S.A., P.O. Box 5-237 06500 Mexico D.F. Mexico; and in Portuguese by Interlivros Edicoes Ltda., Rua Comandante Coelho 1085, CEP 21250, Rio de Janeiro, Brazil; and in Greek by Paschalidis Medical Publications, Athens Greece.

The Surgical Clinics of North America is covered in *MEDLINE/PubMed (Index Medicus)*, *EMBASE/Excerpta Medica*, *Current Contents/Clinical Medicine*, *Current Contents/Life Sciences*, *Science Citation Index*, and *ISI/BIOMED*.

Contributors

CONSULTING EDITOR

RONALD F. MARTIN, MD, FACS
Colonel (ret.), United States Army Reserve, Department of Surgery, York Hospital, York, Maine

EDITOR

JOHN H. BRAXTON, MD, MBA, FACS, FACC
Member, Structural Heart Services, Chief, Section of Cardiothoracic Surgery, Marshfield Clinic, Saint Joseph Hospital, Marshfield, Wisconsin

AUTHORS

JOHN H. BRAXTON, MD, MBA, FACS, FACC
Member, Structural Heart Services, Chief, Section of Cardiothoracic Surgery, Marshfield Clinic, Saint Joseph Hospital, Marshfield, Wisconsin

ROBERT J. CERFOLIO, MD, MBA
Professor, Chief of Thoracic Surgery, JH Estes Endowed Chair for Lung Cancer Research, Division of Cardiothoracic Surgery, University of Alabama-Birmingham Medical Center, University of Alabama at Birmingham, Birmingham, Alabama

ERIC J. CHARLES, MD
Surgery Resident, Department of Surgery, University of Virginia, Charlottesville, Virginia

WASEEM CHAUDHRY, MD
Cardiovascular Institute, Maine Medical Center, Portland, Maine; Tufts University School of Medicine, Boston, Massachusetts

MYLAN C. COHEN, MD, MPH
Cardiac Imaging and Diagnostics, Cardiovascular Institute, Maine Medical Center, Portland, Maine; Tufts University School of Medicine, Boston, Massachusetts

JOHN V. CONTE, MD
Professor, Division of Cardiac Surgery, Johns Hopkins Hospital, Baltimore, Maryland

SARAH J. COUNTS, DO
Fellow, Cardiothoracic Surgery, Yale-New Haven Hospital, Yale School of Medicine, New Haven, Connecticut

TODD C. CRAWFORD, MD
Resident, General Surgery, Hugh R. Sharp Endowed Cardiac Surgery Research Fellow, Division of Cardiac Surgery, Johns Hopkins Hospital, Baltimore, Maryland

ANDREW P. DHANASOPON, MD
Fellow, Cardiothoracic Surgery, Section of Thoracic Surgery, Yale-New Haven Hospital, Yale School of Medicine, New Haven, Connecticut

THOMAS FABIAN, MD
Chief, Thoracic Surgery, Associate Professor, Endowed Chair of Catherine Sheer Britton Chair of Surgery, Department of Surgery, Albany Medical College, Albany, New York

LOIC FABRICANT, MD
University of Vermont Medical Center, Burlington, Vermont

JOHN A. FEDERICO, MD, FACS, FRCSC
Chief, Thoracic Surgery, Department of Surgery, Kalispell Regional Medical Center, Kalispell, Montana

DOUGLAS W. HADEN, MD
Medical Intensivist, Carolinas HealthCare System, Charlotte, North Carolina

ROBERT S.D. HIGGINS, MD, MSHA, FACS
The William Stewart Halsted Professor, Department of Surgery, Chair and Surgeon-in-Chief, Johns Hopkins Medicine, Baltimore, Maryland

AHMET KILIC, MD, FACS
Director, Heart Transplantation and Mechanical Circulatory Support, Co-Director, Advanced Heart Failure Program, Vice Director, Clinical and Academic Affairs, Associate Professor, Division of Cardiac Surgery, The Ohio State University Wexner Medical Center, Columbus, Ohio

ANTHONY W. KIM, MD
Chief and Professor of Clinical Surgery, Division of Thoracic Surgery, Keck School of Medicine, University of Southern California, Los Angeles, California

IRVING L. KRON, MD
Chair, Division of Thoracic and Cardiovascular Surgery, University of Virginia, Charlottesville, Virginia

KEVIN W. LOBDELL, MD
Director of Quality, Sanger Heart and Vascular Institute, Carolinas HealthCare System, Charlotte, North Carolina

JAMES H. MEHAFFEY, MD
Surgery Resident, Department of Surgery, University of Virginia, Charlottesville, Virginia

KSHITIJ P. MISTRY, MD
Intensivisit, Cardiovascular Critical Care, Boston Children's Hospital, Boston, Massachusetts

MITCH NOROTSKY, MD
University of Vermont Medical Center, Burlington, Vermont

JOSEPH J. PLATZ, MD
University of Vermont Medical Center, Burlington, Vermont

KELLY S. RASMUSSEN, MS, RN, NP-C, AACC
Member, Structural Heart Services, Valve Clinic Coordinator, Department of Cardiology, Marshfield Clinic, Saint Joseph Hospital, Marshfield, Wisconsin

JUAN A. SANCHEZ, MD
Associate Professor, Division of Cardiac Surgery, Johns Hopkins Hospital, Baltimore, Maryland

SARAH A. SCHUBERT, MD
Surgery Resident, Division of Thoracic and Cardiovascular Surgery, Department of Surgery, University of Virginia, Charlottesville, Virginia

THOMAS A. SCHWANN, MD, MBA
Department of Surgery, University of Toledo College of Medicine and Life Sciences, Toledo, Ohio

MILIND S. SHAH, MD, FACC, FSCAI
Member, Structural Heart Services, Chief, Section of Cardiology, Marshfield Clinic, Saint Joseph Hospital, Marshfield, Wisconsin

JOHN MICHAEL SMITH, MD, FACS, FACC, FAHA, FACP
Division of Cardiothoracic Surgery, Good Samaritan Hospital, TriHealth Heart Institute, Cincinnati, Ohio

DANIEL G. TANG, MD, FACS, FACC
Assistant Professor, Division of Cardiothoracic Surgery, Virginia Commonwealth University, Richmond, Virginia

BENJAMIN WEI, MD
Assistant Professor, Division of Cardiothoracic Surgery, University of Alabama-Birmingham Medical Center, University of Alabama at Birmingham, Birmingham, Alabama

MUHAMMAD HABIB ZUBAIR, MD
Division of General Surgery, Good Samaritan Hospital, TriHealth Heart Institute, Cincinnati, Ohio

Contents

This article will address common cardiac conditions that require evaluation prior to noncardiac surgery, characterization of urgency and the risk associated with surgical procedures, calculation of preoperative risk assessment, indications for diagnostic testing to quantify cardiac risk, and perioperative strategies to minimize the risk of cardiac complications.

Modalities to detect and characterize lung cancer are generally divided into those that are invasive [endobronchial ultrasound (EBUS), esophageal ultrasound (EUS), and electromagnetic navigational bronchoscopy (ENMB)] versus noninvasive [chest radiography (CXR), computed tomography (CT), positron emission tomography (PET), and magnetic resonance imaging (MRI)]. This chapter describes these modalities, the literature supporting their use, and delineates what tests to use to best evaluate the patient with lung cancer.

Lung cancer screening has demonstrated a reduction in lung cancer mortality by 20%. Annual low-dose computed tomography examination in high-risk individuals is now recommended by multiple national health care organizations and is covered under Medicare and Medicaid services. The impact of this public health intervention is projected to increase the case load for the thoracic surgery workforce.

Many esophageal patients with cancer were undertreated for their malignancy, which played a role in the poor long-term survival rate. Surgeons have been eager to see real change in short-term and long-term outcomes. Dramatic and profound advances continue

Coronary artery disease remains a formidable challenge to clinicians. Percutaneous interventions and surgical techniques for myocardial revascularization continue to improve. Concurrently, in light of emerging data, multiple practice guidelines have been published guiding clinicians in their therapeutic decisions. The multidisciplinary Heart Team concept needs to be embraced by all cardiovascular providers to optimize patient outcomes.

Degenerative mitral valve disease causing mitral regurgitation is the most common organic valve pathology and is classified based on leaflet motion. The "French correction" mitral valve repair method restores normal valvular anatomy with extensive leaflet resection, chordal manipulation, and rigid annuloplasty. The American correction attempts to restore normal valve function through minimal leaflet resection, flexible annuloplasty, and use of artificial chordae. These differing methods of mitral valve repair reflect an evolution in principles, but both require understanding of the valve pathology and correction of leaflet prolapse and annular dilatation. Adhering to those unifying principles and ensuring that no patient leaves the operating room with significant persistent mitral regurgitation produces durable results and satisfactory patient outcomes.

Significant improvement and development have occurred in minimally invasive cardiac surgery over the past 20 years. Although most studies have consistently demonstrated equivalent or improved outcomes compared with conventional cardiac surgery, with significantly shorter recovery times, adoption continues to be limited. In addition, cost data have been inconsistent. Further ongoing trials are needed to help determine the exact roles for these innovative procedures.

 Video content accompanies this article at http://www.surgical. theclinics.com/.

Patients with inoperable, high-risk, and intermediate-risk aortic stenosis can now be treated with transcatheter aortic valve replacement. Centers for Medicare and Medicaid Services and the Food and Drug Administration selectively choose centers based on experience and require a collaborative, multidisciplinary team approach in the treatment and decision making for these patients. The work-up has been streamlined. Gated multislice computed tomography angiogram has emerged as the gold standard for assessment of valve anatomy and sizing of the transcatheter heart valve. Assessment of risk has evolved to include a more comprehensive functional and frailty evaluation. Long term-results are needed before the expansion of transcatheter aortic valve replacement into the low-risk category.

Robert S.D. Higgins, Ahmet Kilic, and Daniel G. Tang

More than 5 million Americans suffer from heart failure and more than 250,000 die annually. Cardiac surgery, as applied to advanced heart failure, has evolved significantly in the past 50 years. Current therapeutic interventions are focused on the appropriate assessment of myocardial dysfunction as a means to select the right patient for the appropriate procedure using state-of-the-art myocardial viability testing and metabolic testing to determine candidacy for conventional interventions, mechanical devices, or transplant. Advances in mechanical circulatory support with more efficient and less morbid ventricular assist devises offer the potential to change the trajectory of this growing epidemiologic dilemma.

SURGICAL CLINICS
OF NORTH AMERICA

THE CLINICS ARE AVAILABLE ONLINE!
Access your subscription at:
www.theclinics.com

Foreword

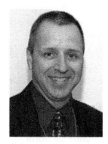

Ronald F. Martin, MD, FACS
Consulting Editor

How we physicians organize ourselves in medicine is an interesting challenge. In the early part of the twentieth century, patient care was progressively becoming hospital-based and became predominantly so as the century progressed. The main groupings of physicians were based on their respective hospital-based functions. Not surprisingly, most were either on the surgical side of the group or on the medical side. As specialization increased, groups of doctors who didn't really belong to one side or the other exclusively started to develop in areas such as anesthesiology, pathology, radiology, transfusion medicine, and so forth. By the end of the century, even these larger groupings were beginning to make less sense.

Subspecialization and hyperspecialization further added to the incongruence of simply being on the surgical side or the medical side of the coin. The more surgery and medicine fragmented, the more necessary it became to forge closer relations across the medical-surgical divide than it did to align closely within either the medicine or the surgery groups.

As we progress toward the end of the first quarter of this century, an even greater divide exists between the hospital-based world of patient care and the outpatient world (medical home, if you will). For many reasons, we are trending to providing as much care and prevention, with emphasis on prevention, outside the hospital-based environment as we can. Laudable as this goal may be, it is creating a group of physicians who will rarely or never see the inside of a hospital anymore, and by corollary, a group of physicians who will never see an outpatient office unless she or he is the patient.

In my opinion, the disconnect between the outpatient and inpatient worlds, while seemingly unavoidable and to a large part beneficial, has one major unintended consequence: it will create by its very structure a widening knowledge gap about what can be done for patients in each "camp." That may make it more likely that some will try to put patients on one side or the other simply because it transfers responsibility for solving the problem to someone else—not always the best reason or choice.

One of the logical extensions of widening the gap between inpatient and outpatient care is that the outpatient portion of patient care will become primarily a

Surg Clin N Am 97 (2017) xiii–xv
http://dx.doi.org/10.1016/j.suc.2017.05.003
0039-6109/17/© 2017 Published by Elsevier Inc.

surgical.theclinics.com

prevention-based process with triage as its main responsibility for patients who are becoming sick—the inbound side. While on leaving the hospital—the outbound side—the main role of outpatient providers will be implementing strategies for recovery based on plans made by inpatient providers, until such a time as prevention becomes the main focus again. Those who work on the inpatient side of the equation will largely be taking care of people with whom they have no prior relationship. Their main responsibility will be fielding triage calls for their services that will have a wide range of validity and then trying to assemble teams with the capacity to solve the immediate problems of the patients until we can safely return them to the outpatient world.

The above proposal guarantees a certain number of handoffs that will all be potential events for degraded health care and unforced errors. The unresolved question is, will it in the long run create fewer problems than our prior system with its sometimes improved continuity but, on average, perhaps decreased expertise in certain areas?

No matter how one feels about the changes we see in health care organization, we are likely going to see greater trends in this direction of fragmentation. As a result, we will see greater numbers of subgroups form and a greater numbers of teams consisting of a wider array of team members (most of whom will not be doctors). This is hardly new to any of us.

Cardiac surgery has been at the forefront of understanding and addressing this concept. Since its earliest days, it has understood the need to concentrate and focus effort. Perhaps better than any other discipline, our cardiac brethren have understood the need to merge patient care with applied science, basic science, biomedical engineering, critical care, image acquisition and analysis, data gathering and analysis, and teamwork.

When I was training as a resident, it was clear to me that our cardiac surgeons, cardiologists, cardiac anesthesiologists, and intensivists had a better understanding of the importance and need for cooperation over competition in order to deliver better care. I can't say that everybody always appeared as if they were enjoying the interdependence, but they all seemed to get the need for it. The willingness to share information among themselves was more evolved at that time than with other disciplines I was aware of. Even the willingness to share information between different institutions was revelatory to me at that time. It came as the complete opposite of a shock when Cardiac Services was the first new department we had created in decades after taking members from cardiac surgery, cardiology, and cardiac anesthesiology and coalescing them into one coherent group. It seemed like the handwriting was on the wall for all of us.

It has been a while since that department was formed. Our Guest Editor for this issue, Dr John Braxton, and I were working together in Maine when all that took place. We later had the opportunity to work together in Wisconsin, where we tried to apply some of what we had learned during our time in Maine there as well. I am deeply indebted to Dr Braxton and his colleagues for providing us with this excellent collection of articles on cardiac and thoracic surgery. Even though many of us general surgeons will have precious little overlap with the direct process of cardiac surgery, we will all operate on patients with varying degrees of cardiac health.

Change to our lives, careers, and the way we practice is coming whether we like it or not. It is always important to remember where we came from, but we should not dwell on it to the exclusion of figuring out where we should be going. We will all need to try to understand our challenges as well as our resources as we make our attempts to change our own organizational structures for the benefit of our patients. Learning the successes and mistakes from those who have gone before us will be better than simply learning by replicating the mistakes or stumbling on the successes. I hope this issue gives every reader a better understanding of not just the clinical issues discussed but also the teamwork of how this information was gathered and brought to us.

Ronald F. Martin, MD, FACS
Colonel (ret.), United States Army Reserve
Department of Surgery
York Hospital
16 Hospital Drive, Suite A
York, ME 03909, USA

E-mail address:
rmartin@yorkhospital.com

Preface

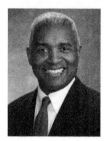

John H. Braxton, MD, MBA, FACS, FACC
Editor

In the last issue dedicated to surgical disease of the chest, the focus was on cardiac and aortic diseases with which the editors sought to create a reference for the general surgeon. After surveying general surgeons, it was decided to create an issue that further built on that reference concept for general surgeons and thoracic surgeons in training. To that end, this issue was born. In order to create a useful reference, we focused this issue on disease of the chest, more specifically disease of the heart and lung.

In the last seven years, the practice of cardiothoracic surgery has undergone exciting changes. New technologies and techniques have been developed and embraced. First, in the field of thoracic surgery, lung cancer screening guidelines have been issued, newer diagnostic modalities have been introduced, and less invasive surgical techniques have shifted the field. In the disease of the heart, catheter-based modalities for aortic valve disease have significantly evolved and changed the landscape. Further understanding of the physiology of mitral valve disease has provided the basis for the American repair. There has also been advancement in the techniques for less invasive cardiac surgery. Finally, changes in team dynamics and intensive care medicine have shifted the cardiothoracic surgeon's daily routine to now include acting as integral members of various team-based care models, such as a valve care team, coronary care group, or intensive care unit team member.

In this issue, we hope to provide the reader with a better understanding of the breadth of changes and a better understanding of the progress that has been made in regards to surgical diseases of the chest. But given these vast changes, a few notable advancements have intentionally been left out of this issue, such as disease

Surg Clin N Am 97 (2017) xvii–xviii
http://dx.doi.org/10.1016/j.suc.2017.05.002
0039-6109/17/© 2017 Published by Elsevier Inc.

surgical.theclinics.com

of the aorta and the burgeoning field of percutaneous mitral valve disease. The reader is encouraged to seek information elsewhere.

John H. Braxton, MD, MBA, FACS, FACC
Section of Cardiothoracic Surgery
Marshfield Clinic/Saint Joseph Hospital
Structural Heart Services
1000 North Oak Avenue, 2C2
Marshfield, WI 54449, USA

E-mail address:
braxton.john@marshfieldclinic.org

Cardiac Screening in the Noncardiac Surgery Patient

Waseem Chaudhry, MD[a,b,*], Mylan C. Cohen, MD, MPH[a,b,c]

KEYWORDS

- Noncardiac surgery • Coronary artery disease • Perioperative cardiac screening
- Myocardial infarction • Risk assessment • Unstable angina

KEY POINTS

- Cardiac conditions in patients undergoing noncardiac surgery confer significant risk of morbidity and mortality, which are largely preventable by implementing appropriate cardiac risk stratification prior to surgery and individually tailoring perioperative therapy to reduce risk.
- A successful surgical outcome requires a team approach and shared decision-making involving the primary care provider, cardiologist, anesthesiologist, surgeon performing the procedure, and the patient.
- With the aging population, increasing number of annual surgeries, and dynamic US health care focused toward cost-effectiveness and appropriate utilization of resources and therapies, the need for evidence-based practice to minimize perioperative surgical morbidity and mortality is of paramount importance.

INTRODUCTION

An estimated 234 million annual noncardiac surgical procedures are performed worldwide, translating to about 1 surgery for every 25 people.[1] In developed countries, the rate of perioperative death and major complications from inpatient surgery has been reported to be 0.4% to 0.8% and 3% to 16%, respectively.[2,3] Up to 42% of these are caused by cardiac complications.[4] Nearly half of the adverse events in these studies were identified as preventable. Similarly, over 50 million surgical procedures are performed annually in the Unites States.[5] The estimated perioperative cardiac complications from these surgical procedures have been reported to be 1.4% to 3.9% in pooled analyses.[6]

Disclosures: None.
[a] Cardiovascular Institute, Maine Medical Center, 22 Bramhall Street, Portland, ME 04102, USA; [b] Cardiovascular Institute, Tufts University School of Medicine, Boston, MA, USA; [c] Cardiac Imaging and Diagnostics, Maine Medical Center, 22 Bramhall Street, Portland, ME 04102, USA
* Corresponding author. Cardiovascular Institute, Maine Medical Center, 22 Bramhall Street, Portland, ME 04102.
E-mail address: COHENM@mmc.org

Surg Clin N Am 97 (2017) 717–732
http://dx.doi.org/10.1016/j.suc.2017.03.010
0039-6109/17/© 2017 Elsevier Inc. All rights reserved.

surgical.theclinics.com

The elderly population requires surgery 4 times as often as the younger population, and the proportion of the elderly population is increasing due in part to improved survival from coronary artery disease. It is estimated that the number of patients undergoing surgery will increase by 25% by 2020, and surgical complications will increase by 100%.[7] Cardiac complications represent about half of total perioperative surgical complications. Therefore, surgical safety represents a substantial global public health concern. Appropriately defining the cardiac risk of noncardiac surgery lays the foundation for successful surgical planning including accurate communication of procedural risk/benefit ratio to the patient and hence facilitating shared decision making, appropriate timing of surgery, identification of high-risk patients, and implementation of preventive medical treatment, thereby leading to positive outcome.

This article will address common cardiac conditions that require evaluation prior to noncardiac surgery, characterization of urgency and the risk associated with surgical procedures, calculation of preoperative risk assessment, indications for diagnostic testing to quantify cardiac risk, and perioperative strategies to minimize the risk of cardiac complications.

CARDIAC CONDITIONS REQUIRING EVALUATION IN PREOPERATIVE RISK ASSESSMENT
Coronary Artery Disease

Perioperative morbidity and mortality due to coronary artery disease (CAD) represent the most common complications of noncardiac surgery. CAD affects an estimated 6.2% of the US adult population, with higher prevalence in men than in women (7.6% and 5%, respectively).[8] Perioperative incidence of major adverse cardiac events (MACE) of death or myocardial infarction (MI) caused by CAD depends on the baseline risk related to prior cardiac events. Patients with chronic stable angina, previous MI, and electrocardiographic signs of ischemia suffer higher rates of perioperative MI and cardiac death.[9] Livhits and colleagues[10] reported a substantial decrease in postoperative MI rate as the length of time from MI to operation increased (0–30 days = 32.8%, 31–60 days = 18.7%, 61–90 days = 8.4%, and 91–180 days = 5.9%); the 30-day mortality rate followed a similar trend. This risk was decreased by prior coronary revascularization performed at the time of MI. Based on these data, American College of Cardiology (ACC)/American Heart Association (AHA) guidelines recommend at least a 60-day interval between an acute coronary syndrome (ACS) and elective noncardiac surgery.[11]

Heart Failure

The prevalence of heart failure (HF) in the United States is 5.7 million cases, and this number is projected to increase to over 8 million cases by 2030.[8] Patients with clinical signs and symptoms of decompensated HF or a history of HF are at significantly higher risk of perioperative complications. Widely used indices of cardiac risk incorporate HF as an independent predictor of perioperative MACE. van Diepen and colleagues[12] studied over 38,000 patients and found that the 30-day postoperative mortality rate was significantly higher in patients with nonischemic HF (9.3%), ischemic HF (9.2%), and atrial fibrillation (AF) (6.4%) than in those with CAD (2.9%), highlighting the higher risk of postoperative death in patients with active HF compared with those with stable CAD.

Preserved Versus Reduced Ejection Fraction and Symptomatic Versus Asymptomatic Heart Failure

Although symptomatic decompensated HF carries the highest perioperative risk, severely decreased (<30%) left ventricular ejection fraction (LVEF) is an independent predictor of perioperative MACE, death, and long-term mortality.[13] Kazmers and colleagues[14] reported significantly worse survival after surgery for those with an LVEF less than 29% than for those with an LVEF greater than 29%. Current guidelines acknowledge limited data on perioperative risk stratification related to diastolic dysfunction. However, the guidelines emphasize that diastolic dysfunction with and without systolic dysfunction has been associated with a significantly higher rate of MACE, prolonged length of stay, and higher rates of postoperative HF.[15] Guidelines also note that the effect of asymptomatic LV dysfunction on perioperative outcome is known, although there is mention only of a single center prospective cohort study reporting evidence of increased perioperative cardiac risk in patients with asymptomatic LV dysfunction. Flu and colleagues[16] followed 1005 patients undergoing elective vascular surgery and found the highest 30-day cardiovascular event rate in patients with symptomatic HF (49%), followed by those with asymptomatic systolic LV dysfunction (23%), asymptomatic diastolic LV dysfunction (18%), and normal LV function (10%).

Valvular Heart Disease

Symptomatic and hemodynamically significant valvular disease confers risk of adverse outcomes to patients undergoing elective noncardiac surgery. ACC/AHA 2014 guidelines make several recommendations to reduce perioperative risk before elective noncardiac surgery[11]:

- Patients with clinically suspected moderate or greater degree of valvular stenosis or regurgitation should undergo perioperative echocardiography within 1 year of the elective noncardiac surgery or earlier if there is a change in clinical status.
- Symptomatic patients with severe valvular stenosis or regurgitation who meet standard indications for valvular intervention consisting of valve replacement or repair should undergo valvular intervention.
- Asymptomatic patients with severe aortic stenosis, severe mitral stenosis, severe aortic regurgitation with normal LVEF and severe mitral regurgitation should be monitored with intraoperative and postoperative invasive hemodynamics monitoring.

Aortic and Mitral Stenosis

The original Cardiac Risk Index published in 1977 incorporated significant valvular stenosis as 1 of the 9 independent predictors of cardiac risk in noncardiac surgical procedures.[17] The mechanism of MACE in severe aortic stenosis is related to the unfavorable hemodynamic alterations (hypotension and tachycardia) associated with the use of anesthetics and surgical stress. Cardiac risk associated with severe aortic stenosis (AS) has declined in recent years because of advancements in anesthetic and surgical approaches. Agarwal and colleagues[18] demonstrated that patients with moderate or severe AS undergoing nonemergency, noncardiac surgery had double the rate of 30-day mortality compared with propensity score-matched patients without aortic stenosis (2.1% vs 1.0%). Patients with AS also suffered postoperative MI 3 times more frequently than patients without AS (3.0 vs 1.1%).[18]

Guidelines recommend aortic valve replacement (AVR) before elective noncardiac surgery for patients with symptomatic or hemodynamically significant AS.[11] For patients who are considered high risk or ineligible for surgical AVR, guidelines delineate 3 options. The first is proceeding with noncardiac surgery with invasive hemodynamic monitoring and optimization of volume status to prevent significant drop in preload, as these patients are preload dependent to maintain adequate cardiac output. The second option includes percutaneous balloon dilation prior to noncardiac surgery with acceptable procedural safety, with the mortality rate being 2% to 3% and the stroke rate being 1% to 2%.[19] This approach is a bridging strategy to AVR, as recurrence and mortality rates approach 50% by 6 months after balloon valvuloplasty.[19] Transcatheter aortic valve implantation (TAVI) is a third option prior to elective noncardiac surgery, as this procedure has been demonstrated to have superior outcomes for patients who are not eligible for surgical AVR, with a 1-year mortality rate of 30.7% versus 50.7% with standard therapy.[20] Similar efficacy has been reported for patients who are at high risk for surgical AVR, with a 1-year mortality rate of 24.2% for TAVI versus 26.8% for surgical AVR.[21]

Furthermore, recent data from PARTNER 2 trial (Placement of Aortic Transcatheter Valves) indicate that TAVI might be a reasonable option in patients with intermediate surgical risk. The trial randomly assigned 2032 intermediate risk patients with severe AS to either SAVR or TAVI (76.3% with transfemoral access and 23.7% with transthoracic access) and found that the primary end points of all-cause death and disabling stroke at 2 years were similar in both groups (19.3% in TAVI vs 21.1% in SAVR group, $P = .25$). The trial also demonstrated that TAVI resulted in larger AV area, lower rates of acute kidney injury, severe bleeding, and new-onset atrial fibrillation than SAVR. Surgery, however, resulted in fewer major vascular complications and less paravalvular artic regurgitation.[22]

Similar to the case of severe AS, patients with severe mitral stenosis are also at increased risk for noncardiac surgery and should be managed similarly. Special attention should be given to intravascular volume to maintain adequate forward cardiac output without excessive rises in left atrial pressure and pulmonary capillary wedge pressure which could lead to pulmonary edema.

Aortic and Mitral Regurgitation

Data indicate that left-sided regurgitant lesions confer increased cardiac risk during noncardiac surgery more than stenotic valvular disease. Lai and colleagues[23] demonstrated that patients with moderate-to-severe aortic regurgitation (AR) and severe AR undergoing noncardiac surgery had 5 times higher in-hospital mortality (9.0% vs 1.8%; $P = .008$) and 3 times higher morbidity (16.2% vs 5.4%; $P = .003$) than case-matched controls without AR. In this study, the significant predictors of in-hospital death included depressed LVEF less than 55% and creatinine greater than 2 mg/dL. Bajaj and colleagues[24] reported patients with moderate-to-severe mitral regurgitation (MR) and severe MR had worse 30-day composite outcomes (death and postoperative MI, HF, and stroke) than patients without MR. In this study, the significant predictors of adverse postoperative outcomes after noncardiac surgery were LVEF less than 35%, ischemic MR, diabetes, and prior carotid endarterectomy.

In the absence of trials regarding perioperative management, guidelines emphasize that patients with moderate-to-severe AR and MR, and severe AR and MR, can be monitored with invasive hemodynamics and echocardiography and can be admitted postoperatively to an intensive care unit setting.[11]

Arrhythmia and Conduction Disorders

Although trials studying the perioperative risk conferred by presence of arrhythmia are lacking, asymptomatic arrhythmias do not appear to be associated with increased risk of postoperative MACE. Mahla and colleagues[25] performed continuous electrocardiographic monitoring and reported that asymptomatic ventricular arrhythmias, including couplets and nonsustained ventricular tachycardia (NSVT), were not associated with increased MACE after noncardiac surgery. In the Original Cardiac Risk Index, supraventricular and ventricular arrhythmia were identified as independent risk factors for perioperative cardiac events.[17] However, subsequent studies indicated a lower level of risk.[26] Although frequent ventricular premature beats and NSVT predispose to development of intraoperative and postoperative arrhythmias, they do not confer increased risk of nonfatal MI or cardiac death perioperatively.[25,27]

Pulmonary Vascular Disease

Data on patients with pulmonary arterial hypertension undergoing noncardiac surgery show consistently high rates of complications. Mortality rates in this cohort range 4% to 26%, and cardiac and/or respiratory failure rates range from 6% to 42%.[28,29] High rates of complications are related to a variety of factors that can occur during the perioperative period, including worsening hypoxia, pulmonary hypertension, and right ventricular dysfunction. Therefore, guidelines recommend continuation of chronic pulmonary vasodilator therapy in the perioperative period (Class I) and preoperative evaluation by a pulmonary hypertension specialist before high-risk, elective, noncardiac surgery (Class IIa).[11] Please see **Fig. 1** for classes of recommendations in guidelines.[11]

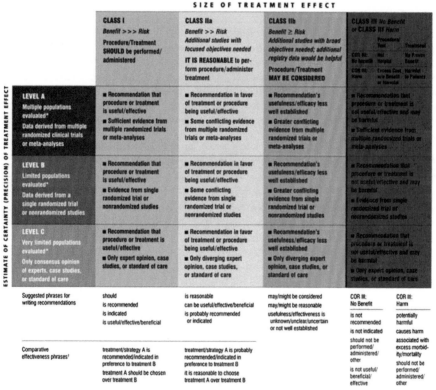

Fig. 1. Treatment recommendations. (*From* Fleisher LA, Fleischmann KE, Auerbach AD, et al. 2014 ACC/AHA guideline on perioperative cardiovascular evaluation and management of patients undergoing noncardiac surgery: a report of the American College of Cardiology/American Heart Association Task Force on practice guidelines. J Am Coll Cardiol 2014;64:e281; with permission.)

CALCULATION OF RISK TO PREDICT PERIOPERATIVE CARDIAC MORBIDITY

Different surgical procedures are associated with different risk of MACE. Guidelines recommend using any of the 3 validated risk prediction tools to predict the risk of MACE in patients undergoing noncardiac surgery (Class IIa).[11] Guidelines do not recommend further preoperative testing for patients with low risk of perioperative MACE (Class III).[11] Following are 3 risk prediction tools that have been recommended in guidelines.

The Revised Cardiac Risk Index

The Revised Cardiac Risk Index (RCRI) is a simple, well-known and easy to use tool in clinical practice to predict perioperative risk of major cardiac events. It was derived and validated in a prospective cohort of 4315 patients and consists of 6 predictors of risk, including high-risk surgery (defined as intrathoracic, intraperitoneal, or suprainguinal vascular surgery), history of ischemic heart disease, history of congestive HF, history of cerebrovascular disease, preoperative treatment with insulin, and preoperative creatinine greater than 2 mg/dL.[26] Patients with at least 2 predictors of risks would have elevated risk of MACE. Presence of at least 2 factors was associated with a MACE rate of 4.0% in a derivation cohort and 7.0% in a validation cohort.[26]

National Surgical Quality Improvement Program Myocardial Infarction and Cardiac Arrest Calculator

The American College of Surgeons created 2 new risk prediction tools by utilizing prospectively collected National Surgical Quality Improvement Program (NSQIP) data on more than 1 million operations performed in over 525 US hospitals.[30] The NSQIP Myocardial Infarction and Cardiac Arrest (MICA) score 200,000 hundred thousand patients in both derivation and validation cohorts. The NSQIP MICA includes adjusted odds ratios for various surgical sites, with inguinal hernia as the reference group, and predicts the risk of cardiac arrest and MI. The derived risk index was found to be robust and outperformed the RCRI in discriminative power.[31]

National Surgical Quality Improvement Program Surgical Risk Calculator

The NSQIP Surgical Risk Calculator predicts procedure-specific risk for a diverse group of outcomes. It was created in 2013 using specific current procedural terminology code of the specific procedure being performed.[30] It incorporates 21 patient-specific variables and calculates the risk of 10 outcomes including MACE and death. This sophisticated risk calculator may provide the most precise estimation of surgery-specific risk despite not being validated in an external population outside the NSQIP. Current guidelines recommend use of either the NSQIP MICA risk index or the NSQIP Surgical Risk calculator, or the RCRI for preoperative risk assessment.

DEFINITIONS OF URGENCY AND PROCEDURE-SPECIFIC RISK

Perioperative risk is substantially impacted by the urgency and the type of procedure a patient will undergo. The guidelines define an emergency procedure as life- or limb-threatening in which there is time for no or very limited or minimal clinical evaluation, typically within less than 6 hours.[11] An urgent procedure is defined as one in which there may be time for limited clinical evaluation and life or limb is threatened if not taken to the operating room between 6 and 24 hours. A time-sensitive procedure is defined as one that will lead to negative outcome if delayed for greater than 1 to 6 weeks to allow for an evaluation and significant changes in management. Finally, an elective procedure is defined as one that can be delayed for up to 1 year.

New from previous versions, the 2014 guidelines characterize risk as either low or high risk and eliminate the previously used intermediate-risk category. A low-risk procedure is defined as one in which the combined surgical and patient characteristics predict a risk of MACE less than 1%. These are generally less invasive procedures that do not involve major fluid shifts and cardiac stress. Examples of low-risk procedures include endoscopy, cataract, and plastic surgery.[32] On the other hand, procedures associated with a risk of 1% or more of MACE are considered to be elevated-risk and typically include open and vascular procedures.[33]

STEPWISE APPROACH TO PERIOPERATIVE CARDIAC TESTING

Guidelines recommend a stepwise approach in determining the appropriateness and utility of perioperative cardiac testing (**Fig. 2**).[11] In case of an emergency surgery (life- or limb-threatening if not operated in <6 hours), proceeding directly to surgery without further cardiac testing is recommended. For elective or time-sensitive surgery, appropriate cardiac testing is recommended for patients who exhibit signs of acute coronary syndrome (ACS), symptomatic arrhythmia, new or decompensated HF, and/or significant valvular heart disease. The goal of cardiac testing in these patients is to appropriately guide their perioperative management to minimize risk by properly characterizing and optimally treating their cardiac condition prior to undertaking of noncardiac surgery. For elective or time-sensitive surgery in patients who do not exhibit signs or symptoms of ACS, calculation of perioperative risk for MACE can be performed by utilizing one of the 3 proposed risk calculators (RCRI, NSQIP MICA, or NSQIP Surgical Risk calculator). Proceeding directly to surgery is reasonable if perioperative risk for MACE is less than 1%.[11] Determination of a patient's functional capacity to aid further risk assessment is recommended if the risk for MACE is greater than 1%.

Assessment of Functional Capacity

A patient's functional capacity is a reliable predictor of his or her ability to tolerate the stress associated with a specific surgery and directly relates to procedural outcome.

Those with poor functional capacity are at higher risk of perioperative complications than those with good functional capacity, and highly functional asymptomatic patients most often safely proceed to planed surgery without further cardiovascular testing. Functional capacity can be estimated from activities of daily living if a patient did not have a recent exercise stress test. Functional capacity is usually expressed in terms of metabolic equivalents (METs), where 1 MET is defined as the amount of oxygen consumed by a 40-year-old, 70 kg man while sitting at rest and is equal to 3.5 mL O_2/kg/min (1.2 kcal/min).[34] Functional capacity is categorized as excellent if someone is able to perform greater than 10 METs, including activities such as racquetball singles or fast running. Good functional capacity is classified as 7 to 10 METs and includes activities such as moderate-to-heavy snow shoveling and woodcutting, ballet dancing, jogging, or alpine skiing. Moderate capacity is defined as 4 to 6 METs and includes activities such as sexual activity (standard missionary position), bicycling, or tennis singles. Poor functional capacity is classified as less than 4 METs and includes light housework, slow ballroom dancing, golfing with a cart, and walking at approximately 2 to 3 mph on flat ground.

Perioperative and long-term cardiac risks are increased in patients unable to perform 4 METs of work during daily activities. In a study of 600 consecutive patients undergoing noncardiac surgery, perioperative MACE were independently associated with poor functional status (defined as the inability to walk 4 blocks or climb 2 flights of stairs).[35]

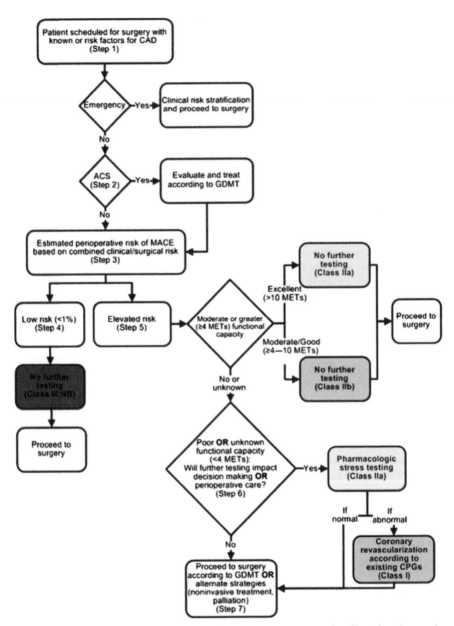

Fig. 2. Stepwise approach in determining the appropriateness and utility of perioperative cardiac testing. (*From* Fleisher LA, Fleischmann KE, Auerbach AD, et al. 2014 ACC/AHA guideline on perioperative cardiovascular evaluation and management of patients undergoing noncardiac surgery: a report of the American College of Cardiology/American Heart Association Task Force on practice guidelines. J Am Coll Cardiol 2014;64:e293; with permission.)

Guidelines recommend proceeding with noncardiac surgery without further exercise testing in patients with elevated risk (MACE >1%) and excellent functional capacity (>10 METs) (Class IIa), and moderate-to-good functional capacity (>4 METs to 10 METs) (Class IIb). On the other hand, if a patient's functional status is unknown, then exercise testing to establish functional capacity is reasonable if it will change perioperative management. Conversely, patients with elevated risk (MACE >1%) and poor functional capacity (METs <4) should undergo additional testing to evaluate for ventricular, coronary, and/or valve status if it would change perioperative management.[11]

Supplemental Perioperative Evaluation

12-Lead electrocardiogram

Guidelines recommend preoperative electrocardiogram (ECG) in patients with known CAD or structural heart disease (Class IIa). A preoperative ECG may also be considered in asymptomatic patients without CAD and structural heart disease (Class IIb), except for those patients undergoing low-risk surgery. These recommendations for a 12-lead ECG have been downgraded from Class I and Class IIa in 2007 guidelines to Class IIa and IIb, respectively. The utility of a preoperative baseline ECG is twofold: (1) it may have prognostic information such as presence of pathologic Q-waves, ST-segment depressions, QTc interval prolongation, and bundle branch blocks relating to short-term and long-term cardiac complications; (2) additionally, it may serve as the baseline against which to assess changes postoperatively.

Assessment of left ventricular function

Guidelines recommend LV function assessment for patients with dyspnea of unknown etiology (Class IIa) or for patients with HF with worsening dyspnea. Reassessment of LV function is also reasonable in patients with clinically stable HF and no prior LV assessment within 1 year (Class IIb). Several studies have demonstrated that the risk of postoperative HF is associated with reduced LV systolic function preoperatively, and the risk of complications is associated with degree of systolic dysfunction.[13,14,16] The greatest incidence of MACE has been observed in patients with LVEF less than 30%.[13]

Stress testing—exercise versus pharmacologic stress

As mentioned in the previous section discussing assessment of functional capacity, patients able to achieve 7 to 10 METs (good functional capacity) have a low risk of perioperative MACE, and those achieving <4 METs (poor functional capacity) have increased risk of perioperative MACE. Electrocardiographic changes with exercise, in the preoperative setting, are not as predictive of MACE as functional capacity in general.[36] Although most data on impact of inducible myocardial ischemia on perioperative outcomes are based on pharmacologic stress testing, guidelines allow exercise stress testing coupled with an imaging modality, either radionuclide myocardial perfusion imaging (MPI) or echocardiography, in patients who are able to exercise. Guidelines recommend patients with elevated preoperative risk with poor functional capacity (<4 METs) who are not able to exercise should undergo pharmacologic stress testing with either radionuclide MPI or dobutamine stress echocardiography (SE) (Class IIa) if results would change perioperative management.[11]

A meta-analysis consisting of 68 studies and over 10,000 patients comparing MPI (thallium imaging) and pharmacologic SE in patients scheduled for noncardiac surgery found that a moderate-to-large defect, seen in 14% of the patients, by either method predicted postoperative MACE.[37] Generally, an abnormal MPI demonstrating moderate-to-large ischemia (reversible perfusion defect) is associated with very high sensitivity for detecting patients at risk for perioperative MI and death, whereas a normal MPI study has a high negative predictive value.[37] Conversely, patients with fixed perfusion defects indicative of prior MI have increased risk of long-term events compared with patients with normal MPI, likely due to the presence of stable CAD. Similarly, a positive dobutamine SE has been reported to have the ability to predict perioperative MACE with a positive predictive value up to 38% and a negative predictive value in the range to 90% to 100%.[38]

Perioperative Coronary Angiography and Revascularization

Guidelines do not recommend routine perioperative coronary angiography (Class III). The indications for perioperative coronary angiography are similar to those in nonoperative settings such as acute coronary syndrome, or presence of significant ischemia on noninvasive stress testing. Coronary revascularization before noncardiac surgery is recommended when indicated according to the 2011 coronary artery bypass grafting (CABG) and percutaneous coronary intervention (PCI) guidelines.[39,40] Conversely, routine prophylactic coronary revascularization primarily to reduce perioperative cardiac events is not recommended even for patients undergoing elective elevated-risk surgery (Class III).[11] This recommendation is driven by the CARP (Coronary Artery Revascularization Prophylaxis) Trial, which demonstrated that patients with stable CAD who underwent preoperative coronary revascularization, PCI, or CABG prior to elective vascular surgery had no difference in mortality and postoperative cardiac events.[33] The preferred revascularization strategy for patients who require PCI prior to a time-sensitive noncardiac surgery is balloon angioplasty or implantation of a bare-metal stent (BMS) if feasible.[11]

Timing of Surgery and Management of Dual Antiplatelet Therapy in Relation to Previous Percutaneous Coronary Intervention

Emergency PCI is often life saving in patients presenting with ST elevation MI, unstable angina, or life-threatening arrhythmia due to ongoing coronary ischemia. After PCI with stent placement, patients require dual antiplatelet therapy (DAPT) with aspirin and a $P2Y_{12}$ platelet receptor inhibitor to prevent stent thrombosis. DAPT significantly reduces the risk of stent thrombosis, and discontinuation of DAPT is one of the strongest risk factors of stent thrombosis and mortality, inversely related to the timing of discontinuation after PCI. Stent thrombosis risk is highest in the first 4 to 6 weeks after stent implantation but remains elevated up to at least 1 year after Drug Eluting Stent (DES) implantation. The urgency of noncardiac surgery and risk of bleeding (if DAPT is continued) and MI due to stent thrombosis (if DAPT needs to be interrupted) associated with surgery in a patient after recent PCI requires thoughtful clinical decision-making. Guidelines recommend postponing elective noncardiac surgery to at least 14 days after balloon angioplasty and at least 30 days after a BMS implantation.[11] In regards to patients treated with DES, the updated 2016 ACC/AHA guidelines on duration of DAPT in patients with CAD have modified the previous Class I and Class IIb recommendations of delaying the elective noncardiac surgery from 1 year to optimally at least 6 months and from 6 months to after 3 months, respectively (**Fig. 3**).[41] These updated recommendations are primarily driven by the data suggesting that the newer-generation DES (second generation) are associated with lower risk of stent thrombosis and require shorter duration of DAPT compared with previous recommendations that were primarily driven by the data on older DES associated with higher risk of stent thrombosis and longer duration of DAPT.[41] Schulz and colleagues,[42] in a randomized, double-blind, placebo-controlled trial comparing 6 months versus 12 months of DAPT after a second-generation DES implantation, found no statistically significant difference in clinical outcome in the 2 groups. Additionally, Palmerini and colleagues,[43] in a patient-level pooled analysis of 4 trials containing over 8000 randomized patients, found that a shorter duration of DAPT (3–6 months) was associated with similar rates of MACE and less major bleeding than DAPT of 1 year duration after second-generation DES implantation. Finally, according to expert opinion expressed in current

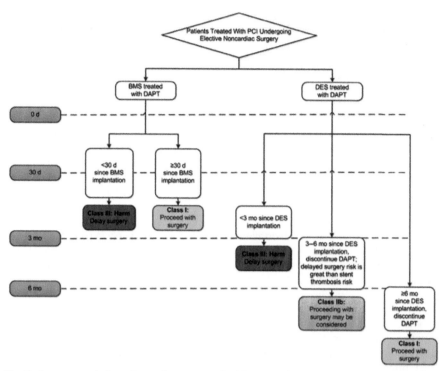

Fig. 3. Recommendations for patients treated with PCI undergoing elective noncardiac surgery. (*From* Levine GN, Bates ER, Bittl JA, et al. 2016 ACC/AHA guideline focused update on duration of dual antiplatelet therapy in patients with coronary artery disease a report of the american college of cardiology/american heart association task force on clinical practice guidelines. J Am Coll Cardiol 2016;68(10):1103; with permission.)

guidelines, aspirin therapy should be continued in the perioperative period if $P2Y_{12}$ inhibitor therapy is held to reduce bleeding risk in the perioperative setting for patients undergoing noncardiac surgery.[41]

PERIOPERATIVE MEDICAL THERAPY
Beta-Blockers

Guidelines recommend continuation of perioperative beta-blockers in patients who have been on beta-blockers chronically.[11] This Class I recommendation is based on observational studies supporting the benefit of continuing beta-blockers in the perioperative period in patients who are on these agents for chronic conditions such as prior MI and congestive heart failure (CHF).[44] In addition, 2014 guidelines incorporate a new Class IIb recommendation for initiating beta-blocker therapy perioperatively (preferably >1 day prior to surgery) in patients with intermediate- or high-risk myocardial ischemia noted on a preoperative risk stratification stress test, or with 3 or more RCRI risk factors.[11] Finally, beta-blocker therapy should not be started on the day of surgery (Class III). Recommendations regarding perioperative beta-blocker therapy are primarily driven by a 2014 systematic review from the ACC/AHA, which found that perioperative beta-blocker therapy started within 1 day of surgery reduced cardiac events overall, but significantly increased the risk of adverse outcomes including bradycardia, stroke, and death.[45] The POISE-1 (Perioperative Ischemic Evaluation Study), a randomized controlled clinical trial consisting of over 8000 patients, found that perioperative use of beta-blocker reduced risk for cardiac events (ischemia, atrial fibrillation, need for coronary intervention) but resulted in higher risk of stroke and death from noncardiac complications.[46] However, POISE-1 was criticized for its use of a high-dose long-acting beta-blocker (metoprolol succinate 100 mg twice daily) and for initiation of the dose immediately before the surgery (2–4 hours). Additionally, the study did not include a titration protocol before or after the surgery. Furthermore, taking into account the controversy surrounding the DECREASE (Dutch Echocardiographic Cardiac Risk Evaluation Applying Stress Echo) studies, related to investigator impropriety,[47] the 2014 ACC/AHA systematic review found that exclusion of POISE-1 and DECREASE studies did not substantially affect estimates of risk or benefits proposed in current guidelines.

Statins

Guidelines recommend (Class I) continuing statins perioperatively in patients who are chronically on statin therapy.[11] In addition, there is a Class IIa recommendation for initiating statin therapy in patients undergoing vascular surgery and a Class IIb recommendation for considering statin therapy for patients who qualify for statin treatment according to 2013 guidelines for treatment of blood cholesterol and are scheduled for elevated-risk noncardiac surgery.[11] A recent randomized controlled trial followed patients on atorvastatin for 6 months after vascular surgery and found significant reduction in MACE in patients treated with atorvastatin 20 mg daily.[48] Additionally, observational trial data consisting of over 780,000 patients found a 5-fold benefit in MACE rates and lower mortality rates following major noncardiac surgery in patients on statin therapy.[49]

Alpha Agonists

Current guidelines do not recommend alpha-2 agonist therapy in patients undergoing noncardiac surgery. The POISE-2 study was a large randomized, blinded, multicenter clinical trial consisting of over 10,000 patients, which demonstrated that administration of clonidine did not reduce perioperative nonfatal MI or death rates, but did increase the rate of nonfatal cardiac arrest and hypotension.[50]

Angiotensin-Converting Enzyme Inhibitors

Guidelines recommend continuation of angiotensin-converting enzyme inhibitors (ACE-I) perioperatively and if held before surgery, that they be restarted postoperatively as soon as clinically feasible (Class IIa).[11] Due to lack of randomized controlled trials studying the impact of ACE-I in the perioperative setting, current evidence is limited to observational studies. In a large retrospective study including 79, 228 patients, with 13% on ACE-I therapy undergoing noncardiac surgery, a matched, nested cohort demonstrated more frequent transient intraoperative hypotension in ACE-I users but no statistically significant difference in other outcomes.[51] Similarly, a meta-analysis of 5 studies consisting of over 400 patients reported hypotension in 50% of patients taking an ACE-I or angiotensin receptor blocker on the day of surgery but no impact on cardiovascular outcomes.[52] Furthermore, 1 study reported discontinuation of ACE-I therapy before surgery resulted in no major adverse outcome.[53]

Antiplatelet Therapy

Guidelines recommend continuing DAPT in patients with recently implanted BMS or DES (within 4–6 weeks) undergoing urgent noncardiac surgery, unless the relative risk of bleeding outweighs the benefit of prevention of stent thrombosis (Class I). If P2Y$_{12}$ platelet inhibitor must be discontinued perioperatively in patients with coronary stents, then guidelines recommend continuing aspirin alone if possible (Class I). Similarly, in patients who are on daily aspirin and who have not had prior coronary stenting, guidelines favor continuing aspirin perioperatively, especially in patients with high-risk CAD, unless the bleeding risk outweighs potential cardiac benefit (Class IIb). On the other hand, guidelines recommend against initiating aspirin therapy preoperatively due to higher risk of bleeding (Class III). This recommendation is based on data from the POISE-2 trial demonstrating no benefit in initiating or continuing aspirin therapy in patients with no previous coronary stenting who were undergoing noncardiac surgery.[50]

SUMMARY

Cardiac conditions in patients undergoing noncardiac surgery confer significant risk of morbidity and mortality, which is largely preventable by implementing appropriate cardiac risk stratification prior to surgery and individually tailoring perioperative therapy to reduce risk. Furthermore, a successful surgical outcome requires a team approach and shared decision-making involving the primary care provider, cardiologist, anesthesiologist, surgeon performing the procedure, and the patient. Finally, with the aging population, increasing number of annual surgeries, and dynamic US health care focused toward cost-effectiveness and appropriate utilization of resources and therapies, the need for evidence-based practice to minimize perioperative surgical morbidity and mortality is of paramount importance.

REFERENCES

1. Weiser TG, Regenbogen SE, Thompson KD, et al. An estimation of the global volume of surgery: a modeling strategy based on available data. Lancet 2008;372: 139–44.
2. Gawande AA, Thomas EJ, Zinner MJ, et al. The incidence and nature of surgical adverse events in Colorado and Utah in 1992. Surgery 1999;126:66–75.
3. Kable AK, Gibberd RW, Spigelman AD. Adverse events in surgical patients in Australia. Int J Qual Health Care 2002;14:269–76.
4. Devereaux PJ, Chan MT, Alonso-Coello P, et al. Association between postoperative troponin levels and 30-day mortality among patients undergoing noncardiac surgery. JAMA 2012;307:2295–304.
5. US Deptartment of Health and Human Services, Centers for Disease Control and Prevention, National Center for Health Statistics. CDC/NCHS National Hospital Discharge Survey, 2010. 2010. Available at: http://www.cdc.gov/nchs/data/nhds/4procedures/2010pro4_numberprocedureage.pdf. Accessed October 24, 2016.
6. Devereaux PJ, Goldman L, Cook DJ, et al. Perioperative cardiac events in patients undergoing noncardiac surgery: a review of the magnitude of the problem, the pathophysiology of the events and methods to estimate and communicate risk. CMAJ 2005;173:627–34.
7. Mangano DT. Peri-operative medicine: NHLBI working group deliberations and recommendations. J Cardiothorac Vasc Anesth 2004;18:1–6.
8. Mozaffarian D, Benjamin EJ, Go AS, et al. American Heart Association Statistics Committee and Stroke Statistics Subcommittee. Heart disease and stroke statistics–2015 update: a report from the American Heart Association. Circulation 2015;131:e29–322.

9. Shah KB, Kleinman BS, Rao TL, et al. Angina and other risk factors in patients with cardiac diseases undergoing noncardiac operations. Anesth Analg 1990; 70:240–7.

10. Livhits M, Ko CY, Leonardi MJ, et al. Risk of surgery following recent myocardial infarction. Ann Surg 2011;253:857–64.

11. Fleisher LA, Fleischmann KE, Auerbach AD, et al. 2014 ACC/AHA guideline on perioperative cardiovascular evaluation and management of patients undergoing noncardiac surgery: a report of the American College of Cardiology/American Heart Association Task Force on practice guide- lines. J Am Coll Cardiol 2014; 64:e77–137.

12. Van Diepen S, Bakal JA, McAlister FA, et al. Mortality and readmission of patients with heart failure, atrial fibrillation, or coronary artery disease undergoing noncardiac surgery: an analysis of 38 047 patients. Circulation 2011;124:289–96.

13. Healy KO, Waksmonski CA, Altman RK, et al. Peri- operative outcome and long-term mortality for heart failure patients undergoing intermediate- and high-risk noncardiac surgery: impact of left ventricular ejection fraction. Congest Heart Fail 2010;16:45–9.

14. Kazmers A, Cerqueira MD, Zierler RE. Perioperative and late outcome in patients with left ventricular ejection fraction of 35% or less who require major vascular surgery. J Vasc Surg 1988;8:307–15.

15. Matyal R, Hess PE, Subramaniam B, et al. Peri-operative diastolic dysfunction during vascular surgery and its association with postoperative outcome. J Vasc Surg 2009;50:70–6.

16. Flu WJ, van Kuijk JP, Hoeks SE, et al. Prognostic implications of asymptomatic left ventricular dysfunction in patients undergoing vascular surgery. Anesthesiology 2010;112:1316–24.

17. Goldman L, Caldera DL, Nussbaum SR, et al. Multifactorial index of cardiac risk in noncardiac surgical procedures. N Engl J Med 1977;297:845–50.

18. Agarwal S, Rajamanickam A, Bajaj NS, et al. Impact of aortic stenosis on postoperative outcomes after noncardiac surgeries. Circ Cardiovasc Qual Outcomes 2013;6:193–200.

19. Ben-Dor I, Pichard AD, Satler LF, et al. Complications and outcome of balloon aortic valvuloplasty in high-risk or inoperable patients. J Am Coll Cardiol Intv 2010;3:1150–6.

20. Leon MB, Smith CR, Mack M, et al. Transcatheter aortic-valve implantation for aortic stenosis in patients who cannot undergo surgery. N Engl J Med 2010; 363:1597–607.

21. Smith CR, Leon MB, Mack MJ, et al. Transcatheter versus surgical aortic-valve replacement in high-risk patients. N Engl J Med 2011;364:2187–98.

22. Leon MB, Smith CR, Mack MJ, et al. Transcatheter or surgical aortic-valve replacement in intermediate-risk patients. N Engl J Med 2016;374(17):1609–20.

23. Lai HC, Lai HC, Lee WL, et al. Impact of chronic advanced aortic regurgitation on the perioperative outcome of noncardiac surgery. Acta Anaesthesiol Scand 2010; 54:580–8.

24. Bajaj NS, Agarwal S, Rajamanickam A, et al. Impact of severe mitral regurgitation on postoperative out-comes after noncardiac surgery. Am J Med 2013;126: 529–35.

25. Mahla E, Rotman B, Rehak P, et al. Perioperative ventricular dysrhythmias in patients with structural heart disease undergoing noncardiac surgery. Anesth Analg 1998;86:16–21.

26. Lee TH, Marcantonio ER, Mangione CM, et al. Derivation and prospective validation of a simple index for prediction of cardiac risk of major noncardiac surgery. Circulation 1999;100:1043–9.

27. O'Kelly B, Browner WS, Massie B, et al. Ventricular arrhythmias in patients undergoing noncardiac surgery. The Study of Perioperative Ischemia Research Group. JAMA 1992;268:217–21.

28. Ramakrishna G, Sprung J, Ravi BS, et al. Impact of pulmonary hypertension on the outcomes of noncardiac surgery: predictors of perioperative morbidity and mortality. J Am Coll Cardiol 2005;45:1691–9.

29. Meyer S, McLaughlin VV, Seyfarth HJ, et al. Outcomes of noncardiac, nonobstetric surgery in patients with PAH: an international prospective survey. Eur Respir J 2013;41:1302–7.

30. Cohen ME, Ko CY, Bilimoria KY, et al. Optimizing ACS NSQIP modeling for evaluation of surgical quality and risk: patient risk adjustment, procedure mix adjustment, shrinkage adjustment, and surgical focus. J Am Coll Surg 2013;217: 336–46.e1.

31. Gupta PK, Gupta H, Sundaram A, et al. Development and validation of a risk calculator for prediction of cardiac risk after surgery. Circulation 2011;124:381–7.

32. Schein OD, Katz J, Bass EB, et al. The value of routine preoperative medical testing before cataract surgery. Study of medical testing for cataract surgery. N Engl J Med 2000;342:168–75.

33. McFalls EO, Ward HB, Moritz TE, et al. Coronary-artery revascularization before elective major vascular surgery. N Engl J Med 2004;351:2795–804.

34. Jette M, Sidney K, Blumchen G. Metabolic equivalents (METS) in exercise testing, exercise prescription, and evaluation of functional capacity. Clin Cardiol 1990;13(8):555–65.

35. Reilly DF, McNeely MJ, Doerner D, et al. Self-reported exercise tolerance and the risk of serious perioperative complications. Arch Intern Med 1999;159:2185–92.

36. Sgura FA, Kopecky SL, Grill JP, et al. Supine exercise capacity identifies patients at low risk for perioperative cardiovascular events and predicts long-term survival. Am J Med 2000;108:334–6.

37. Beattie WS, Abdelnaem E, Wijeysundera DN, et al. A meta-analytic comparison of preoperative stress echocardiography and nuclear scintigraphy imaging. Anesth Analg 2006;102:8–16.

38. Poldermans D, Arnese M, Fioretti PM, et al. Improved cardiac risk stratification in major vascular surgery with dobutamine-atropine stress echocardiography. J Am Coll Cardiol 1995;26:648–53.

39. Hillis LD, Smith PK, Anderson JL, et al. 2011 ACCF/AHA guideline for coronary artery bypass graft surgery: a report of the American College of Cardiology Foundation/American Heart Association Task Force on Practice Guidelines. J Am Coll Cardiol 2011;58:e123–210.

40. Levine GN, Bates ER, Blankenship JC, et al. 2011 ACCF/AHA/SCAI guideline for percutaneous coronary intervention: a report of the American College of Cardiology Foundation/American Heart Association Task Force on Practice Guidelines and the Society for Cardiovascular Angiography and Interventions. J Am Coll Cardiol 2011;58:e44–122.

41. Levine GN, Bates ER, Bittl JA, et al. 2016 ACC/AHA guideline focused update on duration of dual antiplatelet therapy in patients with coronary artery disease. J Am Coll Cardiol 2016;68(10):1082–115.

42. Schulz-Schüpke S, Byrne RA, Ten Berg JM, et al. ISAR-SAFE: a randomized, double-blind, placebo- controlled trial of 6 vs. 12 months of clopidogrel therapy after drug-eluting stenting. Eur Heart J 2015;36:1252–63.

43. Palmerini T, Sangiorgi D, Valgimigli M, et al. Short- versus long-term dual anti-platelet therapy after drug-eluting stent implantation: an individual patient data pairwise and network meta-analysis. J Am Coll Cardiol 2015;65:1092–102.

44. Lindenauer PK, Pekow P, Wang K, et al. Peri-operative beta-blocker therapy and mortality after major noncardiac surgery. N Engl J Med 2005;353:349–61.

45. Wijeysundera DN, Duncan D, Nkonde-Price C, et al. Perioperative beta blockade in noncardiac surgery: a systematic review for the 2014 ACC/AHA guideline on perioperative cardiovascular evaluation and management of patients undergoing noncardiac surgery: a report of the American College of Cardiology/American Heart Association Task Force on practice guidelines. J Am Coll Cardiol 2014; 64:2406–25.

46. POISE Study Group. Effects of extended-release metoprolol succinate in patients undergoing non-cardiac surgery (POISE trial): a randomised controlled trial. Lancet 2008;371:1839–47.

47. Chopra V, Eagle KA. Perioperative mischief: the price of academic misconduct. Am J Med 2012;125:953–5.

48. Durazzo AE, Machado FS, Ikeoka DT, et al. Reduction in cardiovascular events after vascular surgery with atorvastatin: a randomized trial. J Vasc Surg 2004; 39:967–75.

49. Lindenauer PK, Pekow P, Wang K, et al. Lipid-lowering therapy and in-hospital mortality following major noncardiac surgery. JAMA 2004;291:2092–9.

50. Devereaux PJ, Sessler DI, Leslie K, et al, POISE-2 Investigators. Clonidine in patients undergoing noncardiac surgery. N Engl J Med 2014;370:1504–13.

51. Turan A, You J, Shiba A, et al. Angiotensin converting enzyme inhibitors are not associated with respiratory complications or mortality after noncardiac surgery. Anesth Analg 2012;114:552–60.

52. Rosenman DJ, McDonald FS, Ebbert JO, et al. Clinical consequences of withholding versus administering renin-angiotensin-aldosterone system antagonists in the preoperative period. J Hosp Med 2008;3:319–25.

53. Bertrand M, Godet G, Meersschaert K, et al. Should the angiotensin II antagonists be discontinued before surgery? Anesth Analg 2001;92:26–30.

Diagnostic Imaging and Newer Modalities for Thoracic Diseases

PET/Computed Tomographic Imaging and Endobronchial Ultrasound for Staging and Its Implication for Lung Cancer

Sarah J. Counts, DO[a],*, Anthony W. Kim, MD[b]

KEYWORDS

- Chest radiograph • Computed tomography • PET • MRI • Endobronchial ultrasound
- Esophageal ultrasound • Navigational bronchoscopy

KEY POINTS

- Computed tomographic (CT) scanning is the test of choice to identify nodules (ie, low-dose CT scanning) and then to further delineate the abnormality (high-resolution CT scanning).
- Integrated PET/CT imaging is superior to either CT scan or PET imaging by itself in accurately characterizing lung cancers.
- Endobronchial ultrasound and esophageal ultrasound must be used in a strategically advantageous manner relying on their individual strengths to maximize their efficacy in the diagnosis and staging of lung cancer.

INTRODUCTION

Tailoring the optimal diagnostic approach for lung cancer requires that a defined goal be based on the results of any study that is planned. Modalities to detect and characterize lung cancer generally can be divided into those that are invasive versus those that are noninvasive. Aside from the standard chest radiograph (CXR), the noninvasive imaging techniques include computed tomography (CT), PET, and MRI. The invasive

---

The authors have nothing to disclose.
[a] Cardiothoracic Surgery, Yale-New Haven Hospital, Yale School of Medicine, 330 Cedar Street, BB 205, New Haven, CT 06520, USA; [b] Division of Thoracic Surgery, Department of Surgery, Keck School of Medicine, University of Southern California, 1510 San Pablo Street, Suite 514, Los Angeles, CA 90033, USA
* Corresponding author.
E-mail address: sarah.counts@yale.edu

imaging modalities include endobronchial ultrasound (EBUS), esophageal ultrasound (EUS), and electromagnetic navigational bronchoscopy (ENB).

NONINVASIVE MODALITIES
Computed Tomographic Scans

- CT scanning is the test of choice to identify nodules (ie, low-dose CT [LDCT] scanning) and then to further delineate the abnormality (ie, high-resolution CT scanning)

The National Lung Screening Trial (NLST) was the landmark prospective randomized, controlled study that revealed a significant decrease in lung cancer–related mortality of 20% when LDCT scans were used (6.8%) compared with CXR alone (26.7%) in the 53,454 participants who were considered to be at "high risk." High risk was defined in this study as those patients who were current smokers or who were former smokers with a total of 30+ pack-years, aged 55 to 74 years old, as long as they had quit within the past 15 years[1] (**Box 1**). The results of this trial as well as others studies evaluating CXRs for lung cancer screening have led to guidelines recommending its avoidance as a lone screening test for lung cancer because it may miss detecting 4 times as many lung cancers compared with with scans.[2–4] Before the NLST, the International Early Lung Cancer Action Program (I-ELCAP) first demonstrated improvements in screening for smokers at high risk for lung cancer.[5] The I-ELCAP subsequently showed that CT imaging detected 4 times more lung cancers and 6 times more stage I lesions as compared with CXR alone when used in the context of screening a higher-risk population.[3–5] Cumulatively and particularly with the results of the NLST, the observed reduction in lung cancer–related mortality now serves as the backbone for the lung cancer screening recommendations from many organizations, including the US Preventive Services Task Force.[1,2,6–11]

From a technical standpoint, a lung cancer screening CT scan should involve low-dose helical (spiral) images from the thoracic inlet moving caudally to the inferior edge of the liver, ensuring that the adrenal glands are included. CT images must be viewed with less than or equal to 2.5-mm slice thickness and with reconstruction intervals less than or equal to slice thickness.[12,13] Additional imaging data may be acquired and reconstructed at less than or equal to 1.0-mm slice thickness and reconstruction intervals to allow for better characterization of small lung nodules.[12] Advanced technology in current iteration CT scanners allows for a high-resolution, comprehensive evaluation of the thorax in a single, several-second breath-hold.[14] Respiratory and cardiac motion artifacts are reduced with rapid acquisition, thereby allowing for more accurate lung nodule depiction, especially in areas that are harder to investigate such as in the bases of the lungs or in the lung parenchyma immediately adjacent to the mediastinum. Newer visualization techniques include maximum intensity projection, volume rendering, stereographic display, and computer-aided detection, which allow for enhanced lung cancer detection and enable the radiologist to better differentiate small lung nodules from other structures.[14] These technologies have also allowed for multiplanar reconstructions, which can then be used to generate 3-dimensional depictions of vascular and bronchial anatomy for potential future operative planning.

Computed tomographic scans in assessing pulmonary nodules
Pulmonary nodules are one of the most common findings on thoracic imaging, and therefore, it is imperative to make as accurate of a characterization as possible.[15] The size of a pulmonary nodule has been thought to correlate with the prevalence of malignancy: less than 5 mm, 0% to 1%; 5 to 10 mm, 6% to 28%; 10 to 20 mm,

---

Box 1
Key elements of annual lung screening guidelines endorsed by United States Preventative Services Task Force with further modifications endorsed by the other organizations (endorsing organizations in parentheses)

Inclusion Criteria

Age
  55 to 80 years
  55 to 79 years (AATS)
  55 to 74 years (ACCP, ACS, ASCO, NLST, NCCN)

Tobacco History (ACCP, ACS, ASCO, NLST, NCCN)
  Former smoker with a 30+ pack-year smoking
  Former smoker quit within the past 15 years
  Current smoker

Additional (NCCN, AATS)
  Age 50+ years *and* tobacco history of ≥20+ pack-year with at least one additional lung cancer risk factor:
  • Major exposure to arsenic, beryllium, oadmium, chromium, nickel, asbestos, coal smoke, soot, silica, and diesel fumes
  • Other cancers (small cell lung cancer, head cancers, neck cancers, Hodgkin lymphoma)
  • Received radiation treatment to chest for other disease
  • Family member with lung cancer (ie, parent, sibling, or child)
  • History of COPD
  • History of pulmonary fibrosis
  • Second-hand smoke exposure

Exclusion Criteria

Age
  Less than 55 years
  Greater than 80 years

Tobacco History
  Less than 30 pack-years
  Quit greater than 15 years ago

Comorbidities (ASCO)
  Severe comorbidities precluding potentially curative treatment and/or limit life expectancy (ASCO)

Discontinuation of Screening

Once a person has not smoked for 15 years or develops a health problem that substantially limits life expectancy or the ability or willingness to have curative lung surgery

Abbreviations: AATS, American Association for Thoracic Surgery; ACCCP, American College of Chest Physicians; ACS, American Cancer Society; ASCO, American Society for Clinical Oncology; COPD, chronic obstructive pulmonary disease; NCCN, National Comprehensive Cancer Network.

33% to 60%; and greater than 20 mm, 64% to 82%.[16] Although there are variations, the more commonly accepted definition of a pulmonary nodule by CT imaging is a lesion with a diameter less than 30 mm. A pulmonary mass is considered to be a lesion greater than 30 mm.[17]

LDCT identifies small nodules in 10% to 50% of those screened with the vast majority of these being benign.[1–3,18] The wide range seen with nodule detection with CT scanning is not readily explained. Accurate staging for primary lung cancer requires precise demarcation of the tumor margin to assess the primary tumor (T) descriptor, and this delineation is best accomplished with thin-slice high-resolution CT scanning.[13] Therefore, when an LDCT scan identifies a suspicious finding, a dedicated chest high-resolution CT (HRCT) scan should be pursued (**Fig. 1**). LDCT (20–50 mAs) has been shown to be comparable to conventional CT mode (140–300 mAs) in sensitivity and specificity for the detection of pulmonary nodules.[4] There is a significant difference in the radiation in LDCT scanning that ranges from 1.3 to 3.4 mSv, whereas in high-resolution CT imaging, it is 8.5 to 14.0 mSv.[19] In this context, a slice thickness, reconstruction interval of 1.5 to 2.5 mm provides a useful compromise between accurate demarcation of the tumor margin and image noise.[13,20] The noise that is identified typically is an irregular granular pattern in the images, which degrades image information.[21]

Lesions less than 3 mm are extremely difficult to identify on CT imaging because such small abnormalities are difficult to decipher from the lung's normal architecture, especially depending on the location of the presumed nodular finding.[22] The role of nodule location is particularly relevant with small lesions. These lesions are extremely difficult to identify when they are low apparent density or in a central location. Not surprisingly, peripheral lesions are identified more frequently (74%) compared with central (49%) and perihilar lesions (37%), owing to the absence of confounding structures that would be of similar size in the periphery.[22]

Computed tomographic scan in assessing regional lymph nodes

CT scanning has a sensitivity of 47% to 54% and a specificity of 84% to 88% in identifying abnormal hilar and mediastinal lymph nodes with roughly 40% of all nodes thought malignant (as defined by being >1 cm on short-axis diameter) actually being benign and 20% thought benign (as defined by being ≤1 cm on short axis) actually being malignant.[23] Volumetric CT histogram analysis is a relatively new means by which lymph nodes on CT can be evaluated.[24] Flechsig and colleagues[24] demonstrated a significant correlation between lymph node Hounsfield units and benign versus malignant disease with a median CT density being significantly higher for histologically positive lymph nodes (average: 33.2 HU) than for histologically negative lymph nodes (average: 10.1 HU). The incidence of malignancy was 88% above a cutoff value of 20 HU in the 10 fluorine-18 fluorodeoxyglucose (FDG) equivocal lymph nodes, and the incidence of benign findings was 100% in the interval between −20 and +20

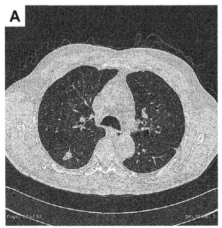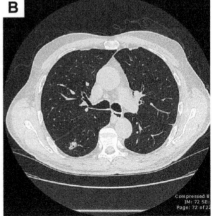

Fig. 1. Differences between low-resolution CT and HRCT scans. (A) LDCT scan of the chest with a grainier image and a (B) HRCT scan with a more refined image.

HU. Others have noted that there is an increased likelihood of lymph node metastasis if the primary lesion: (1) is solid or spiculated, (2) has a peak enhancement greater than 110 HU, (3) has a net enhancement of greater than 60 to 70 HU on CT scan, (4) is centrally located, or (5) is associated with a pleural effusion.[25,26] Cumulatively, these studies demonstrate promise with respect to the ability of CT scans to distinguish benign from malignant disease, but have not allowed CT scanning to definitively determine if a lymph node harbors metastatic disease.

Integrated PET with Computed Tomography

- Integrated PET/CT imaging is superior to either CT scan or PET imaging by itself in accurately characterizing lung cancers

Integrated PET/CT is the most accurate noninvasive imaging modality for the staging of primary lung cancers.[27,28] Integrated PET/CT refers to when PET is fused with CT scanning and is proven to be a superior imaging modality to either obtained as a sole modality (**Fig. 2**). Current recommendations for PET/CT imaging include obtaining

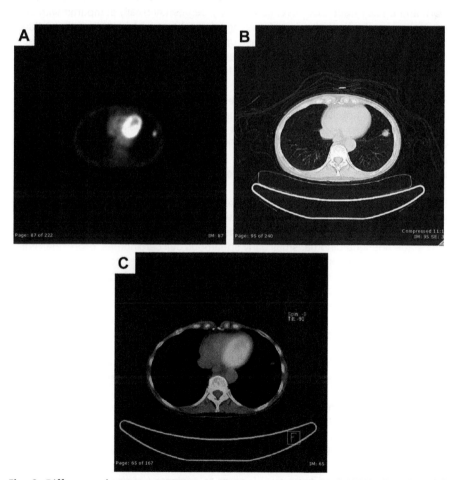

Fig. 2. Differences between a PET scan, CT scan, and integrated PET/CT imaging. (*A*) Attenuation-corrected PET scan, (*B*) CT scan of nodule, (*C*) integrated PET/CT scan of the same nodule.

images from the skull base to the thigh with a slice thickness of 2.5 mm to gain the most accurate demarcation of the tumor margin while maximizing the signal-to-noise ratio.[13] PET imaging alone without CT scan fusion is not adequate as a sole modality because it lacks the spatial resolution to accurately and definitely characterize areas of interest.[18,29,30] The paucity of anatomic landmarks on PET imaging is made up for when the images are fused with that of the anatomic cross-sectional data from CT imaging.[31]

The PET component uses an FDG tracer to depict abnormal metabolic uptake with a sensitivity of 79% to 85% and a specificity of 87% to 92% for identifying malignancy.[32] In order to have the PET component have the highest true yield, patients must fast for 4 to 6 hours before the test as well as avoid strenuous activity for 24 to 48 hours before the examination.[13] The FDG tracer is dosed based on the patient's height and weight. Patients with elevated hemoglobin A1c may not be candidates for PET because this can affect the FDG tracer metabolism, with the upper cutoff number varying by institution.

There are areas of the body that have increased uptake of the FDG tracer that are not pathologic, and these must be known so as to not create undue alarm. The most concentrated areas of normal FDG uptake at 1 hour after injection are the brain, heart, and urinary tract. Low-level activity may be seen normally in the thyroid gland, breast, and mediastinal blood pool. Laryngeal uptake can be identified after talking. Physical activity and anxiety can increase uptake within muscle groups in what should be in a symmetric, and if applicable, bilateral fashion.[18] Therefore, a sound grasp of the context in which a PET/CT scan is performed must be understood.

Integrated PET/computed tomography to evaluate the primary lesion

The standardized uptake value (SUV), defined as the activity per milliliter within the region of interest divided by the injected dose in megabec-querels per kilogram of body weight, of a lesion greater than 2.5 originally was deemed concerning for malignancy.[30] Since then, the maximum SUV (SUVmax) of greater than 2.5 has been used widely as the cutoff value suggestive of malignancy. This threshold, however, is associated with a wide range of sensitivity (40%–97%) and specificity (60%–96%).[33] This observation may be linked, in part, to false negative results in small nodules (<1 cm) because they may not have the necessary critical mass of metabolically active malignant cells for accurate detection.[34] False negatives occur in small early stage adenocarcinoma, small early squamous cell carcinomas, bronchoalveolar cell carcinoma, and some carcinoid tumors.[35] False positives (nonmalignant lesions with a high SUVmax) also can occur in disease states such as tuberculosis, aspergillomas, rheumatoid nodules, Wegener granulomatosis, and amyloidosis.[35] Cerfolio and colleagues[36] showed that patients with a high SUVmax ($\geq$10) were more likely to have poorly differentiated tumors, more likely to have an advanced stage, and less likely to undergo complete resection of their disease. Patients with squamous cell carcinoma also were found to have a higher SUVmax (13.2) than those with other types of non–small cell lung cancer (NSCLC 8.9).[36] Despite the potential ominous findings associated with elevated SUVmax, some investigators have shown no difference in overall survival or progression-free survival between high and low SUVmax groups.[37] This finding may be reflective of the heterogeneity in treatment rather than a direct effect of the SUV value, per se. Outside of a quantitative assessment, qualitatively, a nodule or mass with increased uptake of [18]FDG in 3 planes as compared with the background on a PET scan is also concerning for malignancy.[30]

Integrated PET/computed tomographic scans to evaluate lymph node involvement

Similar to the data for primary lung nodules, an SUVmax of 2.5 or greater has been used to differentiate benign from malignant lymph nodes.[38,39] One prospective, multicenter comparison of CT alone to integrated PET/CT allowed for an 11% increase in accuracy in detecting lymph node metastasis on a per-patient basis.[40] Integrated PET/CT appears to be a better predictor than PET alone for N status.[40] The metabolic characteristics obtained from PET imaging combined with the information regarding lymph node size from CT imaging allows for improved staging accuracy.[41] The risk of mediastinal disease is increased if the SUVmax of the primary lesion is greater than 4.[38]

Integrated PET/CT detects unexpected mediastinal lymph node FDG avidity in 10% of patients originally thought not to have mediastinal disease on other imaging.[41] As with other modalities, there is a risk of false positive findings in mediastinal and hilar lymph nodes. This risk is higher in larger lymph nodes, in those with a higher volume of lymphocytes and macrophages, in reactive lymph nodes, and in those with lymphoid follicular hyperplasia.[40] When the area of concern is small (5–7 mm), the sensitivity of PET drops significantly to only 40% as compared with when investigating larger lymph node stations of concern (8–10 mm) at 78%.[42] Lee and colleagues[43] described lymph node density as an adjunct to FDG avidity in those nodes deemed to have "mild FDG uptake" (SUVmax 2–4), where using density criteria (median HU 25–45) increased the sensitivity (88.3%) and specificity (82.6%) in this subgroup. There are no trials showing a difference in PET/CT imaging between different lung cancer subtypes. A retrospective review by Wang and colleagues[44] found no significant difference in SUVmax on preoperative PET/CT in patients with what was later pathologically proven to be positive lymph node disease between squamous cell carcinoma and other forms of NSCLC.

Integrated PET/computed tomographic scans to delineate metastases
Integrated PET/CT detects unexpected metastases in 10% to 15% of patients with NSCLC.[41] A review of all randomized control trials using PET or PET/CT in the evaluation of patients with lung cancer showed that its greatest benefit was in identifying metastatic disease in patients with a high chance of such involvement.[45] Preoperatively, integrated PET/CT has reduced the total number of thoracotomies including those thoracotomies used for staging in those NSCLC patients presumed to have advanced disease.[30] Integrated PET/CT scans are replacing bone scintigraphy in most cases because it has been shown to be a very sensitive imaging modality to detect osseous disease. One meta-analysis described a higher sensitivity (92%) and specificity (98%) with integrated PET/CT scanning as compared with bone scintigraphy (sensitivity 86%, specificity 87%) in correctly identifying metastatic disease to bone.[46]

Future advances in integrated PET/computed tomographic imaging
Alternative methods to improve upon current integrated PET/CT imaging are on the horizon. One such approach uses respiratory gating of PET/CT scans, whereby data acquisition corresponds to a specific part of the respiratory cycle phase. This unique approach is different than standard PET/CT techniques, whereby patients are allowed to breathe freely during the examination. Respiratory-gated PET/CT scan use has not been proven to be superior at this time, but has the potential to play a role in the management of patients with early stage disease because it shows slightly improved clinical staging accuracy and higher interobserver agreement between nuclear medicine physicians.[47]

PET imaging using other tracer materials to achieve more sensitive and specific imaging than presently available with [18]FDG is under investigation at this time. A fluorine-18-A-methyltyrosine tracer is currently in clinical trial phases.[48] Other tracers such as 11C-methionine (protein metabolism marker), 11C-choline (a marker of the cell membrane component phosphatidylcholine), and 18F-fluorothymidine (a marker of cell proliferation) have also been studied, but the experience is limited, with no clear clinical advantage identified yet.[49]

INVASIVE EVALUATION

Invasive studies allow the clinician to obtain tissue for both diagnosis and staging. Before using an invasive option for either of these purposes, it is recommended that imaging will have afforded the clinician the knowledge of selecting the target that would provide a diagnosis and the highest possible stage in a safe manner.[50] In certain circumstances, such as in those patients who are suggested to have a peripheral stage IA tumor, invasive preoperative evaluation of mediastinal nodes may not be required.[2,51] However, in general, most abnormal imaging should be confirmed by tissue biopsy using the method that will best ensure accurate staging because evidence shows that more complete staging workups improve patient outcomes.[52–54] In fact, most practice guidelines recommend that patients with a peripheral lesion, defined as being in the outer third of the lung parenchyma, concerning for cancer, require tissue diagnosis before further management can be planned.[55] It is recommended that patients with peripheral pulmonary nodules be considered for a CT-guided transthoracic needle aspiration (TTNA) as an initial diagnostic option.[26,56,57]

Computed Tomographic Imaging to Guide Percutaneous Biopsies

Although CT scans are not used to biopsy lesions, per se, CT still allows for real-time guidance in assessing nodules to allow for percutaneous sampling in the same way an endoscope is used.[58] The indication for biopsy put forth by the I-ELCAP protocol was when a solitary nodule measured 15 mm or more in size, was a solid nodule that had grown on follow-up scans, or was a nonsolid or part-solid nodule that persisted in size and did not resolve on 1- or 3-month follow-up scans.[2,59] More recent guidelines are more stringent and recommend that nodules greater than 8 mm in diameter that have either a pretest probability of malignancy $\geq$10%, PET avidity, or when a fully informed patient desires a definitive diagnostic procedure, should have a biopsy performed.[2] Additional guidelines for nodules greater than 8 mm also include undergoing a biopsy if there are any data to support a substantial suspicion of lung cancer.[8,10,60]

Transthoracic needle biopsy (TTNB) may provide more information over only the cellular material obtained by TTNA alone because the core needle provides more material by which information regarding cellular architecture and degree of invasiveness can be obtained. The sensitivity of CT-guided TTNB for malignancy ranges from 74% to 97%, and its specificity ranges from 95% to 100%.[58,61–64] A recent review found that CT-guided TTNB was a reliable procedure associated with an 88% to 91% sensitivity for the diagnosis of lung cancer, specifically with the yield being enhanced to 97% when larger core needles ($\geq$18 gauge) were used.[65] If the sample or results of a biopsy are inadequate or inconclusive, respectively, and the suspicion of malignancy remains high, additional biopsy tests should be attempted.[66] Unfortunately, percutaneous procedures also are associated with a significantly higher pneumothorax rate because the needle traverses the pleura and lung.[40,55] These CT-guided transthoracic lung biopsies are associated with an overall incidence of complications that vary greatly (1.7%–45%).[55]

Endoscopically Directed Biopsies

- EBUS and EUS must be used in a strategically advantageous manner relying on their individual strengths to maximize their efficacy in the diagnosis and staging of lung cancer

The primary advantage of EBUS or EUS over surgical cervical mediastinoscopy is that it can be performed with sedation and rarely requires general anesthesia in skilled hands. Another advantage is that in addition to accessing the mediastinal lymph nodes for sampling, EBUS more so than EUS provides the added advantage of being able to biopsy the hilar lymph nodes and the lung parenchymal lesion itself. EBUS and EUS allow complementary evaluation of almost all mediastinal lymph node levels when combined (**Box 2**).[67]

EUS and EBUS have been shown to be safe techniques with low morbidities and mortalities. Studies of patients undergoing EBUS for peripheral lung nodules have reported an overall low incidence of complication ranging from well under 1%–5%. Specific complications have included pneumothorax (0.8%–2.1%), pulmonary infections (0.5%), and bleeding (1%–5%).[68–72] Deaths due to complications from these procedures are extremely rare (0.04%), with those mortalities occurring in patients with poor preoperative performance status defined by their American Society of Anesthesiologists Physical Status Classification of III or IV.[40]

Advances in on-site tissue sample investigation, referred to as ROSE (ie, Rapid Onsite Evaluation), have also allowed for another advantage with EBUS and EUS in that the biopsies are examined while the patient is undergoing the procedure itself. ROSE of cytology when used with EBUS or EUS sampling has been shown to correlate with 94.8% of lymph nodes having a clear diagnosis on the first pass biopsy as compared with subsequent passes.[73] Therefore, with the addition of

---

Box 2
Indications for endoscopic biopsies

EBUS

1. Sampling tissue from lung nodule or mass
   R-EBUS if peripheral (outer 1/3)
   L-EBUS if central
   Tissue sampling for biomarker testing (use ROSE if possible)
   Peripheral nodule/mass of any size in a patient with poor surgical candidacy and/or if other techniques are higher risk for that particular patient (ie, CT-guided TTNA in severe bullous chronic obstructive pulmonary disease)

2. Staging patients with lung cancer with mediastinal or hilar lymph node involvement
   Clinical hilar (N1) and/or mediastinal (N2 or N3) disease by CT and/or PET/CT scan
   Central tumor
   Peripheral tumor and >3 cm

3. Confirming pathologic diagnosis of enlarged lymph nodes in suspected or confirmed lymphoproliferative or infectious diseases

4. Evaluating tracheobronchial tree
   Biopsy abnormal tissue
   Assess depth of invasion

5. Sampling tissue from mediastinal nodule or mass

6. Sampling abnormal-appearing tissue concerning for malignant infiltration of the mediastinum

EUS

1. Biopsying left adrenal lesion when concerned for metastasis

2. Biopsying levels 5, 8, and 9 lymph nodes

3. Biopsying of celiac and infradiaphragmatic retroperitoneal lymph nodes

ROSE, the need for more than 3 biopsy passes may be unnecessary. The true benefit of ROSE is that the sampled tissue is evaluated in real time to reduce the rate of nondiagnostic sampling. Furthermore, ROSE has been shown to correlate very well with final pathology and may guide the proceduralist in the order and way the tissues are sampled.[74] If no onsite assessment is available, it is recommended that the needles be changed between sampling of N3, N2, and N1 nodes rather than simply flushing the needles in between sampling of different nodal stations to avoid cross-contamination.[32]

Endobronchial Ultrasound

EBUS was introduced in 1990 and has the advantage of being able to obtain sufficient tissue samples for histologic diagnosis, including immunohistochemistry, which is important in many diseases.[74] Masses adjacent to the airway, intrapulmonary nodules, and mediastinal tumors of unknown cause often times require advanced pathologic diagnosis for definitive diagnosis, and EBUS is able to accomplish this.[40,74]

EBUS uses a radial (R-EBUS) or linear (L-EBUS) probe with a bronchoscope and uses frequencies between 5 and 10 MHz with a penetration at 5 MHz to about 6 to 8 cm (**Fig. 3**).[40,74] The current EBUS iteration includes a dedicated biopsy needle (typically 22 gauge) allowing EBUS-TBNA of levels 2R, 2L, 4R, 4L, 7, 10R, 10L, 11R, and

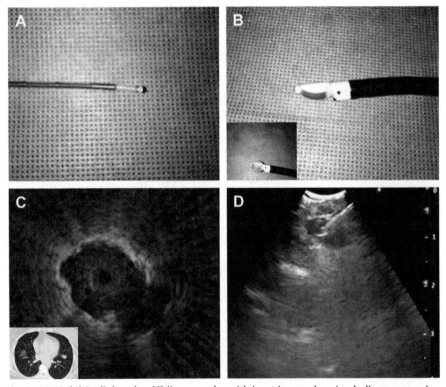

Fig. 3. EBUS. (*A*) Radial probe, (*B*) linear probe with inset image showing balloon expansion, (*C*) ultrasound image of pathologic pulmonary nodule using radial probe with inset showing lesion on CT scan, (*D*) ultrasound image showing needle within a pathologic lymph node using linear probe.

11L.[40,67,74,75] L-EBUS facilitates TBNA of mediastinal lymph nodes, hilar lymph nodes, intrapulmonary lymph nodes, and central lesions under real-time ultrasound guidance.[76,77] The L-EBUS probe typically is larger than a standard flexible bronchoscope and requires oral intubation.[78] R-EBUS allows for evaluation of central airways and their wall structure (ie, defining airway invasion), hilar lymph nodes, mediastinal lymph nodes, intrapulmonary lymph nodes, and peripheral lung lesions.[33,76,77] The more peripheral intrapulmonary lymph node levels 12 to 14 are also accessible if a miniature R-EBUS probe is used.[67] Small R-EBUS probes (miniprobes) allow for the biopsy of peripheral nodules independent of lesion size with sensitivities ranging from 61% to 80%.[26,77] The further development of even smaller probes with guiding catheters and more advanced miniprobes will solve the navigation issue to move farther into the periphery.[77]

The prevalence of positive mediastinal lymph node disease following a negative EBUS-TBNA is reported to be low at 4.9%.[79] On the other hand, one retrospective study using EBUS sampling for negative CT and PET imaging (ie, unsuspected N2 disease) found that there was an incidence of malignancy in 17.6% of the EBUS samples obtained.[80] Generally, EBUS-TBNA is useful in biopsying centrally located, paratracheal and peribronchial tumors with a diagnostic sensitivity of 82% to 94%.[78]

There are no consistent characteristics on EBUS to predict malignancy. One study suggested that a round or oval shape was correlated with malignancy[73]; however, this has not been universally accepted criteria. Consequently, no particular ultrasound shape characteristic should deter the proceduralist from proceeding with a biopsy. Nevertheless, 3 variables have been correlated strongly with false negative EBUS outcomes: (1) central location of the lung tumor, (2) nodal enlargement on CT, and (3) FDG-avidity for mediastinal lymph nodes on PET imaging.[81]

Endoscopic Ultrasound

EUS-guided biopsy gives the proceduralist the ability to sample lymph nodes that are not accessible via an EBUS approach (levels 5, 8, and 9 lymph nodes and the infradiaphragmatic and retroperitoneal lymph nodes).[67] EUS-guided fine-needle aspiration (FNA) uses a curved linear array ultrasound transducer, which allows for real-time ultrasound-guided needle sampling of the lymph node stations accessible from the esophagus as well as lung and pleural lesions.[82,83] The location of the esophagus, which is posterior and to the left of the trachea, makes right-sided visualization and sampling more of a challenge even when the lymph nodes are grossly enlarged.[67] The lymph nodes that can be sampled include some of the paratracheal lymph nodes (levels 2R 2L, 4R, and 4L), although anatomic constraints make it challenging to reliably access these levels especially anterior to and to the right of the trachea. Not surprisingly, EUS is associated with an incidence of false negative biopsies in these areas of 19%.[67,82] EUS is better suited for reaching the lymph nodes in the subcarinal (level 7), aortopulmonary window (level 5), periesophageal (level 8), and inferior pulmonary ligament (level 9) stations as well as the infradiaphragmatic retroperitoneal lymph nodes close to the aorta and celiac trunk.[52,67,75,82] EUS-FNA can use a transgastric approach to biopsy abnormalities of the left adrenal glan.[83,84] It is noted that EUS is inferior to transcutaneous ultrasound in the evaluation of the right adrenal gland due to the esophagus's left-sided location.[67]

EUS-guided FNA has been reported to decrease the need for surgical mediastinoscopy by 68% when used as the initial staging tool.[41,83,85] EUS-guided FNA has a sensitivity of 84% to 92.5%, specificity of 89% to 100%, and positive predictive value of 79% to 100% in confirming suspicious mediastinal lymph nodes for malignancy that are detected by FDG-PET in patients with suspected or proven NSCLC.[86] In patients with negative lymph nodes on CT scan (ie, <1 cm), EUS has been shown to identify malignant mediastinal involvement in 25% of those patients as well as identify invasion or left adrenal involvement in 18.75%.[87] Surgical mediastinoscopy continues to have an important role in working up patients with concern for mediastinal lymph node involvement when EBUS/EUS sampling is negative.[2]

Endobronchial Ultrasound Combined with Esophageal Ultrasound

Accurate staging of the disease may be enhanced through combining the EBUS and EUS (EBUS + EUS) techniques. This approach is supported by the results of the Assessment of Surgical Staging versus Endobronchial and Endoscopic Ultrasound in Lung Cancer prospective randomized trial. This study showed a sensitivity of 79% for detecting mediastinal lymph node metastasis with immediate surgical staging alone versus 85% for EUS + EBUS only.[88] The same study showed that when EUS + EBUS was negative followed by immediate surgical mediastinoscopy to confirm this finding, the sensitivity was 94%.[88] Ultimately, this approach resulted in fewer thoracotomies. It was determined that 11 patients needed to undergo mediastinoscopy in order to detect one single patient with N2 disease missed by combined EBUS + EUS.[88] These findings may represent a point in the evolution of a possible enhanced role in combined endoscopic modalities that may challenge surgical staging in the future.

Electromagnetic Navigational Bronchoscopy

ENB was approved for use in 2004 and is used to evaluate lesions that are peripherally located beyond the depth that a traditional bronchoscope can reach.[89] This technique uses an electromagnetic array to create an electromagnetic field around the patient with a computer system that then uses a preoperative CT scan to provide the bronchoscopic probe location on a screen in 3 dimensions.[90] It combines conventional and virtual bronchoscopy to enable the guidance of bronchoscopic instruments to target areas within the peripheral lung parenchyma.[91] This system is analogous to a Global Positioning System that is used to guide an automobile's navigation. The navigation system shows a "road map" of the bronchial tree on the display screen that the proceduralist can follow. The diagnostic yield of this technique for biopsying these peripheral lesions varies widely and is reported to range from 55.7% to 94%.[91–93]

Other uses for ENB have also included marking peripheral lesions with dye, placing fiducials for nonpalpable lesions before planned thoracoscopic resections, and placing brachytherapy catheters.[91,92] Relatively small series have demonstrated complete success when using ENB for localizing and resecting lung parenchymal lesions.[92] Although promising, refinements to ENB are needed to fully define the scope of its applicability.

DISCUSSION

In terms of noninvasive studies, although CXRs have been the historical workhorse in evaluating patients with lung cancer, CT scanning has become the diagnostic imaging study that has allowed for the greatest anatomic detail. Integrated PET/CT scanning has now emerged as an important adjunct to imaging for lung cancer because of its sensitivity in detecting metabolic activity that would be suggestive of malignancy. Other modalities and advances in imaging either have been shown to be inferior to these 2 imaging modalities or have yet to supplant these 2 modalities as the mainstays in the workup of patients with lung cancer. Nevertheless, more data regarding the refinements in these modalities surely will hone their utility in the diagnosis and staging of lung cancer. With respect to invasive studies, EBUS and EUS techniques are evolving modalities that are approaching the effectiveness, particularly when used in conjunction, that is rivaling more traditional surgical diagnostic and staging proced-ures. Furthermore, advances such as ENB have the potential to steer innovation down new exciting avenues.

SUMMARY

In summary, CXR, although useful in detecting some thoracic abnormalities, should not be part of a formal screening or staging protocol exclusively. Rather, LDCT scan-ning should be used to screen for lung cancer in high-risk patients as defined by na-tional and international guidelines. Once an abnormality is identified by screening LDCT, additional imaging should be performed with HRCT scanning to characterize the abnormality in greater detail. If concern for a malignancy remains, a follow-up PET/CT scan should be used to further delineate the lesion as well as complete nonin-vasive staging through the assessment of the mediastinum and the identification of, or lack thereof, possible metastatic disease. Mediastinal involvement of disease then can be confirmed by minimally invasive techniques such as EBUS and EUS. In experi-enced hands, these techniques are approaching an efficacy similar to that of cervical mediastinoscopy in being the definitive invasive staging procedure. EBUS may pro-vide the additional benefit over cervical mediastinoscopy of allowing the clinician to achieve a tissue diagnosis of the pulmonary lesion during the same setting of medias-tinal staging.

REFERENCES

1. National Lung Screening Trial Research Trial, Aberle DR, Adams AM, et al. Reduced lung-cancer mortality with low-dose computed tomographic screening. N Engl J Med 2011;365(5):395–409.
2. Detterbeck FC, Mazzone PJ, Naidich DP, et al. Screening for lung cancer: diag-nosis and management of lung cancer, 3rd ed: American College of Chest Phy-sicians evidence-based clinical practice guidelines. Chest 2013;143(5 Suppl): e78S–92S.
3. Henschke CI, McCauley DI, Yankelevitz DF, et al. Early Lung Cancer Action Proj-ect: overall design and findings from baseline screening. Lancet 1999;354(9173): 99–105.
4. Midthun DE, Jett JR. Screening for lung cancer: the US studies. J Surg Oncol 2013;108(5):275–9.
5. Henschke CI, Yankelevitz DF, Kostis WJ. CT screening for lung cancer. Semin Ul-trasound CT MR 2003;24(1):23–32.
6. Rocco G, Allen MS, Altorki NK, et al. Clinical statement on the role of the surgeon and surgical issues relating to computed tomography screening programs for lung cancer. Ann Thorac Surg 2013;96(1):357–60.
7. Bach PB, Mirkin JN, Oliver TK, et al. Benefits and harms of CT screening for lung cancer: a systematic review. JAMA 2012;307(22):2418–29.
8. Jaklitsch MT, Jacobson FL, Austin JH, et al. The American Association for Thoracic Surgery guidelines for lung cancer screening using low-dose computed tomography scans for lung cancer survivors and other high-risk groups. J Thorac Cardiovasc Surg 2012;144(1):33–8.
9. Wood DE, Eapen GA, Ettinger DS, et al. Lung cancer screening. J Natl Compr Cancer Netw 2012;10(2):240–65.

10. Wood DE. National Comprehensive Cancer Network (NCCN) clinical practice guidelines for lung cancer screening. Thorac Surg Clin 2015;25(2):185–97.

11. Moyer VA, Force USPST. Screening for lung cancer: U.S. Preventive Services Task Force recommendation statement. Ann Intern Med 2014;160(5):330–8.

12. Fischbach F, Knollmann F, Griesshaber V, et al. Detection of pulmonary nodules by multislice computed tomography: improved detection rate with reduced slice thickness. Eur Radiol 2003;13(10):2378–83.

13. Paul NS, Ley S, Metser U. Optimal imaging protocols for lung cancer staging: CT, PET, MR imaging, and the role of imaging. Radiol Clin North Am 2012;50(5):935–49.

14. Lee WK, Lau EW, Chin K, et al. Modern diagnostic and therapeutic interventional radiology in lung cancer. J Thorac Dis 2013;5(Suppl 5):S511–23.

15. Sieren JC, Ohno Y, Koyama H, et al. Recent technological and application developments in computed tomography and magnetic resonance imaging for improved pulmonary nodule detection and lung cancer staging. J Magn Reson Imaging 2010;32(6):1353–69.

16. Wahidi MM, Govert JA, Goudar RK, et al, American College of Chest Physicians. Evidence for the treatment of patients with pulmonary nodules: when is it lung cancer?: ACCP evidence-based clinical practice guidelines (2nd edition). Chest 2007;132(3 Suppl):94S–107S.

17. Hansell DM, Bankier AA, MacMahon H, et al. Fleischner Society: glossary of terms for thoracic imaging. Radiology 2008;246(3):697–722.

18. Devaraj A, Cook GJ, Hansell DM. PET/CT in non-small cell lung cancer staging-promises and problems. Clin Radiol 2007;62(2):97–108.

19. Ono K, Hiraoka T, Ono A, et al. Low-dose CT scan screening for lung cancer: comparison of images and radiation doses between low-dose CT and follow-up standard diagnostic CT. Springerplus 2013;2:393.

20. Henschke CI, Yankelevitz DF, Smith JP, et al. Screening for lung cancer: the early lung cancer action approach. Lung Cancer 2002;35(2):143–8.

21. Goldman LW. Principles of CT: radiation dose and image quality. J Nucl Med Technol 2007;35(4):213–25 [quiz: 226–8].

22. Naidich DP, Rusinek H, McGuinness G, et al. Variables affecting pulmonary nodule detection with computed tomography: evaluation with three-dimensional computer simulation. J Thorac Imaging 1993;8(4):291–9.

23. Silvestri GA, Gould MK, Margolis ML, et al. Noninvasive staging of non-small cell lung cancer: ACCP evidenced-based clinical practice guidelines (2nd edition). Chest 2007;132(3 Suppl):178S–201S.

24. Flechsig P, Kratochwil C, Schwartz LH, et al. Quantitative volumetric CT-histogram analysis in N-staging of 18F-FDG-equivocal patients with lung cancer. J Nucl Med 2014;55(4):559–64.

25. Tsim S, O'Dowd CA, Milroy R, et al. Staging of non-small cell lung cancer (NSCLC): a review. Respir Med 2010;104(12):1767–74.

26. Detterbeck FC, Jantz MA, Wallace M, et al. Invasive mediastinal staging of lung cancer: ACCP evidence-based clinical practice guidelines (2nd edition). Chest 2007;132(3 Suppl):202S–20S.

27. Schrevens L, Lorent N, Dooms C, et al. The role of PET scan in diagnosis, staging, and management of non-small cell lung cancer. Oncologist 2004;9(6):633–43.

28. Toba H, Kondo K, Otsuka H, et al. Diagnosis of the presence of lymph node metastasis and decision of operative indication using fluorodeoxyglucose-positron emission tomography and computed tomography in patients with primary lung cancer. J Med Invest 2010;57(3–4):305–13.

29. Lardinois D, Weder W, Hany TF, et al. Staging of non-small-cell lung cancer with integrated positron-emission tomography and computed tomography. N Engl J Med 2003;348(25):2500–7.

30. Fischer B, Lassen U, Mortensen J, et al. Preoperative staging of lung cancer with combined PET-CT. N Engl J Med 2009;361(1):32–9.

31. von Schulthess GK, Steinert HC, Hany TF. Integrated PET/CT: current applications and future directions. Radiology 2006;238(2):405–22.

32. Fielding DI, Kurimoto N. EBUS-TBNA/staging of lung cancer. Clin Chest Med 2013;34(3):385–94.

33. Mattes MD, Moshchinsky AB, Ahsanuddin S, et al. Ratio of lymph node to primary tumor SUV on PET/CT accurately predicts nodal malignancy in non-small-cell lung cancer. Clin Lung Cancer 2015;16(6):e253–8.

34. Kitajima K, Doi H, Kanda T, et al. Present and future roles of FDG-PET/CT imaging in the management of lung cancer. Jpn J Radiol 2016;34(6):387–99.

35. Rankin S. PET/CT for staging and monitoring non small cell lung cancer. Cancer Imaging 2008;8 Spec No A:S27–31.

36. Cerfolio RJ, Bryant AS, Ohja B, et al. The maximum standardized uptake values on positron emission tomography of a non-small cell lung cancer predict stage, recurrence, and survival. J Thorac Cardiovasc Surg 2005;130(1):151–9.

37. Kim SJ, Chang S. Limited prognostic value of SUV max measured by F-18 FDG PET/CT in newly diagnosed small cell lung cancer patients. Oncol Res Treat 2015;38(11):577–85.

38. Moloney F, Ryan D, McCarthy L, et al. Increasing the accuracy of 18F-FDG PET/CT interpretation of "mildly positive" mediastinal nodes in the staging of non-small cell lung cancer. Eur J Radiol 2014;83(5):843–7.

39. Hellwig D, Graeter TP, Ukena D, et al. 18F-FDG PET for mediastinal staging of lung cancer: which SUV threshold makes sense? J Nucl Med 2007;48(11):1761–6.

40. Dietrich CF, Annema JT, Clementsen P, et al. Ultrasound techniques in the evaluation of the mediastinum, part I: endoscopic ultrasound (EUS), endobronchial ultrasound (EBUS) and transcutaneous mediastinal ultrasound (TMUS), introduction into ultrasound techniques. J Thorac Dis 2015;7(9):E311–25.

41. Tournoy KG, Carprieaux M, Deschepper E, et al. Are EUS-FNA and EBUS-TBNA specimens reliable for subtyping non-small cell lung cancer? Lung Cancer 2012;76(1):46–50.

42. Reinhardt MJ, Wiethoelter N, Matthies A, et al. PET recognition of pulmonary metastases on PET/CT imaging: impact of attenuation-corrected and non-attenuation-corrected PET images. Eur J Nucl Med Mol Imaging 2006;33(2):134–9.

43. Lee SM, Goo JM, Park CM, et al. Preoperative staging of non-small cell lung cancer: prospective comparison of PET/MR and PET/CT. Eur Radiol 2016;26(11):3850–7.

44. Wang Y, Ma S, Dong M, et al. Evaluation of the factors affecting the maximum standardized uptake value of metastatic lymph nodes in different histological types of non-small cell lung cancer on PET-CT. BMC Pulm Med 2015;15:20.

45. Detterbeck FC, Figueroa Almanzar S. Lung cancer staging: the value of PET depends on the clinical setting. J Thorac Dis 2014;6(12):1714–23.

46. Qu X, Huang X, Yan W, et al. A meta-analysis of (1)(8)FDG-PET-CT, (1)(8)FDG-PET, MRI and bone scintigraphy for diagnosis of bone metastases in patients with lung cancer. Eur J Radiol 2012;81(5):1007–15.

47. Grootjans W, Hermsen R, van der Heijden EH, et al. The impact of respiratory gated positron emission tomography on clinical staging and management of patients with lung cancer. Lung Cancer 2015;90(2):217–23.

48. Kaira K, Oriuchi N, Otani Y, et al. Fluorine-18-alpha-methyltyrosine positron emission tomography for diagnosis and staging of lung cancer: a clinicopathologic study. Clin Cancer Res 2007;13(21):6369–78.

49. Wynants J, Stroobants S, Dooms C, et al. Staging of lung cancer. Radiol Clin North Am 2007;45(4):609–25, v.

50. Evison M, Crosbie P, Booton R. Should all lung cancer patients requiring mediastinal staging with EBUS undergo PET-CT first? J Bronchology Interv Pulmonol 2015;22(2):e5–7.

51. Darling GE, Dickie AJ, Malthaner RA, et al. Invasive mediastinal staging of non-small-cell lung cancer: a clinical practice guideline. Curr Oncol 2011;18(6): e304–10.

52. Silvestri GA, Gonzalez AV, Jantz MA, et al. Methods for staging non-small cell lung cancer: diagnosis and management of lung cancer, 3rd ed: American College of Chest Physicians evidence-based clinical practice guidelines. Chest 2013;143(5 Suppl):e211S–250S.

53. Vilmann P, Clementsen PF, Colella S, et al. Combined endobronchial and oesophageal endosonography for the diagnosis and staging of lung cancer. European Society of Gastrointestinal Endoscopy (ESGE) Guideline, in cooperation with the European Respiratory Society (ERS) and the European Society of Thoracic Surgeons (ESTS). Eur Respir J 2015;46(1):40–60.

54. Novello S, Barlesi F, Califano R, et al. Metastatic non-small-cell lung cancer: ESMO Clinical Practice Guidelines for diagnosis, treatment and follow-up. Ann Oncol 2016;27(Suppl 5):v1–27.

55. Heerink WJ, de Bock GH, de Jonge GJ, et al. Complication rates of CT-guided transthoracic lung biopsy: meta-analysis. Eur Radiol 2016;27(1):138–48.

56. Ost DE, Gould MK. Decision making in patients with pulmonary nodules. Am J Respir Crit Care Med 2012;185(4):363–72.

57. Ettinger D, et al. NCCN Clinical Practice Guidelines in Oncology (NCCN Guidelines), Non-Small Cell Lung Cancer. Version 7.2015. 2015; Version 7.2015: NCCN Clinical Practice Guidelines in Oncology (NCCN Guidelines), Non-Small Cell Lung Cancer. Available at: https://www.tri-kobe.org/nccn/guideline/lung/english/non_small.pdf. Accessed October 31, 2016.

58. Ghaye B, Dondelinger RF. Imaging guided thoracic interventions. Eur Respir J 2001;17(3):507–28.

59. Wagnetz U, Menezes RJ, Boerner S, et al. CT screening for lung cancer: implication of lung biopsy recommendations. AJR Am J Roentgenol 2012;198(2):351–8.

60. Vansteenkiste J, De Ruysscher D, Eberhardt WE, et al. Early and locally advanced non-small-cell lung cancer (NSCLC): ESMO Clinical Practice Guidelines for diagnosis, treatment and follow-up. Ann Oncol 2013;24(Suppl 6): vi89–98.

61. Larscheid RC, Thorpe PE, Scott WJ. Percutaneous transthoracic needle aspiration biopsy: a comprehensive review of its current role in the diagnosis and treatment of lung tumors. Chest 1998;114(3):704–9.

62. Toloza EM, Harpole L, Detterbeck F, et al. Invasive staging of non-small cell lung cancer: a review of the current evidence. Chest 2003;123(1 Suppl):157S–66S.

63. Rivera MP, Mehta AC, Wahidi MM. Establishing the diagnosis of lung cancer: diagnosis and management of lung cancer, 3rd ed: American College of Chest

Physicians evidence-based clinical practice guidelines. Chest 2013;143(5 Suppl):e142S–65S.

64. de Margerie-Mellon C, de Bazelaire C, de Kerviler E. Image-guided biopsy in primary lung cancer: why, when and how. Diagn Interv Imaging 2016;97(10): 965–72.

65. Loubeyre P, Copercini M, Dietrich PY. Percutaneous CT-guided multisampling core needle biopsy of thoracic lesions. AJR Am J Roentgenol 2005;185(5): 1294–8.

66. Fontaine-Delaruelle C, Souquet PJ, Gamondes D, et al. Negative predictive value of transthoracic core-needle biopsy: a multicenter study. Chest 2015;148(2): 472–80.

67. Jenssen C, Annema JT, Clementsen P, et al. Ultrasound techniques in the evaluation of the mediastinum, part 2: mediastinal lymph node anatomy and diagnostic reach of ultrasound techniques, clinical work up of neoplastic and inflammatory mediastinal lymphadenopathy using ultrasound techniques and how to learn mediastinal endosonography. J Thorac Dis 2015;7(10):E439–58.

68. Hayama M, Izumo T, Matsumoto Y, et al. Complications with endobronchial ultrasound with a guide sheath for the diagnosis of peripheral pulmonary lesions. Respiration 2015;90(2):129–35.

69. Dong X, Qiu X, Liu Q, et al. Endobronchial ultrasound-guided transbronchial needle aspiration in the mediastinal staging of non-small cell lung cancer: a meta-analysis. Ann Thorac Surg 2013;96(4):1502–7.

70. Bernasconi M, Casutt A, Koutsokera A, et al. Radial ultrasound-assisted transbronchial biopsy: a new diagnostic approach for non-resolving pulmonary infiltrates in neutropenic hemato-oncological patients. Lung 2016;194(6):917–21.

71. Georgiou HD, Taverner J, Irving LB, et al. Safety and efficacy of radial EBUS for the investigation of peripheral pulmonary lesions in patients with advanced COPD. J Bronchology Interv Pulmonol 2016;23(3):192–8.

72. Zamora FD, Moughrabieh A, Gibson H, et al. An expectorated "stent": an unexpected complication of EBUS-TBNA. J Bronchology Interv Pulmonol 2016. [Epub ahead of print].

73. Memoli JS, El-Bayoumi E, Pastis NJ, et al. Using endobronchial ultrasound features to predict lymph node metastasis in patients with lung cancer. Chest 2011;140(6):1550–6.

74. Nakajima T, Yasufuku K, Yoshino I. Current status and perspective of EBUS-TBNA. Gen Thorac Cardiovasc Surg 2013;61(7):390–6.

75. Gelberg J, Grondin S, Tremblay A. Mediastinal staging for lung cancer. Can Respir J 2014;21(3):159–61.

76. Gomez M, Silvestri GA. Endobronchial ultrasound for the diagnosis and staging of lung cancer. Proc Am Thorac Soc 2009;6(2):180–6.

77. Zaric B, Stojsic V, Sarcev T, et al. Advanced bronchoscopic techniques in diagnosis and staging of lung cancer. J Thorac Dis 2013;5(Suppl 4):S359–70.

78. Anantham D, Koh MS, Ernst A. Endobronchial ultrasound. Respir Med 2009; 103(10):1406–14.

79. Taverner J, Cheang MY, Antippa P, et al. Negative EBUS-TBNA predicts very low prevalence of mediastinal disease in staging of non-small cell lung cancer. J Bronchology Interv Pulmonol 2016;23(2):177–80.

80. Shingyoji M, Nakajima T, Yoshino M, et al. Endobronchial ultrasonography for positron emission tomography and computed tomography-negative lymph node staging in non-small cell lung cancer. Ann Thorac Surg 2014;98(5):1762–7.

81. Talebian Yazdi M, Egberts J, Schinkelshoek MS, et al. Endosonography for lung cancer staging: predictors for false-negative outcomes. Lung Cancer 2015;90(3): 451–6.

82. Khoo KL, Ho KY. Endoscopic mediastinal staging of lung cancer. Respir Med 2011;105:515–8.

83. Colella S, Vilmann P, Konge L, et al. Endoscopic ultrasound in the diagnosis and staging of lung cancer. Endosc Ultrasound 2014;3(4):205–12.

84. Eloubeidi MA. Endoscopic ultrasound-guided fine-needle aspiration in the staging and diagnosis of patients with lung cancer. Semin Thorac Cardiovasc Surg 2007;19(3):206–11.

85. Tournoy KG, Ryck FD, Vanwalleghem L, et al. The yield of endoscopic ultrasound in lung cancer staging: does lymph node size matter? J Thorac Oncol 2008;3(3): 245–9.

86. Eloubeidi MA, Cerfolio RJ, Chen VK, et al. Endoscopic ultrasound-guided fine needle aspiration of mediastinal lymph node in patients with suspected lung cancer after positron emission tomography and computed tomography scans. Ann Thorac Surg 2005;79(1):263–8.

87. Wallace MB, Ravenel J, Block MI, et al. Endoscopic ultrasound in lung cancer patients with a normal mediastinum on computed tomography. Ann Thorac Surg 2004;77(5):1763–8.

88. Annema JT, van Meerbeeck JP, Rintoul RC, et al. Mediastinoscopy vs endosonography for mediastinal nodal staging of lung cancer: a randomized trial. JAMA 2010;304(20):2245–52.

89. Kalanjeri S, Gildea TR. Electromagnetic navigational bronchoscopy for peripheral pulmonary nodules. Thorac Surg Clin 2016;26(2):203–13.

90. Bauer TL, Berkheim DB. Bronchoscopy: diagnostic and therapeutic for non-small cell lung cancer. Surg Oncol Clin N Am 2016;25(3):481–91.

91. Goud A, Dahagam C, Breen DP, et al. Role of electromagnetic navigational bronchoscopy in pulmonary nodule management. J Thorac Dis 2016;8(Suppl 6): S501–8.

92. Awais O, Reidy MR, Mehta K, et al. Electromagnetic navigation bronchoscopy-guided dye marking for thoracoscopic resection of pulmonary nodules. Ann Thorac Surg 2016;102:223–9.

93. Gildea TR, Mazzone PJ, Karnak D, et al. Electromagnetic navigation diagnostic bronchoscopy: a prospective study. Am J Respir Crit Care Med 2006;174(9): 982–9.

Lung Cancer Screening and Its Impact on Surgical Volume

Andrew P. Dhanasopon, MD[a], Anthony W. Kim, MD[b],*

KEYWORDS

- Lung cancer • Lung cancer screening • Thoracic surgery

KEY POINTS

- Screening for lung cancer in high-risk individuals with annual low-dose computed tomography examinations has been shown to reduce lung cancer mortality by 20%.
- Screening for lung cancer by chest radiography or in low-risk individuals is not recommended.
- Lung cancer screening is recommended by multiple health care organizations and is covered by Medicare and Medicaid.
- Lung cancer screening is projected to increase the case volume for the thoracic surgery workforce.

INTRODUCTION

Lung cancer is the leading cause of cancer-related death in the United States, with 1 out of 4 cancer deaths owing to lung cancer.[1] Each year, more people die of lung cancer than of colon, breast, and prostate cancers combined. For 2016, the American Cancer Society estimates about 224,390 new cases of lung cancer leading to about 158,080 deaths. Lung cancer mainly occurs in older people. Approximately 2 out of 3 people diagnosed with lung cancer are 65 years of age or older, and fewer than 2% are younger than 45 years. The average age at the time of diagnosis is about 70 years.

Cigarette smoking is the leading risk factor for developing lung cancer. Although reduced rates of cigarette smoking in the United States have resulted in a reduced incidence of lung cancer, the substantial burden of lung cancer will continue for many years. Smoking cessation has been the most important public health intervention that has reduced this burden. However, owing to its long preclinical phase and

Disclosures: None.
[a] Section of Thoracic Surgery, Yale-New Haven Hospital, Yale School of Medicine, 330 Cedar Street, BB205, New Haven, CT 06520, USA; [b] Division of Thoracic Surgery, Keck School of Medicine, University of Southern California, 1510 San Pablo Street, Suite 514, Los Angeles, CA 90033, USA
* Corresponding author.
E-mail address: Anthony.Kim@med.usc.edu

Surg Clin N Am 97 (2017) 751–762
http://dx.doi.org/10.1016/j.suc.2017.03.006
0039-6109/17/© 2017 Elsevier Inc. All rights reserved.

surgical.theclinics.com

markedly improved outcomes for patients treated at an earlier stage, there is substantial rationale for screening asymptomatic, high-risk individuals to improve the morbidity and mortality from this disease.[2]

Lung cancer screening has been implemented since the early 1960s. Numerous large-scale clinical trials have evaluated the use of chest radiographs, sputum analyses, computed tomography (CT), and most recently low-dose CT (LDCT) scans as screening tools. Coincident with the improvements in imaging technology, there also have been the refinements in surgical techniques for lung resections. With the establishment of lung cancer screening guidelines, the impact on the workforce needed to implement these guidelines are beginning to be studied. This article reviews the lung cancer screening data and its impact on the thoracic surgical workforce.

LUNG CANCER SCREENING TRIALS

Early, large-scale, clinical trials published in the 1980s and 1990s used chest radiographs for lung cancer screening and were disappointing.[3–6] None of the 6 randomized, controlled trials demonstrated any mortality benefit.[3–8] In the PLCO Screening trial (Prostate, Lung, Colorectal, and Ovarian Cancer), 154,942 smokers and nonsmokers from the general population were randomized to the intervention arm with an annual chest radiographs versus the control arm with "usual care," which was standard care as determined by their general health care practitioners.[7] After 13 years of follow-up, only 20% of lung cancers in the screening group were detected by screening, and no mortality benefit was seen in either the general population or the subset determined to be at higher risk of lung cancer based on smoking history and age. The Mayo Clinic conducted a randomized trial of chest radiographs and sputum analysis versus usual care. In a 20-year follow-up of this Mayo Lung Project, significantly more cancers were detected in the screening group; however, there was a higher overall lung cancer death rate, attributed to biased documentation of lung cancer as a cause of death.[8] These studies, along with others, resulted in a recommendation by the US Preventive Services Task Force in 2004 against using chest radiographs for lung cancer screening.[9] With the failure of chest radiography-based screening, centers began evaluating CT-based screening for lung cancer.

Initial studies of LDCT screening were observational, including the ELCAP (Early Lung Cancer Action Project), International ELCAP, the Mayo Clinic CT study, and the COSMOS study (Continuous Observation of Smoking study).[10–13] Owing to the lack of randomization, the studies were subject to lead-time bias and overdiagnosis bias. However, they did demonstrate for the first time the ability of CT to detect lung cancer at an early stage.

The most important randomized, controlled trial to date is the National Lung Screening Trial (NLST) conducted by the National Cancer Institute of LDCT for lung cancer screening.[14,15] To date, it is the only large-scale, randomized trial of LDCT lung cancer screening. Other ongoing randomized trials exist, but may not be adequately powered to detect a mortality benefit. A total of 53,454 high-risk persons at 33 medical centers across the United States were enrolled. Determinants of high risk included age and smoking history: between 55 and 74 years of age with at least 30 pack-years of smoking, and subjects could not have quit smoking more than 15 years before enrollment. Excluded were subjects who had any prior history of lung cancer, unexplained weight loss or symptoms suggestive of lung cancer, other cancers within the past 5 years (other than a nonmelanoma skin cancer), a chest CT scan in the past 18 months, or a medical condition that posed a significant risk of mortality during the trial period.

Subjects were first enrolled in 2002 and randomized to either an annual chest radiographs or annual LDCT for 3 consecutive years. Imaging was completed in 2007, with continued follow-up until the trial was stopped in November 2010 when an interim analysis showed a significant benefit for LDCT screening. At median follow-up of 6.5 years, there were 1060 lung cancers and 247 lung cancer deaths in the LDCT group compared with 941 lung cancers and 309 lung cancer deaths in the chest radiography group. The data demonstrated a 20% reduction in lung cancer mortality and a 6.7% reduction in all-cause mortality. Positive findings were defined as any noncalcified nodule seen on chest radiographs and any nodule at least 4 mm in size seen on LDCT. A total of 24% of subjects in the LDCT arm had a positive result. Of these positive results, 96% ultimately were shown not to be lung cancer and considered false positives. These false positives had been determined based on additional imaging, but also with surgery in 297 subjects. The rate of complications from the evaluation of true or false-positive findings was only 1.4% in the LDCT group (**Table 1**).

Based largely on the strength of the results of the NLST, multiple organizations[16–21] involved in lung cancer and cancer screening now recommend annual lung cancer screening with LDCT for high-risk individuals using the aforementioned definitions or variations thereof. These organizations include the American Cancer Society, the American Association of Thoracic Surgeons, the American College of Chest Physicians, the American Society of Clinical Oncology and the American Thoracic Society, and the US Preventive Services Task Force. In 2015, the Centers for Medicare and Medicaid Services released a decision memorandum on coverage for LDCT and visits for counseling and shared decision making.[22]

A post hoc analysis of the NLST included an application of a lung cancer risk assessment model based on the PLCO screening trial cohort that included smoking history, age, race/ethnicity, education, obesity, chronic obstructive pulmonary disease, and personal or family history of cancer.[23,24] The NLST cohort was divided into quintiles of risk of death from lung cancer over 5 years (**Fig. 1**). Although the

Table 1
National Lung Screening Trial: Potential benefits and risks of low-dose computed tomography screening

Benefits	Events per 1000 Subjects Screened
Diagnosis of stage I or II lung cancer	16
Prevented lung cancer deaths	3
Harms	
False-positive CT	
Nodule size considered abnormal (mm)	
>4	263
>5	155
>6	93
>7	61
Invasive biopsy for benign lesion	41
Surgery for benign lesion	10
Major complication during evaluation of a benign lesion	3
Overdiagnosis of lung cancer	0.6–1.2

Adapted from Deffebach ME, Humphrey L. Lung cancer screening. Surg Clin North Am 2015;95(5):967–78; with permission.

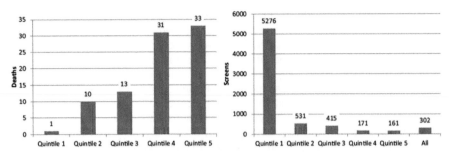

Fig. 1. From the National Lung Screening Trial, screened subjects divided into quintiles of risk of lung cancer death over 5 years. (*Left*) Lung cancer deaths prevented by low-dose computed tomography screening. (*Right*) Number needed to treat to prevent 1 lung cancer death. (*Data from* Kovalchik SA, Tammemagi M, Berg CD et al. Targeting of low-dose CT screening according to the risk of lung-cancer death. N Engl J Med 2013;369(3):245–54.)

20% decrease in lung cancer deaths was observed in all quintiles, only 1% of the prevented lung cancer deaths occurred in the lowest risk quintile. The number needed to screen to prevent 1 lung cancer death varied greatly with lung cancer risk. The lowest risk quintile required 5276 subjects to prevent 1 lung cancer death, whereas in the highest risk quintile, only 161. In addition, the proportion of false-positive results decreased with increasing risk of lung cancer.

There are several ongoing lung cancer screening studies that, although underpowered for determining the effect of LDCT on lung cancer screening mortality, are able to provide important information for the practice of lung cancer screening. The NELSON trial (Dutch-Belgian Lung Cancer Screening Trial) is a randomized trial of LDCT versus usual care (no screening) being conducted in Europe with 7557 subjects undergoing LDCT screening with a baseline CT followed by repeat LDCT at years 1 and 3.[25–29] Unlike the NLST, 5-year lung cancer survivors were eligible for inclusion. From published data thus far, the investigators have demonstrated that interval cancers (diagnosed outside of screening, between rounds of screening, and cancers detected at later rounds of screening) tend to be more aggressive.[30]

RISKS OF LUNG CANCER SCREENING

LDCT screening for lung cancer exposes individuals to radiation, which may include repeated exposure over 20 years. The risks of radiation are often extrapolated from environmental exposures, including atomic bomb survivors.[31] Analyses have suggested that serial imaging may add independently to the risk of developing a malignancy, and consideration of the risks of radiation need to include not only the screening LDCT, but also the radiation exposure from studies of positive (mostly false-positive) findings on follow-up imaging studies.[32] Restricting screening to the appropriate (older) age group, close attention to adherence and monitoring of an LDCT protocol, and judicious use of follow-up imaging are required to minimize the risks of radiation. The reported radiation dose for LDCT in screening studies ranges from 0.61 to 1.5 mSv, with 1 study documenting cumulative doses of up to 7 mSv for the screening and follow-up studies.[33]

Any abnormal finding that might indicate malignancy can cause anxiety, and this has been demonstrated in the context of lung cancer screening. Assessing the definition of abnormal and careful communication are important to reducing the stress and anxiety associated with screening for lung cancer.[34]

In the NLST, 96% of all positive findings were false-positive findings and required some evaluation, and 11% led to an invasive procedure. Many of the procedures carry substantial risks, such as image-guided biopsies, bronchoscopies, and surgery. Judicious use of these tests and expertise in their conduct are required to minimize associated risks.

Overdiagnosis occurs when there is a diagnosis of a cancer or other disease that would otherwise not go on to cause symptoms or death.[35] This result is not a false-positive diagnosis, because these individuals are diagnosed with tumors that meet pathologic criteria for cancer. The challenge is that one currently cannot determine which cancers will progress and which cancers will not progress; therefore, evaluation and treatment typically occur for all of them. However, when a patient is exposed to the risks of evaluation and treatment of disease that would not have become symptomatic during their lifetime, overdiagnosis has occurred with no benefit and undue harm may be incurred to the patient. Only randomized studies with long-term follow-up can determine the actual rate of overdiagnosis. Determinates of overdiagnosis include the aggressiveness of the cancer and the competing comorbidities in patients being diagnosed with cancer. Although lung cancer is generally an aggressive malignancy, it is heterogeneous with many subtypes that are very indolent. Studies have found that very indolent lung cancers, defined as having a doubling time greater than 400 days make up anywhere from 3% to 31% of detected lung cancers.[36] Furthermore, with smoking and age being the major lung cancer risks, patients at risk for developing lung cancer often have significant comorbidities, some of which result in death before development of symptoms.

Using a model of extended lifetime follow-up after LDCT screening in one study, the overdiagnosis rate of LDCT for non–small cell lung cancer was estimated to be less than 4%.[37] It has been suggested that lesions presenting as pure ground-glass nodules and typically associated with bronchoalveolar cell carcinoma or minimally invasive adenocarcinoma, although pathologically classified as cancers, may be candidates for overdiagnosis. Whether these lesions, when detected by screening, can be managed as truly indolent lesions, avoiding invasive procedures, is not yet known.

CHALLENGES FOR THE THORACIC SURGICAL WORKFORCE

As developments in imaging technology afforded the benefits seen in the lung cancer screening trials, similarly, refinements in surgical technique and instruments for lung resections led to improvements in outcomes for patients undergoing surgery.[38] Lung cancer surgery began with the first successful pneumonectomy reported by Graham and Singer in 1933.[39] Lobectomies and segmentectomies were reported in the 1940s and 1950s and the first successful sleeve lobectomy for carcinoma in 1952.[40,41] The introduction and development of surgical sutures and staplers made lung resections safer, faster, and less traumatic, while maintaining sound surgical oncologic principles. With surgeons gaining experience in lung resections and thoracic anesthesia, and intensive care progressing, specialized thoracic units developed in hospitals, and surgeons started extending cancer resections to the chest wall and great vessels.[42] The importance of lymph node involvement (hilar and mediastinal stations) in the prognosis of lung cancer was recognized.[43] The advent of video-assisted thoracic surgery in the 1990s considerably changed the approach to early stage lung cancer.[44–46] More recently, surgeons are gaining experience with robotic approaches to reduce the operative trauma, facilitate the surgical procedure, and reduce the duration of hospital stay.[47] Furthermore, new techniques, such as radiofrequency ablation and stereotactic body radiation therapy, are now offered as an alternative to surgery in patients unfit for lung resection, but are still being evaluated in prospective, randomized trials.[48,49]

Multiple publications have shown that the volume of lung cancer resections performed was associated positively with the survival of patients.[50] Patients operated on at high-volume centers have lower postoperative complication rates and lower 30-day mortality. Outcomes seem to be better in large teaching hospitals[51,52] and the surgeon's subspecialty—thoracic or cardiothoracic surgery versus general surgery—also influences in-hospital mortality.[53,54]

Despite a clear need for thoracic surgeons, the workforce is projected to decrease. A study by Williams and colleagues[55] in 2010 predicted a steady decrease in the number of practicing thoracic surgeons in the United States from about 4000 surgeons in 2000 to about 3000 surgeons in 2050, an approximate 25% decrease (**Fig. 2**). However, owing to continued population growth and increasing life expectancy, there will be an increasing need such that, by 2050, the number of practicing thoracic surgeons will be one-half the number that is needed. Furthermore, not accounting for this increase in the population is the potential impact of lung cancer screening programs throughout the country that will contribute to the increased workload for the thoracic surgery workforce.

CONSEQUENCES OF LUNG CANCER SCREENING IN RELATION TO SURGICAL VOLUME

To date, there has been only one published study examining the potential impact of the implementation of lung cancer screening programs on the thoracic surgery workforce.[56] The authors of this study by Edwards and colleagues[56,57] at the University of Calgary in Alberta, Canada, applied computer modeling techniques to forecast the "demand" for thoracic surgeons (the incidence of operable lung cancers in the Canadian population over time) and the "supply" of Canadian thoracic surgeons in the workforce, after the introduction of LDCT screening.[56,57] The demand component of the model used data from the annual Canadian Community Health Survey to determine smoking rates and smoking history (current, former, never, pack-years, quit time), controlling for age, sex, and location. The supply component of the model used data from the 2009 Canadian Thoracic Manpower and Education survey on the demographics, training history, practice characteristics, and estimated retirement age of thoracic surgeons in Canada.[58] The number of thoracic surgeons entering the workforce was calculated based on the number of Royal College of Physicians and

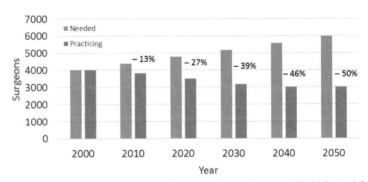

Fig. 2. Predicted number of surgeons practicing and number needed. (*Adapted from* Williams TE Jr, Satiani B, Thomas A, et al. The impending shortage and the estimated cost of training the future surgical workforce. Ann Surg 2009;250(4):590–7; with permission.)

Surgeons accredited programs in Canada (n = 8), with 4 to 8 graduates per year. A typical 7-year duration of training was assumed (5 years for general surgery, 2 years for thoracic surgery) with 0% attrition and emigration. This model was then advanced in 1-year cycles with the future year's projections based on present-day supply, clinical volume, retirement estimates, and the number of new surgeons entering the workforce. A national lung cancer screening program was then introduced into the model, phased in from 2014 to 2016, for the same population to predict changes in the number of operable lung cancers per surgeon.

In their model, the investigators forecasted an increase in the Canadian population from about 3.2 million (in 2006) to 4.6 million (in 2049). Those eligible for lung cancer screening (55–74 years old, >30 pack-years of current or former smoking) increased from 1,118,000 cases (in 2014) to 1,147,700 cases (in 2017) and then progressively decreased to 446,000 (in 2049) as lung cancer screening went into effect. Screening with chest radiographs was applied in 2014 to demonstrate lung cancer incidence and stage distribution in the absence of LDCT screening. With chest radiographs, the overall number of lung cancer diagnoses was forecasted to increase from 23,529 (in 2010) to 32,196 (in 2030) and then decrease to 28,585 cases (in 2040). With CT screening, the incidence of lung cancer diagnoses was projected to increase from 23,928 (in 2010) to 34,189 (in 2030) and then decrease to 30,681 cases (in 2040). When compared with chest radiographs, there was about a 7% increase in lung cancer diagnoses with LDCT for any given year.

Examining by stage, their model forecasted an increase in early stage lung cancer diagnosed with LDCT versus chest radiographs. From 2010 to 2020, the proportion of stage IA lung cancer diagnosed by LDCT underwent a relative increase of 27.2%. For the same period, stage IB diagnosis increases by 2%, and stages II and IIIA remain stable. Stage IIIB lung cancer diagnoses decrease by 5.6% with LDCT screening, and stage IV decreases by 14.7%. Defining stage IA to IIIA as "operable lung cancer," the study also forecasted the incidence of operable lung cancer per surgeon to reach 114 cases per surgeon in 2030.

ESTIMATING THE IMPACT OF LUNG CANCER SCREENING IN THE UNITED STATES: SURGICAL VOLUME AND OTHER SEQUELAE

The American Cancer Society's 2016 estimate of new lung cancer cases (224,390) can be used to extrapolate the Canadian data in the study by Edwards and colleagues to the United States population and obtain estimates in a similar fashion. Assuming the same percentage of change as in the Canadian study, the number of operable (stages IA–IIIA) lung cancer cases in the United States each year steadily increases from 115,323 in 2010, to 148,454 in 2020, to 167,386 in 2030, and then decreases to 146,544 cases in 2040 (**Fig. 3**).

If one were to take into account the decreasing trend of US practicing thoracic surgeons according to the study from Williams and colleagues, the total number of lung cancer cases per surgeon would increase from 30 in 2010, to 42 in 2020, to 53 in 2030, to 49 cases per surgeon in 2040 (**Fig. 4**). However, if one were to assume a fixed number of practicing thoracic surgeons in the United States, the total number of lung cancer cases per surgeon would similarly increase and then decrease: 30 in 2010, to 39 in 2020, peak to 44 in 2030, then decrease to 38 in 2040. The difference at its peak in 2030 will be 9 additional cases per surgeon, followed by a greater difference of 11 additional cases per surgeon in 2040.

In addition to the increased workload for the foreseeable future, there may be a substantial downstream financial impact that may or may not affect the future workforce

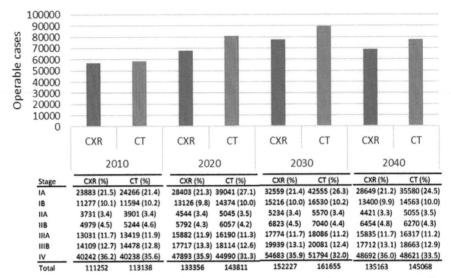

Stage	CXR (%)	CT (%)	CXR (%)	CT (%)	CXR (%)	CT (%)	CXR (%)	CT (%)
IA	23883 (21.5)	24266 (21.4)	28403 (21.3)	39041 (27.1)	32559 (21.4)	42555 (26.3)	28649 (21.2)	35580 (24.5)
IB	11277 (10.1)	11594 (10.2)	13126 (9.8)	14374 (10.0)	15216 (10.0)	16530 (10.2)	13400 (9.9)	14563 (10.0)
IIA	3731 (3.4)	3901 (3.4)	4544 (3.4)	5045 (3.5)	5234 (3.4)	5570 (3.4)	4421 (3.3)	5055 (3.5)
IIB	4979 (4.5)	5244 (4.6)	5792 (4.3)	6057 (4.2)	6823 (4.5)	7040 (4.4)	6454 (4.8)	6270 (4.3)
IIIA	13031 (11.7)	13419 (11.9)	15882 (11.9)	16190 (11.3)	17774 (11.7)	18086 (11.2)	15835 (11.7)	16317 (11.2)
IIIB	14109 (12.7)	14478 (12.8)	17717 (13.3)	18114 (12.6)	19939 (13.1)	20081 (12.4)	17712 (13.1)	18663 (12.9)
IV	40242 (36.2)	40238 (35.6)	47893 (35.9)	44990 (31.3)	54683 (35.9)	51794 (32.0)	48692 (36.0)	48621 (33.5)
Total	111252	113138	133356	143811	152227	161655	135163	145068

Fig. 3. Absolute incidence of operable lung cancer (stages I, II, and IIIA) per year according to screening methodology. CT, computed tomography; CXR, chest radiography. (*Adapted from* Edwards JP, Datta I, Hunt JD, et al. The impact of computed tomographic screening for lung cancer on the thoracic surgery workforce. Ann Thorac Surg 2014;98(2):447–52; with permission.)

trajectory. Based on other publications estimating the hospital margin associated with anatomic resections for lung cancer to be approximately $20,000 per lobectomy,[59] it may be assumed that the gross financial impact of performing about 190 more cases per surgeon from 2010 to 2040 (estimated difference in area under the curves in **Fig. 4**) will be approximately $4,000,000 per surgeon from 2010 to 2040. A financially advantageous position as a result of higher margins may serve as an appealing factor in the pursuit of a career in thoracic surgery. In contrast, the inability to realize greater

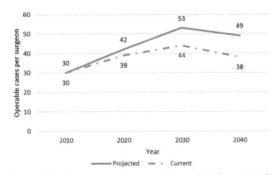

Fig. 4. Incidence of operable lung cancer (stages I, II, and IIIA) per US thoracic surgeon per year. "Projected" curve refers to the estimated cases per surgeon assuming the projected downtrend in thoracic surgeons.[55] "Current" refers to the estimated cases per surgeon assuming the current number of thoracic surgeons is maintained. (*Adapted from* Edwards JP, Datta I, Hunt JD, et al. The impact of computed tomographic screening for lung cancer on the thoracic surgery workforce. Ann Thorac Surg 2014;98(2):447–52; with permission.)

compensation despite increased volume and increased cumulative margin may result in a stagnation or even a continued decrease in the thoracic surgical workforce. Furthermore, health care systems must consider the increasing regionalization of surgical care toward high-volume centers.[60,61]

The Edwards and colleagues[56] Canadian simulation model forecasted that the operative caseload for thoracic surgeons will increase, even with the current number of trainees entering the workforce per year and retiring surgeons leaving the workforce per year. However, an important yet unaccounted consideration is the impact of body radiation therapy for the primary treatment of early stage lung cancer for high-risk surgical patients.[62] The outcomes of stereotactic body radiation therapy seem to be promising, and its impact on operable lung cancer cases and on workforce planning remains to be seen and will become an essential consideration. In the absence of randomized, controlled trials showing equivalence of this radiation therapy modality to surgical therapy, it could be argued that the proportion of patients actually undergoing a nonoperative form of therapy will have not changed.

SUMMARY

Lung cancer is an immense public health burden. Lung cancer screening has demonstrated a reduction in lung cancer mortality by 20%. Annual LDCT screening in high-risk individuals is now recommended by multiple national health care organizations and is covered under Medicare and Medicaid services. The impact of this public health intervention is projected to increase the case load for the thoracic surgery workforce and is incumbent upon the current workforce to continually improve outcomes in this patient population.

REFERENCES

1. American Cancer Society. Cancer facts and figures 2016. Atlanta (GA): American Cancer Society; 2016. p. 1–72.

2. Deffebach ME, Humphrey L. Lung cancer screening. Surg Clin North Am 2015; 95(5):967–78.

3. Kubik A, Parkin DM, Khlat M, et al. Lack of benefit from semi-annual screening for cancer of the lung: follow-up report of a randomized controlled trial on a population of high-risk males in Czechoslovakia. Int J Cancer 1990;45(1):26–33.

4. Friedman GD, Collen MF, Fireman BH. Multiphasic health checkup evaluation: a 16-year follow-up. J Chronic Dis 1986;39(6):453–63.

5. Melamed MR. Lung cancer screening results in the National Cancer Institute New York study. Cancer 2000;89(11 Suppl):2356–62.

6. Berlin NI, Buncher CR, Fontana RS, et al. The National Cancer Institute cooperative early lung cancer detection program. Results of the initial screen (prevalence). Early lung cancer detection: introduction. Am Rev Respir Dis 1984; 130(4):545–9.

7. Oken MM, Hocking WG, Kvale PA, et al. Screening by chest radiograph and lung cancer mortality: the prostate, lung, colorectal, and ovarian (PLCO) randomized trial. JAMA 2011;306(17):1865–73.

8. Marcus PM, Bergstralh EJ. Lung cancer mortality in the Mayo Lung Project: impact of extended follow-up. J Natl Cancer Inst 2000;92(16):1308–16.

9. U.S. Preventive Services Task Force. Lung cancer screening: recommendation statement. Ann Intern Med 2004;140(9):738–9.

10. Henschke CI, McCauley DI, Yankelevitz DF, et al. Early Lung Cancer Action Project: overall design and findings from baseline screening. Lancet 1999;354(9173): 99–105.

11. International Early Lung Cancer Action Program Investigators, Henschke CI, Yankelevitz DF, Libby DM, et al. Survival of patients with stage I lung cancer detected on CT screening. N Engl J Med 2006;355(17):1763–71.

12. Swensen SJ, Jett JR, Hartman TE, et al. Lung cancer screening with CT: Mayo Clinic experience. Radiology 2003;226(3):756–61.

13. Veronesi G, Maisonneuve P, Spaggiari L, et al. Diagnostic performance of low-dose computed tomography screening for lung cancer over five years. J Thorac Oncol 2014;9(7):935–9.

14. National Lung Screening Trial Research Team, Aberle DR, Adams AM, et al. Reduced lung-cancer mortality with low-dose computed tomographic screening. N Engl J Med 2011;365(5):395–409.

15. National Lung Screening Trial Research Team. The National Lung Screening Trial: overview and study design. Radiology 2011;258(1):243–53.

16. Wender R, Fontham ET, Barrera E Jr, et al. American Cancer Society lung cancer screening guidelines. CA Cancer J Clin 2013;63(2):106–17.

17. Jaklitsch MT, Jacobson FL, Austin JH, et al. The American Association for Thoracic Surgery guidelines for lung cancer screening using low-dose computed tomography scans for lung cancer survivors and other high-risk groups. J Thorac Cardiovasc Surg 2012;144(1):33–8.

18. Detterbeck FC, Mazzone PJ, Naidich DP, et al. Screening for lung cancer: diagnosis and management of lung cancer, 3rd edition: American College of Chest Physicians evidence-based clinical practice guidelines. Chest 2013;143(5 Suppl):e78S–92S.

19. Bach PB, Mirkin JN, Oliver TK, et al. Benefits and harms of CT screening for lung cancer: a systematic review. JAMA 2012;307(22):2418–29.

20. Moyer VA. Screening for lung cancer: U.S. preventive services task force recommendation statement. Ann Intern Med 2014;160(5):330–8.

21. Humphrey LL, Deffebach M, Pappas M, et al. Screening for lung cancer with low dose computed tomography. Ann Intern Med 2014;160(3):212.

22. Centers for Medicare and Medicaid Services. Decision memo for screening for lung cancer with low dose computed tomography (LDCT) (CAG-00439N). Available at: https://www.cms.gov/medicare-coverage-database/details/nca-decision-memo.aspx?NCAId=274. Accessed January 11, 2016.

23. Kovalchik SA, Tammemagi M, Berg CD, et al. Targeting of low-dose CT screening according to the risk of lung-cancer death. N Engl J Med 2013;369(3):245–54.

24. Tammemagi MC, Katki HA, Hocking WG, et al. Selection criteria for lung-cancer screening. N Engl J Med 2013;368(8):728–36.

25. Horeweg N, van der Aalst CM, Vliegenthart R, et al. Volumetric computed tomography screening for lung cancer: three rounds of the NELSON trial. Eur Respir J 2013;42(6):1659–67.

26. Horeweg N, van der Aalst CM, Thunnissen E, et al. Characteristics of lung cancers detected by computer tomography screening in the randomized NELSON trial. Am J Respir Crit Care Med 2013;187(8):848–54.

27. van den Bergh KA, Essink Bot ML, Bunge EM, et al. Impact of computed tomography screening for lung cancer on participants in a randomized controlled trial (NELSON trial). Cancer 2008;113(2):396–404.

28. Xu DM, Gietema H, de Koning H, et al. Nodule management protocol of the NELSON randomised lung cancer screening trial. Lung Cancer 2006;54(2): 177–84.
29. van Iersel CA, de Koning HJ, Draisma G, et al. Risk-based selection from the general population in a screening trial: selection criteria, recruitment and power for the Dutch-Belgian randomised lung cancer multi-slice CT screening trial (NELSON). Int J Cancer 2006;120(4):868–74.
30. Horeweg N, Scholten ET, de Jong PA, et al. Detection of lung cancer through low dose CT screening (NELSON): a prespecified analysis of screening test performance and interval cancers. Lancet Oncol 2014;15:1342–50.
31. Brenner DJ. Radiation risks potentially associated with low-dose CT screening of adult smokers for lung cancer. Radiology 2004;231(2):440–5.
32. Berrington de Gonzalez A, Kim KP, Berg CD. Low-dose lung computed tomography screening before age 55: estimates of the mortality reduction required to outweigh the radiation-induced cancer risk. J Med Screen 2008;15(3):153–8.
33. Mascalchi M, Mazzoni LN, Falchini M, et al. Dose exposure in the ITALUNG trial of lung cancer screening with low-dose CT. Br J Radiol 2012;85(1016):1134–9.
34. Slatore CG, Sullivan DR, Pappas M, et al. Patient-centered outcomes among lung cancer screening recipients with computed tomography: a systematic review. J Thorac Oncol 2014;9(7):927–34.
35. Welch HG, Black WC. Overdiagnosis in cancer. J Natl Cancer Inst 2010;102(9): 605–13.
36. Infante M, Berghmans T, Heuvelmans MA, et al. Slow-growing lung cancer as an emerging entity: from screening to clinical management. Eur Respir J 2013;42(6): 1706–22.
37. Patz EF, Pinsky P, Gatsonis C, et al. Overdiagnosis in low-dose computed tomography screening for lung cancer. JAMA Intern Med 2014;174(2):269–74.
38. Lang-Lazdunski L. Surgery for nonsmall cell lung cancer. Eur Respir Rev 2013; 22(129):382–404.
39. Evarts A, Graham MD, Singer JJ. Successful removal of an entire lung for carcinoma of the bronchus. JAMA 1984;251:257–60.
40. Jensik RL, Faber LP, Milloy FJ, et al. Segmental resection for lung cancer. A 15-year experience. J Thorac Cardiovasc Surg 1973;66:563–72.
41. Thomas CP. The present position relating to cancer of the lung. Lobectomy with sleeve resection. Thorax 1960;15:9–11.
42. Locicero J III, Ponn RB, Daly BDT. Surgical treatment of non-small cell lung cancer. In: Shields TW, LoCicero J, Ponn RB, et al, editors. General thoracic surgery. 5th edition. Philadelphia: Lippincott Williams and Wilkins; 2000. p. 1311–41.
43. Martini N, Flehinger BJ, Zaman MB, et al. Results of resection in non-oat cell carcinoma of the lung with mediastinal lymph node metastases. Ann Surg 1983;198: 386–97.
44. Lewis RJ, Caccavale RJ, Sisler GE, et al. Video-assisted thoracic surgical resection of malignant lung tumors. J Thorac Cardiovasc Surg 1992;104:1679–85.
45. Walker WS, Carnochan FM, Pugh GC. Thoracoscopic pulmonary lobectomy. Early operative experience and preliminary clinical results. J Thorac Cardiovasc Surg 1993;106:1111–7.
46. McKenna RJ Jr. Lobectomy by video-assisted thoracic surgery with mediastinal node sampling for lung cancer. J Thorac Cardiovasc Surg 1994;107:879–81.
47. Park BJ, Melfi F, Mussi A, et al. Robotic lobectomy for non-small cell lung cancer (NSCLC): long-term oncologic results. J Thorac Cardiovasc Surg 2012;143: 383–9.

48. Grills IS, Hope AJ, Guckenberger M, et al. A collaborative analysis of stereotactic lung radiotherapy outcomes for early-stage non-small cell lung cancer using daily online cone-beam computed tomography image-guided radiotherapy. J Thorac Oncol 2012;7:1382–93.

49. Donington J, Ferguson M, Mazzone P, et al. American College of Chest Physicians and Society of Thoracic Surgeons consensus statement for evaluation and management for high-risk patients with stage I non-small cell lung cancer. Chest 2012;142:1620–35.

50. Bach PB, Cramer LD, Schrag D, et al. The influence of hospital volume on survival after resection for lung cancer. N Engl J Med 2001;345:181–8.

51. Sioris T, Sihvo E, Sankila R, et al. Effect of surgical volume and hospital type on outcome in non-small cell lung cancer surgery: a Finnish population-based study. Lung Cancer 2008;59:119–25.

52. Cheung MC, Hamilton K, Sherman R, et al. Impact of teaching facility status and high-volume centers on outcomes for lung cancer resection: an examination of 13,469 surgical patients. Ann Surg Oncol 2009;16:3–13.

53. Lien YC, Huang MT, Lin HC. Association between surgeon and hospital volume and in-hospital fatalities after lung cancer resections: the experience of an Asian country. Ann Thorac Surg 2007;83:1837–43.

54. von Meyenfeldt EM, Gooiker GA, van Gijn W, et al. The relationship between volume or surgeon specialty and outcome in the surgical treatment of lung cancer: a systematic review and meta-analysis. J Thorac Oncol 2012;7:1170–8.

55. Williams TE Jr, Satiani B, Thomas A, et al. The impending shortage and the estimated cost of training the future surgical workforce. Ann Surg 2009;250(4):590–7.

56. Edwards JP, Datta I, Hunt JD, et al. The impact of computed tomographic screening for lung cancer on the thoracic surgery workforce. Ann Thorac Surg 2014;98(2):447–52.

57. Statistics Canada. Canadian Community Health Survey. Annual component. Available at: http://www23.statcan.gc.ca/imdb/p2SV.pl?Function=getSurvey&SDDS=3226. Accessed November 1, 2016.

58. Grondin SC, Schieman C, Kelly E, et al. A look at the thoracic surgery workforce in Canada: how demographics and scope of practice may impact future workforce needs. Can J Surg 2013;56:E75–81.

59. Park HS, Detterbeck FC, Boffa DJ, et al. Impact of hospital volume of thoracoscopic lobectomy on primary lung cancer outcomes. Ann Thorac Surg 2012; 93(2):372–9.

60. Smith AK, Shara NM, Zeymo A, et al. Travel patterns of cancer surgery patients in a regionalized system. J Surg Res 2015;199(1):97–105.

61. Sundaresan S, McLeod R, Irish J, et al. Early results after regionalization of thoracic surgical practice in a single-payer system. Ann Thorac Surg 2013; 95(2):472–8 [discussion: 478–9].

62. Nanda RH, Liu Y, Gillespie TW, et al. Stereotactic body radiation therapy versus no treatment for early stage non-small cell lung cancer in medically inoperable elderly patients: a National Cancer Data Base analysis. Cancer 2015;121(23): 4222–30.

The Impact of Minimally Invasive Esophageal Surgery

Thomas Fabian, MD[a],*, John A. Federico, MD, FRCSC[b]

KEYWORDS

• Esophagectomy • Minimally invasive esophagectomy • Esophageal cancer

KEY POINTS

• Esophagectomy is one of the larger more complex surgeries commonly performed on the human body.

• Esophageal cancer is the 18th most common malignancy and accounts for less than 1% of all cancer cases in the United States annually.

• The National Institutes of Health estimates that of the 16,910 new cases diagnosed in the United States in 20,016 there will be 15,690 deaths and only 18.4% of patients will survive 5 years. This is partly attributable to the late presentation of the disease.

INTRODUCTION

To most Americans, esophageal cancer remains a fairly unknown malignancy. According to the National Institutes of Health (NIH) esophageal cancer is the 18th most common malignancy and accounts for less than 1% of all cancer cases in the United States annually. This is despite that adenocarcinomas of the esophagus are increasing at a faster rate than any other malignancies. The annual incidence of esophageal cancer in the United States is 4.3 cases per 100,000. Yet, for physicians caring for these patients, the relative infrequency of the disease provides little solace and even less if the disease has a personal effect.

The NIH estimates that of the 16,910 new cases diagnosed in the United States in 20,016 there will be 15,690 deaths and only 18.4% of patients will survive 5 years. This is attributable in part to the late presentation of the disease. It is estimated by the Surveillance, Epidemiology, and End Results (SEER) database that 30% of tumors are limited to the primary site and nearly three-fourths of patients have regional (31%) and distant (38%) disease. Poor long-term survival is not surprising in advanced

Disclosures: None.
[a] Department of Surgery, Albany Medical College, 47 New Scotland Avenue, Albany, NY 12159, USA; [b] Department of Surgery, Kalispell Regional Medical Center, 310 Sunnyview Ln, Kalispell, MT 59901, USA
* Corresponding author.
E-mail address: tfabs@yahoo.com

Surg Clin N Am 97 (2017) 763–770
http://dx.doi.org/10.1016/j.suc.2017.03.005
0039-6109/17/© 2017 Elsevier Inc. All rights reserved.
surgical.theclinics.com

disease cases but survival among patients with localized disease should be considerably better and perhaps comparable to other malignancies. Regrettably, this is not the case. Again, based on the SEER database, 5-year survival for localized tumor is 41%. This is considerably lower than lung cancer for example (70%).

There are several axioms that are frequently referred to regarding esophageal malignancies. Often it is stated that the tumor is more aggressive, implying worse outcome as a result of disease. Certainly, from an anatomic perspective, it is more likely to spread to lymphatics at an earlier depth of invasion than in other malignancies for the gastrointestinal tract. For example, tumor stage T1b tumors involving the submucosa have a 5% risk of lymph node metastasis and T2 tumors invading the muscularis propria have a 20% risk of metastatic lymphatic involvement. Another perceived adverse predictor of risk is age. The median age at diagnosis is 67 years old (NIH) and nearly 40% of patients diagnosed are less than 65 years old. Others point to lower health care dollars spent on esophageal cancer research. The amount of money spent on esophageal cancer per death is $1542 per patient, which is similar to other less funded diseases, such as lung cancer $1553. These numbers pale in comparison to other malignancies, such as cervical cancer, $18,870; breast cancer, $14,095; and lymphoma, $12,791. These issues may lead to treatment bias, lack of optimism in treatment, and frequently undertreatment of the tumor. This negative outlook is further exacerbated by realistic and unrealistic morbidity and mortality associated with esophagectomy. In fact, many patients who are potentially resectable are either not offered surgery or decline surgery, and are, therefore, less likely cured of their disease. Dubecz and colleagues[1] analyzed multiple databases to review care and outcomes of more than 25,000 esophageal subjects with cancer. This large study found only 44% of subjects with potentially resectable disease underwent surgery in the state of New York. In other words, 56% of subjects with resectable disease were undertreated for their malignancy. This pervasive undertreatment likely plays a role in the poor long-term survival of esophageal patients with cancer.

Surgeons who care for these patients have been eager to see real change in short-term and long-term outcomes. Advances in diagnosis, screening, referral, and treatment of this cancer have been slow in coming and, while waiting for those changes, work continues toward improving surgical outcomes, techniques, and expanding the reach of esophagectomy to deserving patients. To many, these advances have been dramatic and profound. Leading the way to new innovation has been the use of minimally invasive techniques in esophagectomy. This article discusses the surgical innovations that have occurred in the last decade and their impact on patients with esophageal cancer.

THE EVOLUTION OF MINIMALLY INVASIVE ESOPHAGECTOMY

Surgical resection of esophageal malignancy is not novel or unique, and remains a mainstay of the treatment of this malignancy. However, as it relates to morbidity and mortality, it can be argued that esophagectomy is one of the larger more complex surgeries commonly performed on the human body. When comparing esophagectomy mortality to that of other major elective surgery, others may pale in comparison. The mortality in the twenty-first century has been reported as 13% nationwide and as high as 23% at low-volume institutions.[2] The disparity is equally compelling in terms of morbidity. Studies routinely demonstrate morbidity rates in esophagectomy series are above 50%.[3–6] Long-term morbidity, as it relates to dysphagia, weight loss, and quality of life (QoL), can be disappointing.

To the point, it is no surprise that more than 60% of patients who need an esophagectomy are not offered or refuse one.[1] Undertreatment, by not offering surgery, is a major factor in the poor outcomes of this disease. In attempts to improve overall outcomes of esophageal cancer, surgeons were challenged to improve surgical outcomes. Some surgeons embraced minimally invasive techniques, resulting in the evolution of the minimally invasive esophagectomy (MIE). Leading the way was the University of Pittsburgh Medical Center (UPMC). In a seminal paper, Luketich and colleagues[3] published the outcomes of 222 consecutive subjects who underwent MIE. The mortality rate of 1.4% and length of stay of 7 days were remarkable compared with any previously published open series. In addition, this paper demonstrated QOL scores similar to preoperative scores. Although, clearly a landmark paper that opened the eyes of many to MIE, there were many who contributed to the development of this procedure. The first to report thoracoscopic esophagectomy was Cuschieri and colleagues[7] in 1992. In 1994, Cuschieri[8] described reported thoracoscopic mobilization in the prone position. The esophagus was mobilized in the chest and later a cervical anastomosis was created after laparotomy. As minimally invasive surgical techniques evolved, thoracoscopic mobilization was performed more frequently via lateral decubitus position.[3] The appeal of the lateral decubitus approach was easy to understand because it allowed similar orientation to open surgery and simplified conversion to open surgery if necessary. Several studies have demonstrated advantages of prone thoracoscopic mobilization in terms of diminished operative times and reduced blood loss.[9] A recently published meta-analysis demonstrated superiority of the prone position in terms of reduced pulmonary complications, reduced estimated blood loss, and increased lymph node procurement.[10] Despite these results, left lateral decubitus position remains the preferred approach at most institutions.

Laparoscopic mobilization of the neoesophagus was the next advancement in the mid-1990s when surgeons began to report smaller series.[11,12] At that time, the overwhelming approach was cervical anastomosis and either totally laparoscopic or a modified Ivor Lewis, frequently referred to as a McKeown, esophagectomy.

In 2002, Luketich and colleagues[3] reported on several modifications made during the series in the hopes of minimizing morbidity. One of these concerned conduit width. Initially, a narrow gastric conduit was used but, according to the investigators, this resulted in higher than expected anastomotic leaks. The technique was modified by moving toward a wider conduit and the investigators concluded this resulted in an 11.7% decrease in anastomotic leaks. In a different study, 220 subjects undergoing transhiatal or transthoracic esophagectomy were compared. The anastomotic leak rate in the neck was 14% and 16%, respectively,[13] and risk of vocal cord paralysis was 14% and 24%, respectively. These complications are often cited as the driving force in the evolution of minimally invasive Ivor Lewis esophagectomy with intrathoracic anastomosis. Watson and colleagues[14] were the first to report a modified Ivor Lewis approach in 1999 but it was Bizekis and colleagues[15] at the University of Pittsburgh who published the first large series of intrathoracic anastomosis in 50 subjects in 2006. Risk of anastomotic leaks vary greatly in the literature but, again, are generally considered higher in the cervical anastomosis at 15%[13] than in the intrathoracic anastomosis at 6%.[15] These issues have collectively led to more frequent use of the Ivor Lewis MIE. In 2012, Luketich and colleagues[16] published a series of 1033 consecutive MIE subjects with more than half receiving intrathoracic anastomosis. Total operative mortality was now reported as even lower at 1.68%. The Ivor Lewis approach also resulted in a reduction of incidence of recurrent laryngeal nerve injury, which was statistically significant. It should be noted that recurrent laryngeal nerve injuries can occur during intrathoracic anastomosis but the risk is generally considered much lower than in the neck.

Esophageal anastomotic techniques vary widely. For many experienced surgeons, creation of the anastomosis remains a challenge. Even open esophageal anastomosis can be challenging. Creation of the anastomosis seems to be variable based on surgeon preference. The Pittsburgh group prefers an end-to-side circular stapled anastomosis,[3,15] whereas others use side-to-side totally stapled anastomosis.[4] Currently, even robotic handsewn anastomosis exists.[17] In 2016, Harustiak and colleagues[18] looked at 415 esophageal anastomosis at a single institution and reported that stapled anastomosis resulted in fewer leaks, 10% versus 21%, and fewer strictures, 6% versus 20%, when compared with handsewn.

A critique of the Harustiak and colleagues[18] publication is that it was a single surgical center outcome and perhaps not all handsewn anastomosis are similar. Another criticism is of the significant variables that come into play. These include width of conduit, handling of the neoesophagus, technique of handsewn anastomosis, and countless others making surgical technique comparisons difficult. Speaking from the authors' own experiences on creation of an anastomosis, we believe that we have performed virtually every type of anastomosis described and are confident that all anastomosis can fail. The authors' advice is that all techniques have advantages and pitfalls, and likely the best choice is the one that the surgeon feels most comfortable with until data demonstrate otherwise.

Surgical simulation may be used in the future to improve anastomotic techniques. The authors published our experience using a bovine tissue block and creating a simulated intrathoracic thoracoscopic anastomosis.[19] The model allows for recreation of virtually any anastomosis. The study demonstrated that, with repetition, residents could improve their technical skills rapidly and create increasingly successful thoracoscopic anastomosis.

Gastric emptying following esophagectomy remains a critical issue as it relates to short-term morbidity and long-term QoL. Delayed gastric emptying is associated with increased aspiration, increased perioperative morbidity, decreased patient satisfaction, and prolonged hospital stay.[20]

Delayed gastric emptying occurs in 15% to 30%[21,22] of cases and can result from several factors, which can cause problems separately or in conjunction with one another. Causes include rotation of gastric conduit, obstruction at the hiatus, hypertonic pylorus, transection of vagal nerves, or any combination of these. It should be noted that there are likely still other factors that might cause delays in emptying that are less well-defined. Frequently, it is stated that narrow gastric conduits are associated with improved emptying but there are little to no data to support this. If in fact, as some argue, the neoesophagus serves as a passive gravity-dependent conduit and, in physics, a wider tube has less resistance and should empty better. It does seem plausible that the idea of a narrow conduit is a conceptualized surrogate for what is actually redundant intrathoracic stomach, which certainly can be a significant problem.

Pyloric obstruction is considered by most physicians a major cause of delayed gastric emptying, and pyloromyotomy and pyloroplasty have been used to reduce delayed gastric emptying. However, randomized trials evaluating these procedures have shown little benefit.[23,24] In one study, Zieren and colleagues[24] stated that in most circumstances no emptying procedure should be done. A meta-analysis in 2002 by Urshel and colleagues[25] shows that early complications from delayed gastric emptying can be reduced when a pyloroplasty is performed. However, no long-term difference was observed. Generally, there is a lack of significant data to support an emptying procedure in the setting of esophagectomy. However, the difficulties with delayed emptying are so severe that they continue to be performed frequently. Unfortunately, pyloroplasty and pyloromyotomy cannot be done with impunity. These procedures can lead to stricture, leak, and death.[26] As some surgeons chose to forgo this procedure in open esophagectomy (OE) and MIE, others looked for alternatives. In 2007, Kent and colleagues[27] (including the senior author of this article) published a pilot study looking at the use of Botox injection of the pylorus. In 2009, this was followed with a larger study[28] that demonstrated 91% of subjects showed no significant delay on esophagram or clinically. Four (9%) subjects in the study group had significant delay on the esophagram but only 2 (4.5%) had clinically relevant delayed emptying. Botox injection seems a reasonable alternative and seems durable. Three (7%) subjects who were doing well developed delayed emptying at approximately 3.5 months. All responded to retreatment. Only 1 of 48 (2%) patients had an aspiration event postoperatively. More recently, other investigators have suggested balloon dilation.[29] Bakhos and colleagues[30] published a multi-institutional study of 220 esophagectomy subjects and found the omission of a pyloric procedure was directly linked to postoperative pneumonia. Most pyloric procedures in that series included Botox injection.

Oncologic principles of esophagectomy are yet another critical issue in the treatment of esophageal cancer. Any modification in technique must not compromise adequacy of oncologic resection. Complete resection (R0) can be used to define oncologic effectiveness of a surgical technique but may not represent the entire picture. Most MIE series demonstrate high R0 resection rates exceeding 95%[3–5] but most of these studies are published at highly specialized centers. The Eastern Cooperative Oncology Group (ECOG) 2202 study was a multicenter feasibility trial of MIE.[31] R0 was achieved in 96% of subjects and the 30-day mortality was 2.1%. The median follow-up was 35 months and 3-year survival was 58.4%. Another frequently used surrogate for oncologic completeness is lymph node procurement. Although the number of lymph nodes harvested has never shown survival benefit, it is clear that lack of adequate procurement can result in under staging, undertreatment, and worse oncologic outcomes. Several series have shown comparable or superior levels of lymph node procurement between MIE and OE.[4,5] One of the most consistent differences between OE and MIE is intraoperative blood loss.[4] As a surrogate this may be relevant. Blood loss is equated to physiologic strain, although it has not been directly linked to oncologic outcomes. Blood transfusions have been shown to negatively affect survival independent of tumor stage in malignancies.[32]

Some data exist supporting better long-term oncologic survival with MIE versus OE. Palazzo and colleagues[33] reported data of 5-year survival as being statistically superior with MIE 64% versus OE 35%. At the same time, the investigators correctly conceded that several biases may have influenced the results. Despite this, the results are intriguing.

Multiple studies have demonstrated the feasibility of MIE at both academic centers and community settings,[4] as well as improved outcomes of patients undergoing esophagectomy at institutions adopting MIE.[4,5] Data have also demonstrated that the technique is applicable to virtually all patients, including patients following neoadjuvant chemoradiation.[19]

Proponents of MIE argue that it confers advantages for patients by reducing morbidity and mortality. Opponents often point to the lack of data supporting that concept or criticize the source. In the case of retrospective studies, subject selection and selection biases can frequently be cited. Certainly, there are limited data comparing MIE to OE; there is only a single prospective randomized trial.[34] In this study, 5 centers in 3 countries randomized subjects between MIE and OE. This study showed less intraoperative blood loss, less postoperative pneumonia, shorter postoperative length of stay, and improved QoL at 6 weeks. These finding were comparable to what was reported in retrospective comparisons nearly a decade earlier.[4,5] However, not all studies have demonstrated benefits with MIE. A retrospective study comparing OE to MIE using the Society of Thoracic Surgeons database showed little difference between the techniques.[35] Notable publications and advancements in MIE techniques are demonstrated in **Fig. 1.**

Regardless of how reported outcomes of MIE and OE are interpreted, MIE is gaining market share and will likely continue to do so, either as some incarnation described by Luketich or, perhaps, using robotic techniques. By reducing morbidity and mortality through clinically oriented research, the opportunity exists to significantly affect survival with this increasingly common malignancy.

As the techniques have advanced in MIE surgery, so has the expertise of thoracic surgeons using minimally invasive techniques and intraabdominal laparoscopy. Advances have allowed foregut surgeons to reassert their expertise. Foregut surgeons are not limited to the thoracic cavity but are also experts in intraabdominal minimally invasive surgery. Laparoscopic approaches to intrathoracic stomach, shortened esophagus, achalasia, and epiphrenic diverticulum have all evolved during this same time. No better evidence of this assertion exists than the more than 50 publications by Dr. James Luketich at UPMC regarding laparoscopic surgical conditions in these 4 areas. There is no reluctance by thoracic surgeons to enter the chest and there are clearly times when this is appropriate but now there is the realization that the ideal approach to these pathologic conditions is via the abdomen. Not only have these advances helped patients but also helped thoracic surgeons broaden the profession as surgeons of the complete foregut.

Advanced laparoscopic and/or robotic surgeons, at this time, prefer to be in the abdomen reducing the giant hiatal hernia, avoiding a Collis gastroplasty, or enjoying the visualization of muscle fibers of the gastroesophageal junction as they complete the ideal myotomy.

Surgeons stand on the shoulders of those who came before: Ivor Lewis, Belsey, Orringer, and Luketich, who each left an everlasting legacy yet were unable to predict the future of surgical techniques or care. For now that is minimally invasive abdominal and thoracic surgery. However, thoracic surgery has always evolved and will continue

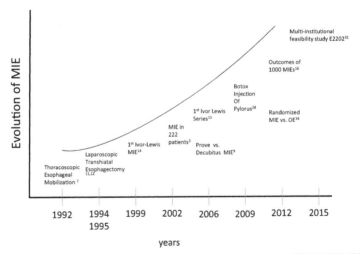

Fig. 1. Technical and notable advancements in MIE. (*Data from* Refs.[3,7,9,11,12,14–16,28,31,34])

on to meet somewhere near the intersection of technology, patient pathologic conditions, and enthusiasm.

REFERENCES

1. Dubecz A, Sepesi B, Salvador R, et al. Surgical resection for locoregional esophageal cancer is underutilized in the United States. J Am Coll Surg 2010;211(6): 754–61.
2. Birkmeyer JD, Siewers AE, Finlayson EV, et al. Hospital volume and surgical mortality in the United States. N Engl J Med 2002;346(15):1128–37.
3. Luketich JD, Alvelo-Rivera M, Buenaventura PO, et al. Minimally invasive esophagectomy: outcomes in 222 patients. Ann Surg 2003;238(4):486–94 [discussion: 494–85].
4. Fabian T, Martin JT, McKelvey AA, et al. Minimally invasive esophagectomy: a teaching hospital's first year experience. Dis Esophagus 2008;21(3):220–5.
5. Nguyen NT, Follette DM, Wolfe BM, et al. Comparison of minimally invasive esophagectomy with transthoracic and transhiatal esophagectomy. Arch Surg 2000;135(8):920–5.
6. Singhal S, Kailasam A, Akimoto S, et al. Simple technique of circular stapled anastomosis in Ivor Lewis esophagectomy. J Laparoendosc Adv Surg Tech A 2017;27(3):288–94.
7. Cuschieri A, Shimi S, Banting S. Endoscopic oesophagectomy through a right thoracoscopic approach. J R Coll Surg Edinb 1992;37(1):7–11.
8. Cuschieri A. Thoracoscopic subtotal oesophagectomy. Endosc Surg Allied Tech 1994;2(1):21–5.
9. Fabian T, Martin J, Katigbak M, et al. Thoracoscopic esophageal mobilization during minimally invasive esophagectomy: a head-to-head comparison of prone versus decubitus positions. Surg Endosc 2008;22(11):2485–91.
10. Markar SR, Wiggins T, Antonowicz S, et al. Minimally invasive esophagectomy: lateral decubitus vs. prone positioning; systematic review and pooled analysis. Surg Oncol 2015;24(3):212–9.
11. DePaula AL, Hashiba K, Ferreira EA, et al. Laparoscopic transhiatal esophagectomy with esophagogastroplasty. Surg Laparosc Endosc 1995;5(1):1–5.
12. Swanstrom LL, Hansen P. Laparoscopic total esophagectomy. Arch Surg 1997; 132(9):943–7 [discussion: 947–9].
13. Hulscher JB, van Sandick JW, de Boer AG, et al. Extended transthoracic resection compared with limited transhiatal resection for adenocarcinoma of the esophagus. N Engl J Med 2002;347(21):1662–9.
14. Watson DI, Davies N, Jamieson GG. Totally endoscopic Ivor Lewis esophagectomy. Surg Endosc 1999;13(3):293–7.
15. Bizekis C, Kent MS, Luketich JD, et al. Initial experience with minimally invasive Ivor Lewis esophagectomy. Ann Thorac Surg 2006;82(2):402–6 [discussion: 406–7].
16. Luketich JD, Pennathur A, Awais O, et al. Outcomes after minimally invasive esophagectomy: review of over 1000 patients. Ann Surg 2012;256(1):95–103.
17. Cerfolio RJ, Bryant AS, Hawn MT. Technical aspects and early results of robotic esophagectomy with chest anastomosis. J Thorac Cardiovasc Surg 2013;145(1): 90–6.
18. Harustiak T, Pazdro A, Snajdauf M, et al. Anastomotic leak and stricture after hand-sewn versus linear-stapled intrathoracic oesophagogastric anastomosis: single-centre analysis of 415 oesophagectomies. Eur J Cardiothorac Surg 2016;49(6):1650–9.

19. Bakhos C, Oyasiji T, Elmadhun N, et al. Feasibility of minimally invasive esophagectomy after neoadjuvant chemoradiation. J Laparoendosc Adv Surg Tech A 2014;24(10):688–92.

20. Aly A, Jamieson GG. Reflux after oesophagectomy. Br J Surg 2004;91(2):137–41.

21. Lee HS, Kim MS, Lee JM, et al. Intrathoracic gastric emptying of solid food after esophagectomy for esophageal cancer. Ann Thorac Surg 2005;80(2):443–7.

22. Lanuti M, de Delva PE, Wright CD, et al. Post-esophagectomy gastric outlet obstruction: role of pyloromyotomy and management with endoscopic pyloric dilatation. Eur J Cardiothorac Surg 2007;31(2):149–53.

23. Chattopadhyay TK, Gupta S, Padhy AK, et al. Is pyloroplasty necessary following intrathoracic transposition of stomach? Results of a prospective clinical study. Aust N Z J Surg 1991;61(5):366–9.

24. Zieren HU, Muller JM, Jacobi CA, et al. Should a pyloroplasty be carried out in stomach transposition after subtotal esophagectomy with esophago-gastric anastomosis at the neck? A prospective randomized study. Chirurg 1995;66(4): 319–25 [in German].

25. Urschel JD, Blewett CJ, Young JE, et al. Pyloric drainage (pyloroplasty) or no drainage in gastric reconstruction after esophagectomy: a meta-analysis of randomized controlled trials. Dig Surg 2002;19(3):160–4.

26. Wang LS, Huang MH, Huang BS, et al. Gastric substitution for resectable carcinoma of the esophagus: an analysis of 368 cases. Ann Thorac Surg 1992;53(2): 289–94.

27. Kent MS, Pennathur A, Fabian T, et al. A pilot study of botulinum toxin injection for the treatment of delayed gastric emptying following esophagectomy. Surg Endosc 2007;21(5):754–7.

28. Martin JT, Federico JA, McKelvey AA, et al. Prevention of delayed gastric emptying after esophagectomy: a single center's experience with botulinum toxin. Ann Thorac Surg 2009;87(6):1708–13 [discussion: 1713–4].

29. Swanson EW, Swanson SJ, Swanson RS. Endoscopic pyloric balloon dilatation obviates the need for pyloroplasty at esophagectomy. Surg Endosc 2012;26(7): 2023–8.

30. Bakhos CT, Fabian T, Oyasiji TO, et al. Impact of the surgical technique on pulmonary morbidity after esophagectomy. Ann Thorac Surg 2012;93(1):221–6 [discussion: 226–7].

31. Luketich JD, Pennathur A, Franchetti Y, et al. Minimally invasive esophagectomy: results of a prospective phase II multicenter trial-the Eastern Cooperative Oncology Group (E2202) study. Ann Surg 2015;261(4):702–7.

32. Reeh M, Ghadban T, Dedow J, et al. Allogenic blood transfusion is associated with poor perioperative and long-term outcome in esophageal cancer. World J Surg 2017;41(1):208–15.

33. Palazzo F, Rosato EL, Chaudhary A, et al. Minimally invasive esophagectomy provides significant survival advantage compared with open or hybrid esophagectomy for patients with cancers of the esophagus and gastroesophageal junction. J Am Coll Surg 2015;220(4):672–9.

34. Biere SS, van Berge Henegouwen MI, Maas KW, et al. Minimally invasive versus open oesophagectomy for patients with oesophageal cancer: a multicentre, open-label, randomised controlled trial. Lancet 2012;379(9829):1887–92.

35. Sihag S, Kosinski AS, Gaissert HA, et al. Minimally invasive versus open esophagectomy for esophageal cancer: a comparison of early surgical outcomes from the Society of Thoracic Surgeons national database. Ann Thorac Surg 2016; 101(4):1281–8 [discussion: 1288–89].

Robotic Lobectomy and Segmentectomy

Technical Details and Results

Benjamin Wei, MD*, Robert J. Cerfolio, MD, MBA

KEYWORDS

- Robotic • Lobectomy • Segmentectomy

KEY POINTS

- Robotic lobectomy and segmentectomy are facilitated by thorough knowledge of the anatomy, preparation, proper port placement, and understanding of the conduct of the operation.
- Robotic lobectomy and segmentectomy can be performed with excellent technical and perioperative results.
- The oncologic efficacy of robotic lobectomy is comparable with video-assisted thoracoscopic surgery and open techniques; the role of robotic segmentectomy remains an active area of investigation.
- Advantages of robotic lobectomy and segmentectomy include improved optics, increased dexterity of instrumentation, and better surgeon economics.
- With a completely portal technique, there is the ability to insufflate the chest, leading to improved view and decreased venous bleeding; disadvantages include cost and complexity.

INTRODUCTION

One of the first published reports of pulmonary lobectomy was by Drs Norman Shenstone and Robert Janes from the Toronto General Hospital, in which they describe "a long incision in the general direction of the ribs, passing just below the scapula," or via a thoracotomy.[1] Since then, practitioners have sought ways to decrease the size of incisions needed and minimize the invasiveness of pulmonary lobectomy and thereby optimize postoperative morbidity, recovery time, and pain. Minimally invasive lobectomy has traditionally been performed using video-assisted thoracoscopic surgery (VATS) techniques. The first robotic lobectomies were reported in 2003 by Morgan and colleagues[2] and Ashton and colleagues.[3] Since then, the use of robotic

Division of Cardiothoracic Surgery, University of Alabama-Birmingham Medical Center, University of Alabama at Birmingham, 703 19th Street South, ZRB 739, Birmingham, AL 352094, USA
* Corresponding author.
E-mail address: bwei@uabmc.edu

Surg Clin N Am 97 (2017) 771–782
http://dx.doi.org/10.1016/j.suc.2017.03.008
0039-6109/17/Published by Elsevier Inc.

surgical.theclinics.com

technology for lobectomy has become increasingly common. In 2015, more than 6000 robotic lobectomies were performed in the United States, and more than 8600 were done worldwide.

INITIAL EVALUATION

The evaluation of candidates for robotic lobectomy includes the standard preoperative studies for patients undergoing pulmonary resection. For patients with suspected or biopsy-proven lung cancer, a whole-body PET-computed tomography scan is currently the standard of care. Pulmonary function testing including measurement of diffusion capacity and spirometry is routine. Mediastinal staging can consist of either endobronchial ultrasound-guided fine-needle aspiration biopsy or mediastinoscopy, depending on expertise. Certain patients may warrant additional testing, including stress test, brain MRI if concern exists for metastatic disease, and/or dedicated computed tomography scan with intravenous contrast or MRI if concern exists for vascular or vertebral/nerve invasion, respectively.

Investigators have shown that thoracoscopic lobectomy is safe in patients with a predicted postoperative forced expiratory volume in 1 second or a diffusion capacity of less than 40% of predicted.[4] We consider robotic lobectomy feasible in these patients as well. At present, we view vascular invasion, locally invasive T4 lesions, Pancoast tumors, and massive tumor (>10 cm) as contraindications for a robotic approach to lobectomy. The need for reconstruction of the airway, chest wall invasion, presence of induction chemotherapy and/or radiation, prior thoracic surgery, and hilar nodal disease are not contraindications for robotic-assisted lobectomy in the hands of experienced surgeons.

RELEVANT ANATOMY AND PHYSIOLOGY

An intimate knowledge of the pulmonary anatomy and, specifically, the relationship between hilar structures and their potential variations, is needed to perform any lobectomy or segmentectomy, whether via thoracotomy, VATS, or robotic techniques. Although a detailed description of this anatomy is beyond the scope and complexity of this article, suffice it to say that the view of the pulmonary hilum is different depending on the angle of approach. Whereas during a thoracotomy the surgeon is viewing the hilum from either the anterior or posterior direction, typically in VATS and robotic lobectomy, the camera approaches the hilum from an inferior direction. Retraction of the lung can change the orientation of structures considerably. That said, the relationship between structures remains the same regardless of how structures are approached and/or retracted. Knowledge of what risk exists when performing particular steps and moves during an operation is critical to avoid injury. Avoiding misidentification of structures and attention to aberrant or variable anatomy are also of paramount importance during robotic lobectomy or segmentectomy, where an injury can force conversion to an open operation and negate the benefit of attempting minimally invasive surgery.

CONDUCT OF OPERATION
Preparation

A well-trained team that communicates effectively is a priority for the successful performance of robotic lobectomy. Criteria for a well-trained team include documented scores of 70% or higher on simulator exercises, certificate of robotic safety training and cockpit awareness, weekly access to the robot, familiarity with the robot and the instruments, and a mastery of the pulmonary artery from both an anterior and posterior approach.

Equipment

The Da Vinci Surgical System is currently the only robotic system approved by the US Food and Drug Administration for lung surgery. The surgeon sits at a console some distance from the patient, who is positioned on an operating table in close proximity to the robotic unit with its 4 robotic arms. The robotic arms incorporate remote center technology, in which a fixed point in space is defined, and about it the surgical arms move so as to minimize stress on the thoracic wall during manipulations. The small proprietary Endowrist instruments attached to the arms are capable of a wide range of high-precision movements. These are controlled by the surgeon's hand movements, via "master" instruments at the console. The master instruments sense the surgeon's hand movements and translate them electronically into scaled-down micromovements to manipulate the small surgical instruments. Hand tremor is filtered out by a 6-Hz motion filter. The surgeon observes the operating field through console binoculars. The image comes from a maneuverable high-definition stereoscopic camera (endoscope) attached to one of the robot arms. The console also has foot pedals that allow the surgeon to engage and disengage different instrument arms, reposition the console master controls without the instruments themselves moving, and activate electric cautery. A second optional console allows tandem surgery and training. Da Vinci currently offers both the Xi and Si systems. The Xi system is newer and features an overhead beam that permits rotation of the instrument arms, allowing for greater flexibility in terms of direction of approach of the robot to the patient. Compared with the Si system, the Xi system also has thinner instrument arms, longer instruments themselves, and the option to switch the camera to any arm/port.

Proper location of the robot should be established before the operation. If using an Xi system, the patient can remain with their head oriented toward the anesthesia station, and the robot can be driven in perpendicular to the patient's body. If using the Si system, the robot is driven from over to patient shoulder at a 15° angle off the longitudinal access of the patient. The patient will need to be turned so that the axis of the patient is 90° away from the typical position (ie, head near the anesthesia workstation) to facilitate this. The third robotic arm will need to be located so that it will approach the patient from the posterior. The use of long ventilator tubing and wrapping up this and other monitoring lines with a towel secured to the side of the bed is helpful to minimize interference with the surgeon/assistant.

Patient Positioning and Port Placement

The patient is positioned in the lateral decubitus position. Precise placement of the double lumen endotracheal tube and the ability to tolerate single lung ventilation should be established before draping the patient, because repositioning the tube will be virtually impossible once the robot is docked. Axillary rolls and arm boards are unnecessary (**Fig. 1**). The robotic ports are inserted in the seventh intercostal space for upper/middle lobectomy and in the eighth intercostal space for lower lobectomy. Typical port placement is shown in **Fig. 2** for a right robotic lobectomy. The ports are marked as follows: robotic arm 3 (5-mm port) is located 1 to 2 cm lateral from the spinous process of the vertebral body, robotic arm 2 (8 mm) is 10 cm medial to robotic arm 3, the camera port (we prefer the 12-mm camera) is 9 cm medial to robotic arm 2, and robotic arm 1 (12 mm) is placed right above the diaphragm anteriorly.

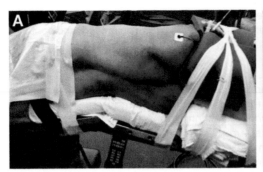
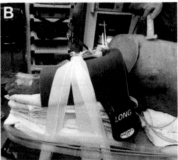

Fig. 1. (*A*) Posterior view of patient in lateral decubitus positioned with only foam and tape. (*B*) Anterior view of patient in lateral decubitus positioned with only foam and tape.

The assistant port is triangulated behind the camera port and the most anterior robotic port, and as inferior as possible without disrupting the diaphragm. We use a zero-degree camera for this operation. Insufflation of the camera or assistant port with carbon dioxide is used to depress the diaphragm, decrease bleeding, and compress the lung.

MEDIASTINAL LYMPH NODE DISSECTION

After examining the pleura to confirm the absence of metastases, the next step during our performance of robotic lobectomy is removal of the mediastinal lymph nodes, for staging and also to help expose the structures of the hilum.

- *Right side:* The inferior pulmonary ligament is divided. Lymph nodes at stations 8 and 9 are removed. Robotic arm 3 is used to retract the lower lobe medially and anteriorly to remove lymph nodes from station 7. Robotic arm 3 is used to retract the upper lobe inferiorly during dissection of stations 2R and 4R, clearing the space between the superior vena cava anteriorly, the esophagus posteriorly, and the azygos vein inferiorly. Avoiding dissection too far superiorly can prevent injury to the right recurrent laryngeal nerve that wraps around the subclavian artery.

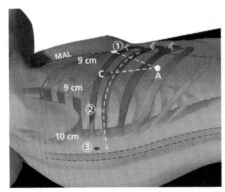
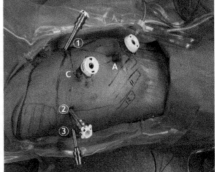

Fig. 2. Total port approach with 4-port placement for right-sided pulmonary lobectomy with da Vinci Si robotic arms 1, 2, 3, camera (C), and access port (A). MAL, mid axillary line.

- *Left side:* The inferior pulmonary ligament is divided to facilitate the removal of lymph node station 9. The nodes in station 8 are then removed. Station 7 is accessed in the space between the inferior pulmonary vein and lower lobe bronchus, lateral to the esophagus. The lower lobe is retracted medially/anteriorly with robotic arm 3 during this process. Absence of the lower lobe facilitates dissection of level 7 from the left. Finally, robotic arm 3 is used to wrap around the left upper lobe and pressed it inferior to allow dissection of stations 5 and 6. Care should be taken while working in the aortopulmonary window to avoid injury to the left recurrent laryngeal nerve. Station 2L cannot typically be accessed during left sided mediastinal lymph node dissection owing to the presence of the aortic arch, but the 4L node is commonly removed.

Wedge Resection

Wedge resection of a nodule may be necessary to confirm the presence of cancer before proceeding with lobectomy. Because the current iteration of the robot does not offer tactile feedback, special techniques may be necessary to identify a nodule that is not obvious on visual inspection. An empty ring forceps may be used via the assistant port to palpate the nodule. Alternatively, preoperative marking of the nodule with a dye marker injected via navigational bronchoscopy can help to facilitate location of the nodule. Preoperative confirmation of a cancer diagnosis with tissue biopsy is helpful to avoid being unable to locate the nodule intraoperatively. In addition, near-infrared imaging of intravenously administered indocyanine green can be used to detect lung nodules; this capability is integrated into the da Vinci Xi platform.[5]

The Five Lobectomies

A certain degree of adaptability is necessary for performance of robotic lobectomy. Structures may be isolated and divided in the order that the patient's individual anatomy permits. What follows is a description of an outline of the typical conduct of each lobectomy.

Right upper lobectomy

- Retraction of the right upper lobe laterally and posteriorly with robot arm 3 helps to expose the hilum.
- The bifurcation between the right upper and middle lobar veins is developed by dissecting it off the underlying pulmonary artery.
- The 10R lymph node between the truncus branch and the superior pulmonary vein should be removed or swept up toward the lung, which exposes the truncus branch.
- The superior pulmonary vein is encircled with the vessel loop and then divided. The truncus branch is then divided.
- The right upper lobe is then reflected anteriorly to expose the bifurcation of the right main stem bronchus. There is usually a lymph node here that should be dissected out to expose the bifurcation. The right upper lobe bronchus is then encircled and divided. Care must be taken to apply only minimal retraction on the specimen to avoid tearing the remaining pulmonary artery branches.
- Finally the posterior segmental artery to the right upper lobe is exposed, the surrounding N1 nodes removed, and the artery encircled and divided.
- The upper lobe is reflected again posteriorly, and the anterior aspect of the pulmonary artery is inspected to make sure that there are no arterial branches remaining. If not, then the fissure between the upper and middle lobes, and the

upper and lower lobes, is divided. This is typically done from anterior to posterior, but may be done in the reverse direction if the space between the pulmonary artery and right middle lobe is already developed. During completion of the fissure, the right upper lobe should be lifted up to ensure that the specimen bronchus is included in the specimen.

Right middle lobectomy

- Retraction of the right middle lobe laterally and posteriorly with the accessory robot arm helps to expose the hilum.
- The bifurcation between the right upper and middle lobar veins is developed by dissecting it off the underlying pulmonary artery. The right middle lobe vein is encircled and divided.
- The fissure between the right middle and lower lobes, if not complete, is divided from anterior to posterior. Care should be taken to avoid transecting segmental arteries to the right lower lobe.
- The right middle lobe bronchus is then isolated. It will be running from left to right in the fissure. Level 11 lymph nodes are dissected from around it. It is encircled and divided, taking care to avoid injuring the right middle lobar artery that is located directly behind it.
- Dissection of the fissure should continue posteriorly until the branches to the superior segment are identified. Then the 1 or 2 right middle lobar segmental arteries are isolated and divided.
- Stapling of middle lobar structures may be facilitated by passing the stapler from posterior to anterior, to have a greater working distance.
- The fissure between right middle and upper lobes is then divided.

Right lower lobectomy

- The inferior pulmonary ligament should be divided to the level of the inferior pulmonary vein.
- The bifurcation of the right superior and inferior pulmonary veins should be dissected out. The location of the right middle lobar vein should be positively identified to avoid inadvertent transection.
- A subadventitial plane on the ongoing pulmonary artery should be established. If the major fissure is not complete, then it should be divided. The superior segmental artery and the right middle lobe arterial branches are identified. The superior segmental artery is isolated and divided. The common trunk to right lower lobe basilar segments may be taken as long as this does not compromise the middle lobar segmental artery or arteries; otherwise, dissection may have to extend further distally to ensure safe division.
- The inferior pulmonary vein is divided.
- The right lower lobe bronchus is isolated, taking care to visualize the right middle lobar bronchus crossing from left to right. The surrounding lymph nodes, as usual, are dissected and the bronchus divided. If there is any question of compromising the right middle lobe bronchus, the surgeon can ask the anesthesiologist to hand ventilate the right lung to confirm that the middle lobe expands.

Left upper lobectomy

- Retraction of the left upper lobe laterally and posteriorly with robot arm 3 helps to expose the hilum.

- The presence of both superior and inferior pulmonary veins is confirmed, and the bifurcation dissected.
- The lung is then reflected anteriorly with robotic arm 3 and interlobar dissection is started, going from posterior to anterior.
- If the fissure is not complete, then it will need to be divided. Reflecting the lung posteriorly again and establishing a subadventitial plane will be helpful. The branches to the lingula are encountered and divided in the fissure during this process. The posterior segmental artery is also isolated and divided. Division of the lingular artery or arteries can be done before or after division of the posterior segmental artery.
- The superior pulmonary vein is isolated then divided. Because the superior pulmonary vein can be fairly wide, it may require that the lingular and upper division branches be transected separately.
- Often the next structure that can be divided readily will be the left upper lobar bronchus, as opposed to the anterior and apical arterial branches to the left upper lobe. The upper lobe bronchus should be encircled and divided, often passing the stapler from robotic arm 1 to avoid injuring the main pulmonary artery.
- Finally, the remaining arterial branches are encircled and divided.

Left lower lobectomy

- The inferior pulmonary ligament should be divided to the level of the inferior pulmonary vein. The lower lobe is then reflected posteriorly by robotic arm 3.
- The bifurcation of the left superior and inferior pulmonary veins should be dissected out.
- The lung is reflected anteriorly by robotic arm 3. The superior segmental artery is identified. The posterior ascending arteries to the left upper lobe are frequently visible from this view also. The superior segmental artery is isolated and divided. The common trunk to left lower lobe basilar segments may be taken as long as this does not compromise the middle lobar segmental artery/arteries; otherwise, dissection may have to extend further distally to ensure safe division. If the fissure is not complete, this will need to be divided to expose the ongoing pulmonary artery to the lower lobe.
- After division of the arterial branches, the lung is reflected again posteriorly. The inferior pulmonary vein is divided.
- The left lower lobe bronchus is isolated. The surrounding lymph nodes, as usual, are dissected and the bronchus divided.
- For left lower lobectomy, it may be simpler to wait until after resection is performed before targeting the subcarinal space for removal of level 7 lymph nodes.
- The superior segment may be spared during lower lobectomy. The superior segment artery, vein, and bronchus are isolated as in performance of superior segmentectomy. Instead of dividing those structures, however, the ongoing vein, artery, and bronchus to the remainder of the lower lobe are divided.

SEGMENTECTOMIES
Posterior Segmentectomy of the Right Upper Lobe

- For a posterior segmentectomy of the right upper lobe and for a superior segment of the right lower lobe, the triangle between the bronchus intermedius and the right upper lobe bronchus is identified.
- The No. 11 lymph node is removed and the posterior segmental artery to the right upper lobe is identified. Robotic arm 3 is then used to retract the upper lobe

- inferiorly while robotic arms 1 and 2 are used to dissect out stations 2R and 4R, clearing the space between the superior vena cava anteriorly and the azygos vein.
- The 10R lymph node between the right main stem bronchus and the pulmonary artery is then removed.
- The appropriate interlobar lymph nodes are removed, especially the ones that are adjacent to the bronchus to be removed. In patients with non–small cell lung cancer, these are sent for frozen section analysis and, if results are positive, a lobectomy is performed.
- If a posterior segmentectomy is performed, the posterior segmental artery is dissected free, taking care not to injure the posterior segmental vein of the right upper lobe that courses just under the artery in the posterior fissure.
- Once the artery is stapled or ligated, the posterior segmental vein is dissected free, staying superior near the bronchus. It is encircled and then stapled or clipped.
- Now the bronchus can be dissected and the posterior segment and apical and anterior segments easily identified. The posterior bronchus is encircled and stapled and it is then retracted cephalad by robotic arm 3. This affords the pulmonary artery to the middle lobe and the lower lobe to be seen and preserved as the parenchyma is stapled to complete the segmentectomy.

Superior Segmentectomy

- If a superior segmentectomy on the right side is to be performed, the triangle between the bronchus intermedius and right upper lobe is identified. Blunt dissection is carried down on the bronchus intermedius until the No. 11 lymph node is identified and removed.
- The superior segmental artery is seen medially under the No. 12 lymph node. The superior segmental artery is encircled and stapled after the posterior superior segmental bronchus is bluntly dissected.
- Before stapling the superior segmental bronchus, the lung should be retracted medially using robotic arm 3, identifying the inferior pulmonary vein. The superior segmental branch of the inferior pulmonary vein is the most cephalad branch of the inferior pulmonary vein. It can be individually encircled and should be stapled or ligated first.
- The staple can then more easily pass around the superior segmental bronchus and be ligated now that the vein has been ligated.
- On the left side, the superior segmental bronchus is generally accessible after the superior segmental vein (or artery) is isolated and divided. The superior segmental artery can be approached via the fissure. The superior segmental vein is the cranial-most branch of the inferior pulmonary vein, and is isolated while retracting the lung anteriorly.
- There is not infrequently a second superior segmental artery found in the left lower lobe.

Lingula-Sparing Upper Lobectomy

- A lingular artery–sparing trisegmentectomy (lingula-sparing upper lobectomy) is performed by removing the N2 lymph nodes and finding the pulmonary artery posteriorly, just cephalad to the inferior pulmonary vein after removal of the level 9, 8, and 7 lymph nodes.
- A complete fissure can be approached from the back by identifying the posterior segmental artery to the left upper lobe and dividing the artery and then working

along the pulmonary artery to identify the other branches and stapling the posterior fissure along the way.

- The lingular artery is identified and preserved, as is the lingular bronchus.
- The 11L lymph node is removed and sent for frozen section analysis to ensure it is free of cancer.
- The lingular vein is identified and preserved and the remaining pulmonary vein is then stapled. The left upper bronchus is now readily visible and the lingular bronchus is easily identified and preserved. The remaining bronchial branches can be stapled while carefully avoiding the anterior-apical trunk of the pulmonary artery.
- Once the anterior-apical and posterior bronchi are all stapled concomitantly, the anterior-apical pulmonary arterial trunk can be stapled, often with 1 firing. The operation is finished by stapling the pulmonary parenchyma from robotic arm 1.

Lingulectomy

- Lingulectomy can be performed with either a vein-first or artery-first technique.
- If performing a vein-first approach, the lung is retracted posteriorly and the lingular vein is identified and divided. Then the lingular bronchus, which often is located fairly distally, is isolated and divided. Finally, the lingular arteries are then isolated and divided.
- The fissure may also be approached first during a lingulectomy. This provided the advantage of being able to assess the level 11 lymph node first because, if it is positive, a lobectomy is a better oncologic operation if able to be tolerated by the patient. If negative, then the vein-first approach can be taken. Alternatively, the lingular arteries can be accessed via the fissure and divided first. Then the bronchus is divided, and finally the vein.

RESULTS

Robotic lobectomy can be performed with excellent perioperative and long-term outcomes. Our median duration of stay after robotic lobectomy is 3 days.[6] We have demonstrated a 30-day mortality rate of 0.25%, 90-day mortality rate of 0.5%, and major morbidity rate of 9.6% in patients undergoing robotic lobectomy and segmentectomy.[7] Similar to VATS, robotic lobectomy is associated with decreased rates of blood loss, blood transfusion, air leak, chest tube duration, duration of stay, and mortality compared with thoracotomy.[8–10] Conversion rates of less than 1% to thoracotomy may be achieved, although 3% to 5% is reported more typically.[6] Vascular injury is rare, and when it does occur, can occasionally be repaired without converting to a thoracotomy.[11] Lymph node upstaging rates and 5-year survival for robotic lobectomy are comparable with lobectomy via thoracotomy and possibly improved versus VATS.[12,13] **Table 1** shows resulted reported in series of robotic-assisted lobectomies.

Robotic segmentectomies have been considered a more demanding technical operation than robotic lobectomy. One investigator found longer operative times (219 minutes vs 175 minutes; $P<.01$) for robotic segmentectomy compared with robotic lobectomy.[15] They found that patients undergoing robotic segmentectomies were more likely to have an effusion or empyema, and pneumothorax after chest tube removal, than patients undergoing robotic lobectomy. We have demonstrated that robotic segmentectomy can be performed with excellent technical and perioperative results (100 patients, 88 minutes median operative time, 7% conversion rate, 10% major postoperative complication rate, 0% 30-day and 90-day mortality rates).[20] Two other series of 21 and 17 patients also support the safety and feasibility of robotic segmentectomy; both author groups commented on the subjective advantages of

Table 1
Results reported in series of robotic-assisted lobectomies

Year	n	Conversion Rate	Morbidity	Perioperative Mortality	Median LOS	Notes
Cerfolio et al,[6] 2016	520	12% (first 100 cases) → 3.3% (last 120 cases)	50% (first 100 cases) → 4.2% (last 120 cases)	0.19% (30-d), 0.57% (90-d)	3 d	
Yang et al,[14] 2016	172	9%	26%	0%	4 d	Equivalent OS and DFS at 5 y to VATS
Veronesi et al,[15] 2009	54	13%	20%	0%	4.5 d	
Gharagozloo et al,[16] 2009	100	—	21%	3%	4 d	
Echavarria et al,[17] 2016	208	9.6%	40.4%	1.44% (in hospital)	5 d	
Louie et al,[10] (STS database) 2016	1220	Not reported	No difference from VATS	0.3% (in hospital), 0.6% (30-d)	4 d	8.44% nodal upstaging
Toker et al,[18] 2016	102 (53% lobectomy)	4%	24%	2% (60-d)	5 d (mean)	104 min (mean operative time)
Adams et al,[8] 2014	116	3.3%	No difference from VATS	0% (30-d)	4.7 d (mean)	
Melfi et al,[19] 2014	229	10.5% (first 69 cases), 5.6% (next 160 cases)	22% and 15%	1.4% and 0%	4.4 d and 3.8 d (mean)	

Abbreviations: DFS, disease-free survival; LOS, length of stay; OS, overall survival; QOL, quality of life; VATS, video–assisted thoracoscopic surgery.
Data from Refs.[6,8,10,14–19]

lymphadenectomy using robotic techniques.[21,22] The oncologic sequelae of and indications for performing segmentectomy as opposed to lobectomy remain active areas of study for both VATS and robotic techniques.

One disadvantage of robotic lung resection compared with VATS lung resection is cost. On average, a robotic lobectomy can cost an additional $3000 to $5000 per case owing to the use of disposable instruments, the additional sunk cost of the robot itself, and the maintenance plans required for using the robot.[23,24] Even with this additional cost, however, each robotic lobectomy yields an estimated median profit margin of around $3500 per patient.[25]

SUMMARY

Robotic lobectomy and segmentectomy have been demonstrated to be safe operations that can be done expeditiously and with low conversion rates. Perioperative morbidity and mortality is similar to VATS lobectomy/segmentectomy, and improved compared with lung resection via thoracotomy. Long-term oncologic outcomes for robotic lobectomy mirror those demonstrated after VATS and open lobectomy. Improved optics, increased dexterity of the instruments, and better ergonomics can yield subjective advantages to the surgeon. With proper training and experience, robotic lobectomy can become part of the fundamental armamentarium of the modern thoracic surgeon.

REFERENCES

1. Shenstone NS, Janes RM. Experiences in pulmonary lobectomy. Can Med Assoc J 1932;27:138–45.
2. Morgan JA, Ginsburg ME, Sonett JR, et al. Advanced thoracoscopic procedures are facilitated by computer-aided robotic technology. Eur J Cardiothorac Surg 2003;23:883–7.
3. Ashton RC, Connery CP, Swistel DG, et al. Robot-assisted lobectomy. J Thorac Cardiovasc Surg 2003;126:292–3.
4. Burt BM, Kosinski AS, Shrager JB, et al. Thoracoscopic lobectomy is associated with acceptable morbidity and mortality in patients with predicted postoperative forced expiratory volume in 1 second or diffusing capacity for carbon monoxide less than 40% of normal. J Thorac Cardiovasc Surg 2014;148:19–28.
5. Okusanya OT, Holt D, Heitjian D, et al. Intraoperative near-infrared imaging can identify pulmonary nodules. Ann Thorac Surg 2014;98:1223–30.
6. Cerfolio RJ, Cichos KH, Wei B, et al. Robotic lobectomy can be taught while maintaining quality patient outcomes. J Thorac Cardiovasc Surg 2016;152:991–7.
7. Cerfolio RJ, Bryant AS, Skylizard L, et al. Initial consecutive experience of completely portal robotic pulmonary resection with 4 arms. J Thorac Cardiovasc Surg 2011;142:740–6.
8. Adams RD, Bolton WD, Stephenson JE, et al. Initial multicenter community robotic lobectomy experience: comparisons to a national database. Ann Thorac Surg 2014;97:1893–8.
9. Kent M, Want T, Whyte R, et al. Open, video-assisted thoracic surgery, and robotic lobectomy: review of a national database. Ann Thorac Surg 2014;97: 236–42.
10. Louie BE, Wilson JL, Kim S, et al. Comparison of video-assisted thoracoscopic surgery and robotic approaches for clinical stage I and stage II non-small cell lung cancer using the Society of Thoracic Surgeons database. Ann Thorac Surg 2016;102:917–24.

11. Cerfolio RJ, Bess KM, Wei B, et al. Incidence, results, and our current intraoperative technique to control major vascular injuries during minimally invasive robotic thoracic surgery. Ann Thorac Surg 2016;102:394–9.

12. Toosi K, Velez-Cubian FO, Glover J, et al. Upstaging and survival after robotic-assisted thoracoscopic lobectomy for non-small cell lung cancer. Surgery 2016;160:1211–8.

13. Park BJ, Melfi F, Mussi A, et al. Robotic lobectomy for non-small cell lung cancer (NSCLC): long-term oncologic results. J Thorac Cardiovasc Surg 2012;143: 383–9.

14. Yang H, Woo KM, Sima CS, et al. Long-term survival based on the surgical approach to lobectomy for clinical stage I nonsmall cell lung cancer: comparison of robotic, video-assisted thoracic surgery, and thoracotomy lobectomy. Ann Thorac Surg 2016;265(2):431–7.

15. Veronesis G, Galetta D, Maisonneuve P, et al. Four-arm robotic lobectomy for the treatment of early-stage lung cancer. J Thorac Cardiovasc Surg 2010;140:19–25.

16. Gharagozloo F, Margolis M, Tempesta B, et al. Robot-assisted lobectomy for early-stage lung cancer: report of 100 consecutive cases. Ann Thorac Surg 2009;88:380–4.

17. Echavarria MF, Cheng AM, Velez-Cubian FO, et al. Comparison of pulmonary function tests and perioperative outcomes after robotic-assisted pulmonary lobectomy vs segmentectomy. Am J Surg 2016;212(6):1175–82.

18. Toker A, Ozyurtkan MO, Kaba E, et al. Robotic anatomic lung resections: the initial experience and description of learning in 102 cases. Surg Endosc 2016; 30:676–83.

19. Melfi FM, Fanucchi O, Davini F, et al. Robotic lobectomy for lung cancer: evolution in technique and technology. Eur J Cardiothorac Surg 2014;46:626–31.

20. Cerfolio RJ, Watson C, Minnich DJ, et al. One hundred planned robotic segmentectomies: early results, technical details, and preferred port placement. Ann Thorac Surg 2016;101:1089–96.

21. Pardolesi A, Park B, Petrella F, et al. Robotic anatomic segmentectomy of the lung: technical aspects and initial results. Ann Thorac Surg 2012;94:929–34.

22. Toker A, Ayalp K, Uyumaz E, et al. Robotic lung segmentectomy for malignant and benign lesions. J Thorac Dis 2014;6:937–42.

23. Deen SA, Wilson JL, Wishire CL, et al. Defining the cost of care for lobectomy and segmentectomy: a comparison of open, video-assisted thoracoscopic, and robotic approaches. Ann Thorac Surg 2014;9:1000–7.

24. Swanson SJ, Miller DL, McKenna RJ, et al. Comparing robot-assisted thoracic surgical lobectomy with conventional video-assisted thoracic surgical lobectomy and wedge resection: results from a multihospital database. J Thorac Cardiovasc Surg 2014;147:929–37.

25. Nasir BS, Bryant AS, Minnich DJ, et al. Performing robotic lobectomy and segmentectomy: cost, profitability, and outcomes. Ann Thorac Surg 2014;98:203–8.

Thoracic Trauma
Injuries, Evaluation, and Treatment

Joseph J. Platz, MD*, Loic Fabricant, MD, Mitch Norotsky, MD

KEYWORDS

- Thoracic trauma • Penetrating • Blunt • Primary survey
- Emergency department thoracotomy

KEY POINTS

- A focused primary survey is essential in the diagnosis and rapid treatment of life-threatening injuries in thoracic trauma.
- Thoracic trauma can uniquely benefit from bedside procedures (eg, tube thoracostomy, emergency airway creation, emergency department thoracotomy) to alleviate immediate threat of mortality and allow further definitive treatment.
- Patient stabilization is necessary before definitive surgical intervention is attempted.
- A thorough secondary survey in combination with diagnostic laboratory and radiologic studies will uncover most traumatic injuries.

INTRODUCTION

Thoracic injury is a common and potentially devastating component of acute trauma care. The incidence of such injury is 14% in blunt trauma and 12% in penetrating. Yet, thoracic injuries account for up to a quarter of early trauma-related mortality, second only to head and neck insults.[1,2] Despite the often serious nature of thoracic trauma, many of these injuries are can be quickly diagnosed, and at times mitigated, in the trauma bay.[3]

PRIMARY SURVEY

The first priority in management of thoracic trauma is evaluation and stabilization of airways, breathing, and circulation (ABC).[4] This initial primary survey encompasses urgent assessment of the airway, quality of respiration, and stability of circulatory status. When any of these factors is insufficient, urgent intervention must be performed and the primary survey reassessed. Although many trauma victims can benefit from basic

The authors have nothing to disclose. They have no funding sources, or commercial or financial conflicts of interest regarding the authorship and publication of this article.
University of Vermont Medical Center, 111 Colchester Avenue, Burlington, VT 05401, USA
* Corresponding author.
E-mail address: Joseph.platz@uvmhealth.org

Surg Clin N Am 97 (2017) 783–799
http://dx.doi.org/10.1016/j.suc.2017.03.004
0039-6109/17/© 2017 Elsevier Inc. All rights reserved.

surgical.theclinics.com

interventions, emergent bedside surgical intervention is uniquely beneficial in thoracic trauma if performed promptly and appropriately (**Table 1**).

Airway

Assessment and stabilization of the airway is always the first priority in the management of all trauma patients. A great deal of assessment can be based on basic patient appearance and verbalization. However, in the presence of severe injury or diminished mental status, evaluation can be more difficult and should be focused on a combined assessment of oxygenation, ventilation, and airway protection.[4] Because the mortality of direct airway injury is so high, most of these patients do not reach the emergency room. As such, loss of airway in hospitalized trauma patients is generally due to secondary failure. Diminished mental status, head injury, cervical spine injury, soft tissue neck trauma, facial wounds, and clavicle fractures can all indirectly lead to loss of adequate airway protection.[2] Initial treatment must include cervical stabilization and proper head positioning with eventual definitive control by endotracheal intubation. If direct airway injury is suspected on primary survey, laryngoscopy can be considered; however, only with the understanding that it is time intensive. If the airway is truly compromised in the setting of suspected injury, an emergency airway is required. The standard method is via cricothyroidotomy due to its speed and ease. The technique can be used in a variety of settings with as little as a scalpel, clamp or bougie, and endotracheal tube. The primary contraindication to this procedure is direct neck injury at the position of the cricothyroid membrane. In this setting, tracheostomy is preferred because its distal location avoids an incision through traumatized soft tissue and reduces the risk of worsening a tracheal disruption.[3]

Breathing

Following, or paralleling, airway evaluation, the patient's respiratory status must be assessed. In the setting of traumatic thoracic injury, this step is of particular importance because significant compromise may be present and emergent bedside intervention may be indicated. Basic evaluations of respiratory rate, chest wall motion, oxygenation, and breath sounds are performed, as in any trauma. The physician must have a suspicion for pneumothorax in the setting of thoracic injury; in particular, there is concern for a life-threatening tension pneumothorax.

Table 1	
Primary survey: life-threatening injuries and emergent treatments	
Injury	**Intervention**
Airway obstruction or rupture	Intubation if possible and safe, consideration of cricothyroidotomy vs tracheostomy
Tension pneumothorax	Initial needle decompression followed by definitive tube thoracostomy
Open pneumothorax	Initial 3-sided occlusive dressing followed by wound closure and tube thoracostomy
Massive hemothorax	Volume resuscitation, tube thoracostomy, consideration of emergency thoracotomy
Pericardial tamponade	Pericardiocentesis if the patient is stable, consideration of emergency thoracotomy

A list of the common life-threatening thoracic traumatic injuries that can be diagnosed during the primary survey. If identified or even strongly suspected, the corresponding emergent intervention must be strongly considered.

Tension pneumothorax is the progressive accumulation of gas within the thoracic cavity to a point that positive pressure is exerted on the mediastinal and intrathoracic structures.[5] This circumstance can be secondary to chest wall trauma, a large bronchial or parenchymal injury, or a smaller lung injury exacerbated by positive pressure ventilation. Regardless of cause, the end result is the development of a 1-way valve; air enters the thoracic cavity without egress. By Boyle's law, the increased volume of air results in increased thoracic pressure, causing ipsilateral lung collapse, contralateral lung compression, mediastinal shift, and decreased venous return to the heart.[2] Tension pneumothorax can progress rapidly and diagnosis should not be delayed for imaging but rather made by clinical examination. As with all pneumothoraces, primary survey may reveal absent breath sounds, unequal chest rise, and hypoxia. However, signs unique to the tension variety include tracheal deviation (away from injury), jugular venous distension, and hypotension.[3] Many of the signs of tension pneumothorax are vague and nonspecific in the presence of other injuries. However, there is substantial morbidity if the pathologic condition is missed, so any suggestion of tension pneumothorax necessitates intervention during the primary survey. Initially, a partially occlusive dressing can be placed (open chest wall wounds) and needle decompression should be performed. This maneuver will allow time for reassessment of the ABCs; however, definitive treatment requires tube thoracostomy once the primary survey is complete.

Circulation

The final element of the primary survey is assessment of circulatory status. Again, with thoracic trauma, circulatory compromise can be profound and rapid. If any trauma patient presents with hypotension, the general assumption is that massive hemorrhage is the cause. However, in thoracic trauma, obstructive shock must also be considered. The deadly circulatory pathologic conditions that are associated with the most immediate morbidity and, therefore, must be dealt with promptly, are massive hemothorax and pericardial tamponade. Analysis of vital signs, pulse pressure, neck veins, and breath sounds may help identify life-threatening injuries. Increased suspicion should be present with near-midline trauma (between the nipples or, posteriorly, the medial scapular borders).[2]

Similar to the abdomen, pelvis, and lower extremities, the thoracic cavity provides a potential space large enough for patient exsanguination. Furthermore, massive hemothorax into this space is not only worrisome for potential large volume blood loss but also for possible tension effects on central venous return. Initial treatment of hemothorax is chest tube placement. This intervention is rapidly decompressive and allows for direct evaluation of hemorrhage volume. General teaching is that if the immediate chest tube output exceeds 1500 mL, or 200 mL per hour for 2 to 4 successive hours, the patient should proceed to the operating room for thoracotomy.[3] A rare but deadly complication associated with hemothorax is bronchovenous air embolism. When direct penetrating pulmonary trauma occurs, injury to both parenchyma and vasculature can result. The already low pulmonary venous pressures exacerbated by hemorrhage allows potential air uptake from injured parenchyma and subsequent air embolism into the left heart. Risk of this phenomenon increases as airway pressures increase. Although air embolism is rare, it should be suspected when rapid circulatory collapse occurs following the initiation of positive pressure mechanical ventilation.[6]

Pericardial tamponade may also produce rapid circulatory collapse following thoracic trauma. For hemothorax to cause significant compromise, substantial blood loss is required. In contrast, tamponade can occur with very little blood in the pericardial space. As this closed space progressively fills and applies pressure on the pericardial contents, preload is initially compromised. If allowed to progress, end diastolic volume is impaired by means of ventricular compression. Signs of pericardial tamponade characteristically present in 3 phases. First observed is tachycardia and increased systemic vascular resistance, followed by decreased cardiac output, and finally complete circulatory collapse.[7] In the setting of severe injury, pericardial filling can be rapid and, therefore, collapse can occur without warning. Along with the previously described changes in vital signs, examination findings of muffled heart sounds, jugular venous distension, and pulsus paradoxus (large decrease in systolic blood pressure during inspiration) may be present in the setting of tamponade. However, though considered standard symptoms, all 3 are only present concurrently 15% of the time and individually are too vague to be accurately predictive.[8] Similarly, elevated intracranial pressure or pulseless electrical activity may be foretelling but are nonspecific. The increased use of ultrasound (US) in the emergency room has helped to alleviate some of the ambiguity in diagnosis, with a sensitivity of 96% and a specificity of 98% in detection. Though, even at bedside, the study requires valuable time and expertise.[9] It is critical, therefore, to have a high suspicion for pericardial tamponade any time thoracic trauma is present, particularly penetrating, in the setting of circulatory collapse.

If pericardial tamponade is recognized early enough (in the first 2 phases), pericardiocentesis can be performed as temporary decompression before definitive repair. If, however, the patient is already in obstructive shock, the patient requires an emergency department thoracotomy (EDT).

Whether for tamponade or hemorrhage, EDT consists of a left anterolateral thoracotomy in approximately the 5th intercostal space with or without extension across the sternum. Once the chest is open, the pericardium should be opened, hemothorax evacuated, lung distracted, and descending aorta clamped if appropriate (**Box 1**). The primary objectives are to release tamponade, control hemorrhage, evacuate air embolization, perform cardiac massage, and allow adequate resuscitation. Hemorrhage from proximal pulmonary vascular injury can be temporized by twisting the lung on its hilum until an appropriate clamp is placed. EDT is potentially life-saving but not without risk, so should only be performed for very specific indications. EDT only demonstrates significant benefit for those patients with a reasonable chance of neurologic

---

Box 1
Emergency department thoracotomy: important steps

- Fifth intercostal space incision from sternum to bed (when the patient is supine)
- Placement and opening of a rib spreader, dial, or crank on the posterior blade
- Evacuation of the thorax and identification or control of the hemorrhagic source
- Craniocaudal (parallel to bed) incision in pericardium with pericardial evacuation and delivery of the heart
  - Control of hemorrhage if appropriate
- Distraction of the lung with hilar torsion
- Incision of the pulmonary ligament, aortic isolation via blunt dissection, clamping of the aorta at the level of the diaphragm
- Internal cardiac massage, if appropriate
- Consideration of extension of the thoracotomy across the sternum (with the Lebsche knife) if concerned for right-sided injury.

recovery; therefore, it is used for patients who become pulseless in the trauma bay or those who continue to demonstrate pupillary response, spontaneous movement, organized electrocardiograph patterns, or cardiac activity on US despite pulseless-ness.[2] Furthermore, EDT is of highest benefit in penetrating trauma with an immediate survival rate of 35% for cardiac injury and 15% for all-comer penetrating injury. Conversely, patient outcomes are poor with EDT for blunt trauma, with only 2% sur-vival for those in shock and 1% for those with loss of vital signs.[10,11] Regardless of the scenario, for an EDT to be effective it must be used as a damage control procedure with rapid pericardial decompression or hemorrhage control followed by expedited transfer to the operating room. Even after stability is obtained, patients with a high injury severity score will often benefit from simple packing, vacuum therapy, and delayed closure.[12]

SECONDARY SURVEY

Once immediately life-threatening injuries have been managed and the patient's ABCs have stabilized, a thorough head-to-toe examination must be performed. A full set of hematologic and metabolic laboratory studies should be sent. This secondary survey not only allows for a more complete picture of the patient's condition but also for the discovery of other nonemergent but possibly life-threatening injuries (**Box 2**).

Imaging

In addition to a thorough but expedited head-to-toe examination, a key component of the secondary survey is imaging. In most trauma situations, especially thoracic trauma, a portable chest radiography (CXR) is recommended. This rapid test can eval-uate chest wall injuries, mediastinal trauma, pneumothorax, hemothorax, pulmonary contusion, and pleural effusions, as well as guide further management without the need to transport a potentially unstable patient. For similar reasons, US has become ever more prevalent in the trauma bay. The effectiveness of focused assessment with sonography for trauma (FAST) has been well-documented.[13] The emergence of extended-FAST (eFAST) makes US all the more useful in thoracic trauma. This bedside imaging study can diagnose pericardial effusions and aortic injuries in addi-tion to the previously mentioned pathologic conditions. Studies have suggested that

---

Box 2
Secondary survey

Components

- Evaluation of glasgow coma scale
- Head-to-toe examination
- Basic laboratory studies
- CXR
- Consideration of eFAST
- Further imaging based on clinical suspicion

Injuries

- Potential life-threatening injuries: simple pneumothorax, hemothorax, rib fractures, sternal fracture, cardiac injury, aortic or major vessel trauma, pulmonary injury, tracheobronchial tree disruption, esophageal trauma, diaphragm rupture.

the effectiveness of US rivals computed tomography (CT) with certain injuries, sensitivity, and specificity nearing 100%. However, there are certainly disadvantages to this modality. First, US depends on the identification of fluid, or the effects of an injury, rather than the injury itself. Therefore, its guidance in treatment is not always clear. Furthermore, though some studies extol the predictive value of US, others cite sensitivities and specificities of less than 50%. This discrepancy is likely due to several factors associated with the modality, including variations in provider technique, imaging analysis not done by a radiologist, and no standardization of anatomic landmarks. Additionally, air in the thoracic or subcutaneous spaces can significantly limit effectiveness.[13]

The definitive imaging modality in chest trauma is CT. It does not offer the cost-effectiveness or speed of radiography or US but provides far superior resolution and scope, allowing the diagnosis of injuries that would otherwise fail to be recognized. With the use of intravenous (IV) or by mouth contrast agents, CT can further identify luminal trauma that formerly required angiography or endoscopy. The drawbacks of CT include the cost, radiation exposure, examination duration, and need for patient travel. If used only when injuries are suspected and imaging is likely to affect management, the first 3 disadvantages are negligible. The latter concern, however, can be significant and careful consideration of the patient's stability must be made before their removal from the trauma bay.

INJURIES AND MANAGEMENT
Pneumothorax

One of the most common pathologic conditions encountered with thoracic trauma is the nontension pneumothorax, with an estimated incidence of 20%.[14] Simple pneumothoraces occur as air slowly leaks from the lung parenchyma. Such leaks often occur as the result of direct penetration by missiles or fractured ribs. Pneumothorax can also occur secondary to alveolar rupture during rapid intrathoracic pressure changes. Findings of tachycardia, hypoxia, decreased breath sounds, or crepitus arise with pneumothorax. If the patient is symptomatic, tube thoracostomy is indicated. Minor pneumothoraces are often asymptomatic and often diagnosed on initial radiography or US. Given the 20% to 35% false-negative rate of supine CXR, small pneumothoraces are frequently only discovered after thoracic CT scan (**Fig. 1**).[2] The

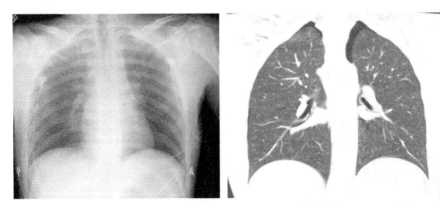

Fig. 1. Demonstration of a seemingly normal portable CXR (*left*) after motor vehicle collision but with evidence of occult bilateral apical pneumothoraces discovered on chest CT (*right*).

treatment of occult pneumothoraces, which occur in 2% to 8% of blunt traumas, is controversial.[15] Some studies conclude that tube thoracostomy is required for pneumothoraces with volumes greater than 5 times 80 mm, those involving more than 2 rib fractures, or in patients requiring positive pressure ventilation.[16,17] However, other studies argue that there is no correlation between these factors and the need for procedural intervention.[18] Aspiration has been described for the treatment of spontaneous pneumothorax and is being adopted in the trauma setting, whereas other physicians use oxygen therapy to aid in intrathoracic air reabsorption.[19] Although this latter treatment has been used for decades, it has been suggested that high oxygen tension therapy (>60%) is no more beneficial than standard low-flow nasal cannula.[20] It is unclear, therefore, what the optimal treatment regimen for small pneumothoraces should be. No matter the intervention, the most important step in management is close clinical monitoring for pneumothorax expansion.

Hemothorax

Intrathoracic hemorrhage often occurs in concurrence with pneumothorax. Nonmassive hemothorax occurs by injury to lung parenchyma, intercostal vessels, or other chest wall vessels. Hemorrhage is rarely large enough to cause immediate patient instability; however, failure to treat early can lead to interval development of empyema or fibrothorax. Small amounts of bleeding (<200–300 mL) are rarely detectable on physical examination or portable supine CXR. If there is concern for hemorrhage, CT allows for the identification of source, estimation of hemothorax volume, and evaluation for associated injuries.[21] Because of the complications associated with retained hemothorax, treatment requires drainage with tube thoracostomy. Although even early chest tube placement fails to evacuate the thorax in 5% of cases, this failure rate increases dramatically when treatment is delayed more than 24 hours after injury; prompt intervention is crucial.[22] For retained hemothoraces failing chest tube drainage, instillation of tissue plasminogen activator and deoxyribonuclease has been found 65% to 90% successful. This treatment does take multiple days, however, and is associated with reported fevers and pleuritic pain. The ultimate treatment of undrained hemothoraces is surgical decortication, whether by thoracotomy or video-assisted thoracoscopic surgery (VATS). Under direct visualization, surgical intervention allows for not only hematoma drainage but also thorough removal of organized collections and loculation debridement. VATS decortication has largely replaced traditional thoracotomy due to decreased long-term cost, length of stay, and chest tube days. However, these benefits are only reliable with careful patient selection. For patients with previous empyema, those who have undergone previous ipsilateral thoracic surgery, those who are hemodynamically unstable, those who cannot tolerate single-lung ventilation, or those who have an organized fibrothorax, open thoracotomy is still recommended.[23]

Rib Fractures

One of the most common injuries from blunt thoracic trauma is rib fracture. Though often considered minor and rarely requiring surgical intervention, these fractures can cause direct trauma to lung parenchyma or intra-abdominal organs. Rib fractures can also cause respiratory complications because significant pain impairs adequate pulmonary toilet. The presence of fractures is an independent risk factor for pneumonia and death in trauma patients.[24] Traditional treatment of rib fractures is supportive, consisting of respiratory therapy and multimodal analgesia, including epidural or paravertebral blocks. Rib plating or stabilization is controversial for most fracture patterns but has demonstrated some benefit when performed in the management of flail chest. A flail segment occurs by disassociation of a portion of the chest from the surrounding chest wall. Diagnosis requires the fracture of 2 or more adjacent ribs in 2 or more locations. This disassociation leads to pain and disrupted respiratory mechanics but also indicates a high-energy traumatic mechanism that should raise suspicion for other injuries, particularly pulmonary contusions (**Fig. 2**).[3] The suggested treatment of flail chest has fluctuated throughout the years. Initially, external stabilization was recommended but high rates of complications pushed treatment toward internal fixation. As positive pressure mechanical ventilation improved and was able to provide effective internal splinting, surgical fixation fell out of favor.[2] However, over the past decade, several studies have demonstrated that, although surgical stabilization of flail chest does not improve overall mortality, there may be benefit for patients with refractory pain or respiratory compromise. Data show reduced length of stay, intensive care unit days, and time on mechanical ventilation.[25,26] Furthermore, longitudinal studies have suggested that patients have improved quality of life, pulmonary function, and pain control over the first year after traumatic flail chest if rib fixation was performed.[27]

Pulmonary Contusion

When it comes to primary respiratory compromise, though pneumothorax may produce the most immediately profound symptoms following thoracic trauma, pulmonary contusion may be the most destructive injury. Contusions are associated with 5% to 30% mortality and are directly causative in many of these deaths.[28] The diffuse energy dissipation of trauma across the pulmonary parenchyma and chest wall causes a combination of intraparenchymal hemorrhage, atelectasis, and consolidation. This form of injury is indolent, not noticeable on initial CXR or examination. Contusion begins to progress at 4 to 6 hours after trauma and develops maximal effect within 24 to 48 hours.[29] Radiography and CT imaging may help with initial diagnosis and allow for monitoring but they rarely change outcomes or allow prediction of eventual severity. Assessment of the patient's pressure of arterial oxygen to fractional inspired oxygen concentration ratio (Pao_2/Fio_2) is helpful in demonstrating the clinical severity of injury and guiding the need for mechanical ventilation but is not necessarily predictive.[2] Management of pulmonary contusion is supportive and consists of oxygen therapy, aggressive pulmonary toilet, fluid restriction, careful pain management, and appropriate diuresis. Early intubation and antibiosis have been studied but at this time are

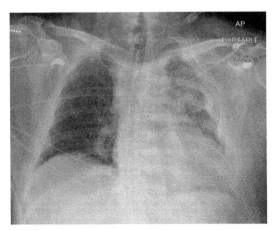

Fig. 2. Portable CXR after motorcycle crash displaying multiple left-sided rib fractures, including a flail segment, as well as the commonly underlying pulmonary contusions.

not recommended unless otherwise indicated. Unlike with penetrating trauma, surgical intervention for blunt pulmonary contusion is rarely indicated. In circumstances when parenchymal contusion is severe enough to produce large regions of necrosis, lobectomy can be performed to prevent infection or improve shunt; however, even after intervention, mortality is as high as 50%.[11]

Blunt Cardiac Injury, Pulmonary Vessel Injury, and Sternal Fractures

Blunt cardiac injuries are generally caused by direct sternal impact or rapid thoracic deceleration. Sheer forces, direct compression, and abrupt alterations in thoracic pressure all contribute to cardiac damage.[30] In its most severe form, free cardiac or, even less commonly, aortic valve rupture may occur. Though most patients with uncontained cardiac rupture die before reaching the hospital, it is important to be aware of the pathologic condition and its signs.[31] Because rupture most commonly occurs in the right heart, hemorrhage correlates to preload. Therefore, in the setting of hypotension, massive hemorrhage or tamponade may not be obvious but will present rapidly with initial trauma resuscitation. A similar presentation can occur when the neighboring proximal pulmonary vessels are injured. Trauma to this low-pressure vasculature may lead to either rapid hemorrhage into the pleural or pericardial space or, contrastingly, may produce few to no symptoms if contained. In severe cases, in which the patient is hemodynamically unstable, EDT and subsequent surgical repair is required; whereas, for stable ruptures and pseudoaneurysms, nonoperative management may be appropriate. Though pulmonary vessel injury can be devastating, it is relatively rare and there is, therefore, little consensus about its ideal treatment. Though complete cardiac and/or pulmonary vessel disruption can occur, most blunt cardiac trauma is milder and more insidious, only being discovered because of subtle secondary signs, such as new arrhythmia, murmur, or abnormal pulse pressure. The most common traumatic cardiac injury is cardiac contusion, a vague pathologic state describing focal myocardial hematoma or edema. Echocardiography may be helpful in diagnosis; however, electrocardiography is more sensitive, and able to detect associated arrhythmias or ST changes. Seventy-six percent of cardiac contusions are associated with sternal fractures. Because of this high correlation, if a fracture is present, the patient should be treated as if cardiac injury is also present.[32] Unless there is an associated effusion that would benefit from pericardiocentesis, treatment is supportive and primarily involves 24 to 48 hours of telemetry monitoring.[3] Cardiac biomarkers are of little value in the initial assessment of a cardiac injury; however, in trending, they may uncover coronary damage. Whether or not cardiac injury is present, sternal fractures are associated with high patient morbidity because of the force required to create such an injury. The degree of sternal displacement is correlated with the risk for further thoracic injury.[33] As with that of rib fractures, management is primarily supportive. However, if the fracture is unstable, pain is uncontrolled, or sternal infection is present, surgical intervention is required. Infected bone necessitates debridement and sternal closure can be achieved by sternal wires, plating, or both. If a significant defect remains, soft tissue flap coverage may be required.[2]

Blunt Aortic Injury

Although penetrating aortic trauma is notably deadly, blunt traumatic aortic injury (BTAI) can be similarly devastating. Second only to head trauma, aortic injury carries 1 of the highest associated mortality rates in all of blunt traumas.[34] Furthermore, incidence is not low; it is estimated that anyone who suffers more than a 10 foot fall or motor vehicle crash (MVC) at more than 40 mph is at risk for aortic trauma.[2] Eighty percent of aortic trauma occurs due to MVCs and can range from small intimal tears to total aortic transection, from which 80% of patients suffer immediate death.[35] Disruption of the aorta in blunt trauma is generally due to rapid patient deceleration. Because the aortic arch is relatively free-floating in contrast to the tethered descending aorta, deceleration imparts significant sheer force at the site of transition, the ligamentum arteriosum. Hence, most blunt aortic injury occurs just distal to the left subclavian artery (**Fig. 3**).[36] Unless the injury is severe, signs and symptoms are often vague and aortic disruption is instead suspected based on the mechanism of trauma or the associated injury pattern, and is confirmed by radiographic studies. Chest CXR may suggest aortic disease through findings of hemorrhage such as hemothorax or mediastinal widening. Thoracic CT scan with IV contrast remains the gold standard, preferably using a trauma or angiogram protocol. In the unstable patient, transesophageal echocardiography (TEE) is also an option and further provides the opportunity for cardiac and valvular evaluation.

If aortic injury is confirmed, the initial goals of treatment are stabilization and prevention of further propagation. Anti-impulse therapy is the first line of treatment and is achieved using such agents as beta and calcium channel blockers. The functional effect is a decreased change in aortic pressure over time (dP/dT). Goals of therapy are based on maximal heart rate reduction while maintaining systemic perfusion.[37] Adequate anti-impulse therapy not only serves as definitive treatment in select patients but also decreases operative mortality should they subsequently require intervention for the aortic injury.[38] This subsequent intervention remains controversial. Traditionally, expeditious surgical repair was the standard of care. Surgical intervention remains the appropriate immediate treatment of an unstable trauma patient with aortic injury but is associated with up to 31% mortality and 9% incidence of paralysis.[39,40] Timing of intervention in the hemodynamically stable patient is less clear.[41] Decision-making is largely based on the risk of aortic free rupture (**Table 2**). Although this risk has been correlated with the size of intramural hematoma or contained rupture, injury propagation remains unpredictable (**Box 3**).[42] Regardless, recent analysis has demonstrated that delayed operative intervention is not only safe but is associated with a decreased mortality. Over the past decade, the average delay to intervention has gone from 15 hours to 55 hours with a 65% decrease in 30-day mortality.[43] The Eastern Association for the Surgery of Trauma (EAST) has supported these findings by formally endorsing delayed aortic intervention.[44]

In the past, a second controversy in the management of BTAI has been open versus endovascular surgical intervention. Currently, thoracic endovascular aortic repair

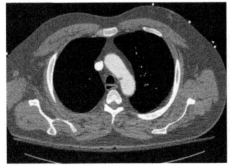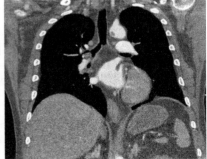

Fig. 3. Axial (*left*) and coronal (*right*) slices of a thoracic CT scan demonstrating a small thoracic aortic lesion after patient fall. Note that this lesion is in the classic location, adjacent to the left subclavian takeoff (seen best in the coronal slice).

Table 2
Classification of traumatic aortic injury

Grade	Description
I	Intimal tear
II	Intramural hematoma
III	Pseudoaneurysm
IV	Rupture

Graded classification of traumatic aortic injury severity. Treatment based on these grades continues to evolve. However, in general, low-grade injuries may be treated medically, moderate grade with delayed endovascular intervention, and high-grade with more urgent surgery.

(TEVAR) is the recommended treatment if anatomically feasible.[34] TEVAR demonstrates decreased rates of paraplegia, heparin-associated hemorrhage, and immediate mortality compared with open aortic repair (3.1% vs 17.8%).[45] Endovascular intervention, however, is not without its own risks. Despite a low early mortality, studies have confirmed late deaths with TEVAR, no decrease in the need for operative reintervention, closer required follow-up, and an overall complication rate nearing 20%. These complications are primarily stent infolding due to oversizing, endoleaks, and cerebrovascular accidents (CVAs).[35] Some of these complications are due to the 50% need for left subclavian coverage during stent placement. There are conflicting data on the risk of subclavian occlusion and, similarly, inconsistent opinions on management.[46] If staged intervention is feasible, pre-TEVAR carotid to subclavian bypass or subclavian transposition is possible. However, their benefit is questionable without clear improvement in post-TEVAR CVA or spinal cord ischemia. Furthermore, most analyses of subclavian coverage addresses nontraumatic injuries and so the applicability with aortic trauma is unclear.[47] With the increasing utility of TEVAR, enthusiasm about the possible use of resuscitative endovascular balloon occlusion of the aorta (REBOA) in BTAI has emerged. REBOA refers to the insertion of a balloon catheter into the aorta via the femoral artery. The balloon is inflated proximal to the aortic injury, halting further distal blood flow and hemorrhage. This new technology is promising; however, indications and criteria for REBOA still need to be better defined.[48]

Penetrating Cardiovascular Trauma

Penetrating cardiac, aortic, and other large vessel trauma can be devastating with rapid hemodynamic compromise. When not immediately fatal, severe injuries often

Box 3
Aortic rupture: risk score criteria

- Lactate >4 mM/L

- Mediastinal hematoma greater than 10 mm

- Lesion to normal aortic diameter ratio greater than 1.4

High risk for aortic rupture after initial traumatic nonrupture injury when more than 1 factor is present.

From Harris DG, Rabin J, Kufer JA, et al. A new aortic injury score predicts early rupture more accurately than clinical assessment. J Vasc Surg 2015;61:532–3; with permission.

result in massive hemothorax or tamponade and require EDT followed by prompt transfer to the operating room. However, in a minority of patients, penetrating trauma causes occult injuries that are only identified during diagnostic workup. Pericardial effusion or hemothorax on radiography may suggest cardiovascular injury but are nonspecific. FAST, TEE, and multidetector CT, on the other hand, are able to identify even stable or contained injuries.[49] Although the management of injury to thin-walled vasculature, such as the inferior vena cava and pulmonary vessels, is controversial, treatment of nonexpanding aortic injuries in the stable patient can be managed non-surgically. These insults can treated similarly to small blunt cardiovascular injuries, with hemodynamic stabilization, anti-impulse therapy, close monitoring, and none-mergent endovascular intervention.

Tracheobronchial Tree Disruption

Major tracheobronchial injury in trauma is rare but when present is associated with an 80% mortality in the field. Penetrating tracheal injury is often cervical in location and easily detected. In contrast, most tracheobronchial injury suffered from blunt trauma is near the carina and can be more difficult to diagnose.[50,51] Patients may demonstrate dyspnea, dysphonia, pneumomediastinum, pneumothorax, or subcutaneous emphysema (**Fig. 4**). Although these signs can also be attributed to other pathologic conditions, together these findings should raise suspicion for tracheobronchial tree injury.[52] Initial diagnostic studies should include CT scan to evaluate for mediastinal hematoma, pneumomediastinum, or tracheal deviation; however, a negative study does not obviate bronchoscopy if tracheobronchial trauma is suspected.[53] If injury is discovered, treatment depends on the severity. Nonoperative management is appropriate for injuries less than 4 cm, with viable airway tissue and an absence of associated esophageal damage or respiratory compromise.[54] For those injuries that do not meet nonoperative criteria, surgical intervention depends on location and extent of disruption. The proximal two-thirds of the tracheobronchial tree can be approached via a low collar incision, which can be extended through the manubrium for improved

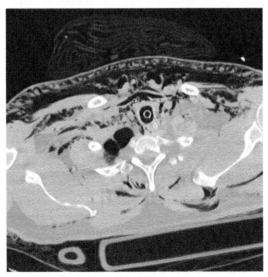

Fig. 4. CT chest of a trauma victim with evident subcutaneous emphysema and mediastinal air tracking superiorly into the anterior chest wall and neck.

distal access. The distal third of the trachea and the intramediastinal main stem bronchi, on the other hand, are more easily exposed by right posterolateral thoracotomy.[55] Once adequate exposure is obtained and nonviable tissue is debrided, simple lacerations can be repaired directly with interrupted absorbable sutures. Larger defects, however, may require pedicle flap closure from the pericardium, parietal pleura, intercostal muscles, or infrahyoid muscles. To further protect the newly repaired tracheobronchial tree, some surgeons use a guardian stitch, or stitch from the chin to the chest, to ensure neck flexion and, therefore, decreased tracheal tension for the first postoperative week.[2] Despite all efforts, complications after tracheobronchial surgery are not infrequent with stenosis and/or dehiscence occurring in 3% to 6% of cases.[56,57] Symptoms of these complications are often subtle, consisting of dyspnea, wheezing, and stridor, and are regularly not discovered until 2 to 4 weeks postoperatively. If symptoms necessitate urgent intervention, bronchoscopic dilation can relieve stenoses but definitive surgical reconstruction may be required in a more elective manner.[58]

Esophageal Trauma

Esophageal injury is rare, occurring in 2% of penetrating and well less than 1% of blunt traumas; however, it is associated with a mortality rate of 20% to 40%.[59] Management follows that of more common nontraumatic causes; however, location of injury is typically more proximal and diagnosis is often delayed. Symptoms can be subtle and often overlap with other cervical injuries. Signs of abscess and mediastinitis are more specific but often slow to present.[60] Similarly, initial CXR and CT scan may demonstrate subcutaneous emphysema or pneumomediastinum but are not sensitive modalities for diagnosing esophageal injury. The gold standard diagnostic modality is the complementary use of esophagram (fluoroscopic or CT) and esophagoscopy, each alone missing 15% of injuries but achieving near 100% sensitivity in combination. Traditionally, surgical intervention was recommended if the injury was diagnosed within 24 hours, whereas medical therapy was recommended for delayed diagnoses. This protocol is changing, however, and early intervention with source control and debridement is recommended.[2] Furthermore, primary repair should be attempted not based on timing but rather tissue viability. Pleural, pericardial, diaphragmatic, or muscle flap reinforcement can be used to aid in tissue protection as can endoscopically placed negative pressure therapy.[61] When the esophageal injury is truly too large to repair, resection and diverting esophagostomy may be required until definitive interposition or conduit creation can be performed. Endoscopically placed esophageal stent therapy is also emerging as a viable treatment modality. Stents have demonstrated 90% effectiveness with iatrogenic esophageal injuries; however, it is unclear if these data are applicable to traumatic disruptions.[62]

Diaphragmatic Injury

Diaphragmatic injury is among the most difficult diagnoses to make in a traumatic setting. Incidence is unclear but is estimated to be anywhere from 0.6% to 24%.[2] Diaphragmatic trauma can be direct from a rib or weapon but can also be due to rapid pressure changes in the abdomen and thorax. Occasionally, diagnosis is aided when bowel is discovered in the thorax on diagnostic imaging. However, the liver and spleen commonly prevent acute herniation of the hollow viscus. Because of this, diagnostic imaging is considered inaccurate, exemplified by sensitivities of CT scan of 78% and 50% with left and right diaphragmatic injuries, respectively.[63] Additionally, symptoms are often vague, relating to injuries of neighboring structures, such as the lungs, spleen, and liver. Often the diagnosis of diaphragmatic trauma is made intraoperatively when intervening for another cause. When an injury is discovered, primary repair can usually be accomplished, and can be performed either from an abdominal or a thoracic approach. If the defect is too large to close primarily, placement of mesh, or cadaveric or bovine graft, is appropriate.

SUMMARY

Thoracic injury is common in both high-energy and low-energy trauma and is associated with significant morbidity and mortality. As with the management of all traumas, thoracic trauma evaluation requires a systematic approach, first prioritizing airway, respiration, and circulation, followed by a focused secondary survey. Unlike other forms of trauma, chest injuries have the potential to progress rapidly and require prompt procedural intervention in the emergency room. Because of this urgency, physicians must have a high level of situational awareness and pay close attention to physical examination findings. Once the primary survey is complete and stable, the secondary survey is crucial in uncovering most thoracic injuries and guiding effective care. The specifics of this care have undergone evolution throughout the recent decades, but an overarching emphasis remains on patient stabilization before definitive surgical repair.

REFERENCES

1. Nathens AB, Meredith JW. National trauma data bank 2009: Annual Report. Chicago: American College of Surgeons; 2009.
2. Varghese TK Jr. Greenfield's surgery: scientific principles and practice. Chapter 22: Chest Trauma. 5th edition. Philadelphia: Lippincott Williams & Wilkins; 2011.
3. Martin RS, Meredith JW. Sabiston textbook of surgery: the biological basis of modern surgical practice. Chapter 18: Management of Acute Trauma. Saunders: Elsevier; 2012.
4. Rotondo MF. ATLS: advanced trauma life support, student course manual. 9th edition. Chicago: American College of Surgeons; 2012.
5. Gaillard F. Tension Pneumothorax. 2005-2016. Available at: https://radiopaedia. org/articles/tension-pneumothorax. Accessed October 23, 2017.
6. Graham JM, Beall AC, Mattox KL, et al. Systemic air embolism following penetrating trauma to the lung. Chest 1977;72:449.
7. Shoemaker WC, Carey JS, Yao ST, et al. Hemodynamic alterations in acute cardiac tamponade after penetrating injuries to the heart. J Thorac Cardiovasc Surg 1974;68:847.
8. Knott-Craig CJ, Dalton RP, Rossouw GJ, et al. Penetrating cardiac trauma: management strategy based on 129 surgical emergencies over 2 years. Ann Thorac Surg 1992;53:1006–9.
9. Mandavia DP, Hoffner RJ, Mahaney K, et al. Bedside echocardiography by emergency physicians. Ann Emerg Med 2001;38:377–82.
10. Beall AC Jr, Dietrich EB, Crawford HW, et al. Surgical management of cardiac injuries. Am J Surg 1996;112:686.
11. Cothren CC, Moore EE. Trauma, chapter: emergency department thoracotomy. 6th edition. New York: McGraw-Hill; 2008.
12. O'Connor JV, DuBose JJ, Scalea TM. Damage-control thoracic surgery: management and outcomes. J Trauma Acute Care Surg 2014;77(5):660–5.
13. Governatori NJ, Saul T, Siadecki SD, et al. Ultrasound in the evaluation of penetrating thoraco-abdominal trauma: a review of the literature. Med Ultrason 2015; 17(4):528–34.

14. Di Bartolomeo S, Sanson G, Nardi G, et al. A population-based study of pneumo-thorax in severely traumatized patients. J Trauma 2001;51:677.

15. Neff M, Monk JJ, Peters K, et al. Detection of occult pneumothoraces on abdom-inal computed tomographic scans in trauma patients. J Trauma 2000;49:281.

16. Garramone RJ, Jacob L, Sahdev P. An objective method to measure and manage occult pneumothorax. Surg Gynecol Obstet 1991;173:257.

17. Enderson BL, Abdalla R, Frame SB, et al. Tube thoracostomy for occult pneumo-thorax: a prospective randomized study of its use. J Trauma 1993;35:726.

18. Brasel K, Satfford R, Weigelt J, et al. Treatment of occult pneumothorax from blunt trauma. J Trauma 1999;46:987.

19. Pasquier M, Hugli O, Carron PN. Videos in clinical medicine. Needle aspiration of primary spontaneous pneumothorax. N Engl J Med 2013;368(19):e24.

20. England G, Hill R, Timberlake G, et al. Resolution of experimental pneumothorax in rabbits by graded oxygen therapy. J Trauma 1998;45:333.

21. Velmahos GC, Demetriades D, Chan L, et al. Predicting the need for thoraco-scopic evacuation of residual traumatic hemothorax: chest radiograph is insuffi-cient. J Trauma 1999;46:65–70.

22. Eddy AC, Luna GK, Copass M. Empyema thoracis in patients undergoing emer-gent closed tube thoracostomy for thoracic trauma. Am J Surg 1989;157:494–7.

23. Meyer DM, Jessen ME, Wait MA, et al. Early evacuation of traumatic retained he-mothoraces using thoracoscopy: a prospective, randomized trial. Ann Thorac Surg 1997;64:1396–400.

24. Brasel K, Guse C, Layde P, et al. Rib fractures: relationship with pneumonia and mortality. Crit Care Med 2006;34:1642–6.

25. Tanaka H, Yukioka T, Yamaguti Y, et al. Surgical stabilization of internal pneumatic stabilization? A prospective randomized study of management of severe flail chest patients. J Trauma 2002;52:727–32.

26. Granetzny A, Abd El-Aal M, Emam E, et al. Surgical versus conservative treat-ment of flail chest: evaluation of the pulmonary status. Interact Cardiovasc Thorac Surg 2005;4:583–7.

27. Caragounis EC, Fagevik Olsen M, Pazooki D, et al. Surgical treatment of multiple rib fractures and flail chest in trauma: a one-year follow-up study. World J Emerg Surg 2016;11:27.

28. Cohn SM. Pulmonary contusion: review of the clinical entity. J Trauma 1997;42: 973–9.

29. Tranbaugh RF, Elings VB, Christensen J, et al. Determinants of pulmonary inter-stitial fluid accumulation after trauma. J Trauma 1982;22:820–6.

30. Schultz J, Trunkey D. Blunt cardiac injury. Crit Care Clin 2004;20(1):57–70.

31. Leavitt BJ, Meyer J, Morton J, et al. Survival following nonpenetrating traumatic rupture of cardiac chambers. Ann Thorac Surg 1987;44(5):532–5.

32. Turk E, Tsokos M. Blunt cardiac trauma caused by fatal falls from height: an autopsy-based assessment of injury pattern. J Trauma 2004;57(2):301–4.

33. von Garrel T, Ince A, Junge A, et al. The sternal fracture: radiographic analysis of 200 fractures with special reference to concomitant injuries. J Trauma 2004;57(4): 837–44.

34. Harris DG, Rabin J, Starnes BW, et al. Evolution of lesion-specific management of blunt thoracic aortic injury. J Vasc Surg 2016;64(2):500–5.

35. Brinster DR. Endovascular repair of blunt thoracic aortic injuries. Semin Thorac Cardiovasc Surg 2009;21:393–8.

36. Feczko J, Lynch L, Pless J, et al. An autopsy case review of 142 nonpenetrating (blunt) injuries of the aorta. J Trauma 1992;33(6):846–9.

37. Fabian TC, Davis K, Gavant M, et al. Prospective study of blunt aortic injury: helical CT is diagnostic and antihypertensive therapy reduces rupture. Ann Surg 1998;227(5):666–77.

38. Maggisano R, Nathens A, Alexandrova N, et al. Traumatic rupture of the thoracic aorta: should one always operate immediately? Ann Vasc Surg 1995;9(1):44–52.

39. Neschis DG, Scalea TM, Flinn WR, et al. Blunt aortic injury. N Engl J Med 2008; 359(16):1708–16.

40. Fabian TC, Richardson JD, Croce MA, et al. Prospective study of blunt aortic injury: multicenter trial of the American Association for the Surgery of Trauma. J Trauma 1997;42:374–80.

41. Demetriades D, Velmahos G, Scalea T, et al. Blunt traumatic thoracic aortic injuries: early or delayed repair-results of an American Association of the Surgery of Trauma prospective study. J Trauma 2009;66(4):967–73.

42. Harris DG, Rabin J, Kufer JA, et al. A new aortic injury score predicts early rupture more accurately than clinical assessment. J Vasc Surg 2015;61:532–3.

43. de Mestral C, Dueck A, Sharma SS, et al. Evolution of the incidence, management, and mortality of blunt thoracic aortic injury: a population-based analysis. J Am Coll Surg 2013;16(6):1110–5.

44. Fox N, Schwartz D, Salazar JH, et al. Eastern association for the surgery of trauma guidelines: blunt aortic injury, evaluation and management of. J Trauma 2015;78(1):136–46.

45. Doss M, Wood J, Balzer J, et al. Emergency endovascular interventions for acute thoracic aortic rupture: four-year follow-up. J Thorac Cardiovasc Surg 2005; 129(3):645–51.

46. Peterson BG, Eskandari MK, Gleason TG, et al. Utility of left subclavian artery revascularization in association with endoluminal repair of acute and chronic thoracic aortic pathology. J Vasc Surg 2006;43:433–9.

47. Cooper DG, Walsh SR, Sadat U, et al. Neurological complications after left subclavian artery coverage during thoracic endovascular aortic repair. J Vasc Surg 2009;49:1594–601.

48. Joseph B, Ibraheem K, Haider AA, et al. Identifying potential utility of REBOA: an autopsy study. J Trauma Acute Care Surg 2016;81(5):S128–32.

49. Shergill AK, Maraj T, Barszczyk M, et al. Identification of cardiac and aortic injuries in trauma with multi-detector computed tomography. J Clin Imaging Sci 2015;5:48.

50. Velly JF, Martigne C, Moreau JM, et al. Post traumatic tracheobronchial lesions. Eur J Cardiothorac Surg 1991;5:352–5.

51. Kiser AC, O'Brien SM, Detterbeck FC. Blunt tracheobronchial injuries: treatment and outcomes. Ann Thorac Surg 2001;71:2059–65.

52. Reece GP, Shatney CH. Blunt injuries of the cervical trachea: review of 51 patients. South Med J 1988;81(12):1542–8.

53. Altinok T, Can A. Management of tracheobronchial injuries. Eur J Med 2014;46(3): 209–15.

54. Gomez-Caro A, Ausin P, Moradiellos FJ, et al. Role of conservative medical management of tracheobronchial injuries. J Trauma 2006;61(6):1426–34.

55. Wood D. Thoracic trauma and critical care. Chapter: tracheobronchial trauma. Boston: Kluwer Academic Publishers; 2002.

56. Grillo HC, Zannini P, Michelassi F. Complications of tracheal reconstruction. Incidence, treatment, and prevention. J Thorac Cardiovasc Surg 1986;91(3):322–8.

57. Jones WS, Mavroudis C, Richardson JD, et al. Management of tracheobronchial disruption resulting from blunt trauma. Surgery 1984;95:319–23.

58. Stephens KEJ, Wood DE. Bronchoscopic management of central airway obstruction. J Thorac Cardiovasc Surg 2000;119:473-7.
59. Asensio JA, Chahwan S, Forno W, et al. Penetrating esophageal injuries: multicenter study of the American Association for the Surgery of Trauma. J Trauma 2001;50:289-96.
60. Gill S, Dierking J, Nguyen K, et al. Seatbelt injury causing perforation of the cervical esophagus: a case report and review of the literature. Am Surg 2004;70(1): 32-4.
61. Leeds SG, Burdick JS, Fleshman JW. Endoluminal vacuum therapy for esophageal and upper intestinal anastomotic leaks. JAMA Surg 2016;151(6):573-4.
62. Verlaan T, Voermans RP, van Berge Henegouwen MI, et al. Endoscopic closure of acute perforations of the GI tract: a systematic review of the literature. Gastrointest Endosc 2015;82(4):618-28.
63. Kileen K, Mirvis S, Shanmuganathan K. Helical CT of diaphragmatic rupture caused by blunt trauma. AJR Am J Roentgenol 1999;173(6):1611-6.

Team-Based Care
The Changing Face of Cardiothoracic Surgery

Todd C. Crawford, MD, John V. Conte, MD, Juan A. Sanchez, MD*

KEYWORDS

- Teamwork • Collaborative care • Clinical microsystems • Team-based
- Patient care • Patient safety • Multidisciplinary approaches

KEY POINTS

- Effective collaboration and teamwork are essential to providing high-quality care and critical to avoiding adverse events and errors.
- An interdisciplinary environment where every member of the team is valued and can significantly contribute toward common goals and objectives is essential to achieving superior results.
- Well-designed multidisciplinary teams, structured conferences and rounds, and strong nontechnical skills by team leaders significantly reduce the rate of adverse events, lower lengths of stay, and reduce costs.

INTRODUCTION

An increasing awareness is emerging of the beneficial impact of a multidisciplinary, team-based approach to the management of several high-risk, complex clinical conditions as demonstrated by improved outcomes and greater patient, family, and staff satisfaction.[1–5] As patient acuity and complexity increase, health care providers will frequently need to draw on the expertise of various types of health care professionals to optimize patient care. This disposition is especially relevant in cardiothoracic surgery, whereby older and sicker patients are increasingly being referred for surgery. Here, the multidisciplinary team must function cohesively, aligning provider initiatives with patient goals in order to achieve the best outcomes. By drawing on a variety of methods and perspectives from different disciplines, these multidisciplinary teams create a synergized environment that improves outcomes by creating something greater than the sum of its parts.

Division of Cardiac Surgery, Johns Hopkins University School of Medicine, 1800 Orleans Street, Zayed 7107, Baltimore, MD 21287, USA
* Corresponding author.
E-mail address: jsanch25@jhmi.edu

Surg Clin N Am 97 (2017) 801–810
http://dx.doi.org/10.1016/j.suc.2017.03.003
0039-6109/17/© 2017 Elsevier Inc. All rights reserved.

TEAM-BASED SURGICAL CARE

Given the technical complexity and high-risk nature of cardiothoracic surgical care, hospital-based teams can demonstrate their value on several dimensions. Such an approach facilitates better decision making, improved diagnostic accuracy, and adherence to clinical practice guidelines, thereby reducing variation in clinical practice and avoiding errors. Well-structured clinical teams ensure the appropriateness and timeliness of treatment plans and the open discussion of risks in a patient-centered environment, where each member, including the patient, is able to contribute independently to the diagnostic and treatment decisions about the patient.[6]

Multidisciplinary care has been part of established clinical practice in many specialties such as transplantation and oncology. An early example of interdisciplinary collaboration in medicine was the institution of the "tumor board," where, based on the final pathologic diagnosis, medical and surgical specialists were able to develop a comprehensive treatment plan. Today, more than 80% of all patients with cancer are managed in the context of organ-specific multidisciplinary cancer conferences, ensuring an evidence-based approach.[7] Modern multidisciplinary teams are able to evaluate and discuss all available treatment strategies and the associated risks of each throughout the entire course of care.

The degree of integration and coordination of clinical teams has been highly variable and highly dependent on the individuals involved and the organizations in which they function. With the evolution of hybrid therapies for cardiovascular diseases and the emphasis on quality improvement, patient safety, and shared governance models, the practice of cardiothoracic surgery has evolved quite dramatically to a paragon of interprofessional and multidisciplinary collaboration and coordination. This shift has been enhanced by emerging evidence supporting improved outcomes, reduced costs, and a positive impact on the health care workforce. Health systems with a strong teamwork orientation, for example, simply exhibit better surgical outcomes following coronary artery bypass grafting (CABG).[8]

Like an orchestra, the coordination, communication, and teamwork performance of such teams can enhance the effectiveness and efficiency of care while protecting patients from harm and ensuring continuity across the entire spectrum of care. Leadership is crucial, and full commitment to placing the patient at the center is essential in their success. Teams are the antidote to the "silos" created by specialization and compartmentalization, which impair the ability to share philosophic approaches to treatment plans and are rife with communication failures and breakdowns. The shared accountability provided by these teams result in a cohesive service delivery model with high levels of clinical effectiveness, workforce satisfaction, and an enhanced patient experience. Hospital-based teams can be configured in a variety of ways but, at their core, consist of individuals across a variety of disciplines, professions, and functions committed to achieving the best possible outcome for the patient.

Cardiothoracic surgery lends itself to following a team-based approach. Preoperatively, cardiothoracic surgeons rely on physiologic and imaging data, such as pulmonary function tests and echocardiography, which are provided by subspecialists and other health professionals to guide treatment strategies. Primary care providers are instrumental in risk stratification and management of comorbidities before surgery. In all, a set of carefully coordinated steps requiring specific expertise and skill is required to restore the patient to health. During the perioperative phase, multidisciplinary approaches to extubation, blood management, and acute rehabilitation have been shown to be superior to the traditional fragmented and isolated process of patient care.[9–11]

Intraoperatively, nurses, technicians, perfusionists, anesthesiologists, and surgeons must function cohesively to ensure that every component of the operation runs smoothly and safely. Sax[12] has proposed 9 interventions to facilitate effective communication and align the goals of all team members in the operating room (**Box 1**). The amalgamation of knowledge and skill among those comprising the operative team should be harnessed to achieve far better results than individuals making isolated decisions. However, to accomplish this, individuals must be willing and able to anticipate and identify opportunities for adding value in an environment of shared accountability, team commitment, and mutual respect.[13]

THE MODERN ERA OF CARDIAC SURGERY

Among the many contemporary complex cardiothoracic operations, transcatheter aortic valve replacement (TAVR) requires precise coordination and collaboration among many professional disciplines. The TAVR team, composed of dedicated nurses, imaging specialists, anesthesiologists, interventional cardiologists, and cardiac surgeons, executes complex percutaneous valve deployments under fluoroscopic guidance, often with the patient awake and spontaneously breathing.[14] Before the intervention, potential candidates are intensely scrutinized to delineate anatomic and physiologic constraints and determine the optimal course of therapy. TAVR is the culmination of weeks, even months, of preoperative optimization of patient comorbidities and careful technical planning. The impact of such teams on mortality after TAVR has been substantial.[15,16] The incredible success of this intervention in a population of patients who otherwise would not be suitable candidates for corrective surgery is a reflection of the close collaboration across medical disciplines, combining knowledge, skill, and determination to improve the quality of life of patients.[17]

Although an efficient and safe operation sets the stage for an uncomplicated recovery, the cardiothoracic intensive care unit (ICU) plays an important role in the path to convalescence.[18] Here, the multidisciplinary ICU team plays an integral role in

---

Box 1
Strategies for effective teamwork and communication in the operating room

- Establish clear expectations for team member behaviors and orient new employees to institutional goals and culture

- Align incentives with desired behaviors

- Create multidisciplinary process improvement teams coupled with expanded morbidity and mortality conference

- Solicit active feedback to suggestions for change

- Establish friendly competition among teams

- Rapidly and consistently address disruptive behavior

- Hire for attitude; train for aptitude

- Identify informal leaders, even if they are not in leadership positions

- Assure that there is institutional support for team building initiatives with prompt responses to identified issues

Adapted from Sax HC. Building high-performance teams in the operating room. Surg Clin North Am 2012;92(1):17–8; with permission.

optimizing patient and environmental factors, and nonsurgical health care providers are increasingly tasked with the day-to-day challenge of managing these complex patients. Team members can provide expert critical care and serve as a liaison between surgeon, patients, and families as well as manage mechanical ventilation and lung protection, nutritional repletion, volume optimization, and glucose management. In consultation with the surgeon, the team is able to set expectations that will help to quickly identify deviations from expected recovery pathways and to intervene when deviations are noted.

The surge in mechanical-circulatory support modalities for patients suffering from heart failure has expanded the role of perfusionists and other members of the operating room team, requiring their presence outside of the operating room. The intricacies of these complex modalities, including ventricular-assist devices, artificial hearts, and extracorporeal membrane oxygenation, require an enormous amount of effort on the part of many health professionals that care for these patients.

Efforts to improve risk assessment and preoperative decision making for patients undergoing CABG continue to be refined. The success of such efforts is reflected in the improvement seen year after year in the reported outcome measures for this procedure. Guidelines developed jointly by multiple professional organizations such as the American Heart Association, the American College of Cardiology, the Society of Thoracic Surgeons and others have strongly endorse the "heart team" approach to complex revascularization decisions, designating this component of care a class I recommendation, particularly in patients with unprotected left main or complex coronary artery disease and those with coexisting carotid artery stenosis.[19]

The multidisciplinary heart team approach seeks to accomplish 3 main goals during the process of clinical decision making: (1) to delineate the coronary anatomy and review the clinical status of the patient; (2) to discuss safety, feasibility, and technical challenges unique to both percutaneous coronary intervention (PCI) and CABG; and (3) to present both revascularization options to the patient and discuss the relevant risks and benefits of each procedure. Evidence supporting the team approach comes from various trials where survival in patients with complex coronary artery disease referred for either PCI or CABG was shown to be superior in comparison to patients randomly assigned to undergo either PCI or CABG.[20,21] One approach to the patient with severe ischemic heart disease and complex anatomy involves completing a diagnostic coronary angiography but delaying any interventions until all revascularization options have been considered and discussed with the patient.

MULTIDISCIPLINARY CONFERENCES AND ROUNDS

Frequent formal meetings to discuss patients prospectively in anticipation of an operation can add considerable value to the treatment plan, particularly when such conferences include a variety of perspectives, including nursing care, physical therapy, and other health professions. The ability of each member to actively participate in the discussion is particularly important given the cognitive biases and unique perspectives each treating specialty and profession bring to the table. Moreover, as a result of power gradients and other behaviors that stifle opinions and dissuade the challenging of assumptions, active participation by all team members should be strongly encouraged.

Multidisciplinary conferences bring together experts from different disciplines with the aim of protecting patients by considering all relevant information and seeking the broadest possible views and opinions before making a decision as to whether to proceed with surgery and what particular approach is best. For example, in discussing patients under consideration for coronary revascularization and transcatheter valve procedures, perspectives from interventional cardiology, cardiac surgery, nursing, and others are essential. These discussions must include a comprehensive risk assessment of the patient and a robust discussion as to the appropriateness of the intended procedure. Guidelines and several risk stratification protocols are available to support the discussion. In addition, case conferences should make liberal use of prospective risk-scoring algorithms, such as the Society of Thoracic Surgery's National Cardiac Database.[22]

In cancer care, obligatory discussion of each patient at a multidisciplinary conference aims to ensure appropriateness and timely treatment in order to achieve the best possible outcome. In this fashion, a clear and agreed-upon management plan can be provided to the patient, thus streamlining and facilitating the coordination among all health care providers. Multidisciplinary conferences also permit the assessment of comorbidities in order to explore opportunities to mitigate risks and prepare the patient psychologically and physiologically ("prehabilitation") along with a consensus as to whether it would be appropriate to operate on certain patients or not.

Multidisciplinary rounding builds on the benefits of case conferences and has been shown to improve clinical outcomes and patient satisfaction. The Concord Collaborative Model, for example, has been shown to reduce surgical mortality following cardiac surgery.[23] This model uses a team-based, collaborative rounds process along with a structured communications protocol, based on human factors science, in conducting daily rounds at each patient's bedside. The entire care team agrees to meet at the same time each day to share information and develop a plan of care for each patient, with patient and family members present and actively involved. Following implementation of collaborative rounds, mortality in cardiac surgery patients was seen to decline significantly from expected rates, and patient satisfaction increased. A quality of work life survey indicated that members of the health care team expressed greater job satisfaction.

A timely, well-coordinated discharge process in which the expectations for how the patient will continue to receive health care as an outpatient is essential to improving outcomes and preventing preventable readmissions, avoiding medication errors, and ensuring adequate follow-up. A multidisciplinary approach to the discharge process involves early and thorough medication reconciliation with patient education about new medications and their side effects. Multidisciplinary discharge rounds and a well-coordinated, timely process facilitate "early in the day" discharge and shorten the length of hospital stays while improving patient flow.[24,25]

NONTECHNICAL SKILLS

The traditional focus on developing excellent technical skills by surgeons does not appear to be sufficient in the modern era of surgical practice. Nontechnical skills, such as communication and teamwork, along with evidence-based practice, an emphasis on lifelong learning, the monitoring of one's own outcomes, and an organizational framework that supports high-performing teams, are essential.[26] These critical cognitive and interpersonal skills complement a surgeon's technical proficiency. As such, surgeons must develop these skills so as to optimize team performance and maximize patient safety in the operating room.

Multidisciplinary teams make fewer mistakes than individuals particularly in environments in which psychological safety of all team members for speaking up is valued. Edmondson[27] studied teams adopting Port Access minimally invasive cardiac operations and found that leadership and team dynamics were more important than factors such as the skill and experience of the team. The degree to which members felt safe in raising issues depended on the leadership style of the attending surgeon. Adoption of new technology occurred faster and more effectively when the team leader exhibited high levels of emotional intelligence, allowing for better communication and coordination. In contrast, surgical teams in which team members were reluctant to transmit information as result of rigid hierarchical team behaviors experienced inferior scores on measures of team performance and patient outcomes.

The perceptions of surgeons regarding their degree of communication and teamwork may not always be in alignment with those of their team. For example, Attitude Surveys demonstrate discrepancies between attending surgeons and other team members in various dimensions of teamwork and leadership.[28] Surgeons tend to rate the quality of their interactions with others much more positively than what others actually see.[29] These differences indicate that considerable opportunities exist to improve teamwork among members of surgical teams.

The increasing specialization of health care requires an approach to patient care that values the input of many different types of professionals. Creating opportunities to discuss and learn from each other should be a fundamental value of clinical teams regardless of specialty, discipline, or level of training in order to work in concert to provide the best possible care for each patient. High levels of emotional intelligence, situational awareness, and communication skills are essential to lead clinical teams effectively. The impact of these characteristics is well documented in many other industries in which safety and reliable results are critical. In health care, deficiencies in these "nontechnical" skills have been associated with an increase in adverse events.[30]

The impact that failures in teamwork have on adverse events and medical errors has been highlighted in several observational and retrospective studies.[31] Communication and teamwork failures are frequently cited as the most important factors contributing to adverse events. However, teamwork is not solely a consequence of colocating individuals with the expectation that the value is added spontaneously. Rather, it is dependent on structure, composition, and leadership of the team such that coordination, communication, and cooperation are emphasized, and hierarchies are downplayed while focusing on common goals. These goals are then sustained by a commitment to a shared set of knowledge, skills, and attitudes.

The intergroup dynamics of teams play an important impact on decision making and improved outcomes. An element of psychological safety wherein all team members feel safe to voice concerns and offer opinions to improve care is strongly desirable. Team discussion tends to be dominated by certain individuals who may forcefully put their views across in an environment where all team members may not be considered equal in terms of the weight of their input and decision making. There is evidence, for example, suggesting that nurses have limited participation in multidisciplinary conferences and clinical teams.[32] This gap may reflect longstanding hierarchies, stereotypes, and perceptions favoring certain specialties and diminishing the value of others in decision making. In a patient-centered model of health care, all contributions are valuable and create synergies that complement the work of all others.

OTHER MODELS OF TEAM-BASED CARE

Several models of clinical care delivery have emerged as organizations have struggled to design operational units that can take full advantage of the collaborative nature of team-based care. The Clinical Microsystem is a model design consisting of a group of people who provide care to a defined set of patients and for a particular purpose.[13] In this concept, the team has both clinical and business aims with tightly coupled processes in an environment in which information is broadly shared in real time. Team members within microsystems are versatile and share ownership jointly in all processes and outcomes. Members of high-performing clinical microsystems have strong teamwork and communication skills. The concept emphasizes robust information tracking, collection, and sharing as well as timely and effective feedback. Clinical, operational, and financial outcomes are measured frequently with a view toward continuous improvement and system-based thinking. Performance improvement measures are focused directly on patient outcomes by identifying processes that enhance or impair the efficiency and effectiveness of the team. Team meetings, multidisciplinary conferences, and collaborative thinking are the drivers of systems improvement in an environment of mutual respect and understanding of each individual's roles.

The Perioperative Surgical Home approach proposes a single team-care model, nested within primary care and designed to optimize patients for surgery in order to improve outcomes and reduce costs.[33] In this model, a team leader coordinates a patient's care using a greater emphasis on shared decision making with the patient a more active member of the team. It allows for better standardization of patient care plans, reduction of practice variation, improved preoperative risk assessment, and "prehabilitation" of the patient to optimize the readiness for surgery.

TEAM-BASED CARE AND THE PATIENT EXPERIENCE

The introduction of multidisciplinary teams appears to have a positive impact on the patient's perception of the quality of care, particularly when patients are encouraged to participate in their care using in a shared decision-making approach.[34] Unfortunately, treatment recommendations by some multidisciplinary teams do not take into account the patients' preferences nor the wider context of psychological and social issues. In the United Kingdom, the National Health System has emphasized its commitment to patient-centered care in its pledge: "no decision about me without me," recognizing this approach as integral to delivering high-quality health services.[35] Optimal decisions are reached when teams incorporate patient-centered, nonclinical information to their decision making, thereby improving not only clinical results but also the patient's experience of the quality of care they receive.[36,37]

SUMMARY

Delivering the best surgical care for patients with cardiac and thoracic diseases is a "team sport." Multidisciplinary teams add value by making better decisions, making more accurate diagnoses, and ensuring appropriate care, particularly in the high-risk patient. In addition, high-performing teams minimize risks and prevent adverse events from reaching the patient, improve patient, family, and staff satisfaction, and reduce costs. All health care professionals and administrators involved in the care of cardiothoracic surgical patients should be cognizant of these benefits and promote and support the establishment and maintenance of these well-designed efforts.

Accumulating evidence for the benefits of multidisciplinary teams is supported by a strong consensus that effective team performance is highly dependent on specific group dynamics and characteristics in order to achieve improved clinical decision making, better coordination, and improved effectiveness of patient care. Best-practice, contemporary cardiothoracic surgical care involves high-functioning multidisciplinary teams, which exemplify the characteristics described in earlier discussion.

REFERENCES

1. Dutton RP, Cooper C, Jones A, et al. Daily multidisciplinary rounds shorten length of stay for trauma patients. J Trauma 2003;55(5):913–9.

2. Leape LL, Cullen DJ, Clapp MD, et al. Pharmacist participation on physician rounds and adverse drug events in the intensive care unit. JAMA 1999;282(3):267–70.

3. O'Mahony S, Mazur E, Charney P, et al. Use of multidisciplinary rounds to simultaneously improve quality outcomes, enhance resident education, and shorten length of stay. J Gen Intern Med 2007;22(8):1073–9.

4. Rosen P, Stenger E, Bochkoris M, et al. Family-centered multidisciplinary rounds enhance the team approach in pediatrics. Pediatrics 2009;123(4):e603–8.

5. Wahr JA, Prager RL, Abernathy JH, et al. Patient safety in the cardiac operating room: human factors and teamwork: a scientific statement from the American Heart Association. Circulation 2013;128:1139–69.

6. Hong NJ, Wright FC, Gagliardi AR, et al. Examining the potential relationship between multidisciplinary cancer care and patient survival: an international literature review. J Surg Oncol 2010;102(2):125–34 [review].

7. Griffith C, Turner J. United Kingdom National Health Service, cancer services collaborative 'improvement partnership', redesign of cancer services: a national approach. Eur J Surg Oncol 2004;30(Suppl 1):1–86.

8. Hollingsworth JM, Funk RJ, Garrison SA, et al. Association between physician teamwork and health system outcomes after coronary artery bypass grafting. Circ Cardiovasc Qual Outcomes 2016;9:641–8.

9. Cove ME, Ying C, Taculod JM, et al. Multidisciplinary extubation protocol in cardiac surgical patients reduces ventilation time and length of stay in the intensive care unit. Ann Thorac Surg 2016;102(1):28–34.

10. Ad N, Holmes SD, Patel J, et al. The impact of a multidisciplinary blood conservation protocol on patient outcomes and cost after cardiac surgery. J Thorac Cardiovasc Surg 2017;153(3):597–605.e1.

11. Raz DJ, Sun V, Kim JY, et al. Long-term effect of an interdisciplinary supportive care intervention for lung cancer survivors after surgical procedures. Ann Thorac Surg 2016;101(2):495–502.

12. Sax HC. Building high-performance teams in the operating room. Surg Clin North Am 2012;92(1):15–9.

13. Sanchez JA, Barach PR. High reliability organizations and surgical microsystems: re-engineering surgical care. Surg Clin North Am 2012;92(1):1–14.

14. Dworakowski R, MacCarthy PA, Monaghan M, et al. Transcatheter aortic valve implantation for severe aortic stenosis-a new paradigm for multidisciplinary intervention: a prospective cohort study. Am Heart J 2010;160(2):237–43.

15. Martinez EA, Shore A, Colantuoni E, et al. Cardiac surgery errors: results from the UK national reporting and learning system. Int J Qual Health Care 2011;23:151–8.

16. Hong SJ, Hong MK, Ko YG, et al. Multidisciplinary team approach for identifying potential candidate for transcatheter aortic valve implantation. Yonsei Med J 2014;55(5):1246–52.

17. Leon MB, Smith CR, Mack M, et al, PARTNER Trial Investigators. Transcatheter aortic-valve implantation for aortic stenosis in patients who cannot undergo surgery. N Engl J Med 2010;363(17):1597–607.

18. Katz NM. The emerging specialty of cardiothoracic surgical critical care: the leadership role of cardiothoracic surgeons on the multidisciplinary team. J Thorac Cardiovasc Surg 2007;134(5):1109–11.

19. Hillis LD, Smith PK, Anderson JL, et al, American College of Cardiology Foundation, American Heart Association Task Force on Practice Guidelines, American Association for Thoracic Surgery, Society of Cardiovascular Anesthesiologists, Society of Thoracic Surgeons. 2011 ACCF/AHA Guideline for Coronary Artery Bypass Graft Surgery. A report of the American College of Cardiology Foundation/American Heart Association Task Force on Practice Guidelines. Developed in collaboration with the American Association for Thoracic Surgery, Society of Cardiovascular Anesthesiologists, and Society of Thoracic Surgeons. J Am Coll Cardiol 2011;58(24):e123–210.

20. Feit F, Brooks MM, Sopko G, et al. Long-term clinical outcome in the Bypass Angioplasty Revascularization Investigation Registry: comparison with the randomized trial. BARI Investigators. Circulation 2000;101(24):2795–802.

21. King SB 3rd, Barnhart HX, Kosinski AS, et al. Angioplasty or surgery for multivessel coronary artery disease: comparison of eligible registry and randomized patients in the EAST trial and influence of treatment selection on outcomes. Emory Angioplasty versus Surgery Trial Investigators. Am J Cardiol 1997;79(11):1453–9.

22. Grover FL, Shahian DM, Clark RE, et al. The STS national database. Ann Thorac Surg 2014;97:S48–54.

23. Uhlig PN, Brown J, Nason AK, et al. Eisenberg Patient Safety Awards—system innovation: Concord Hospital. Jt Comm J Qual Improv 2002;28(12):666–72.

24. Durvasula R, Kayihan A, Del Bene S, et al. A multidisciplinary care pathway significantly increases the number of early morning discharges in a large academic medical center. Qual Manag Health Care 2015;24(1):45–51.

25. Chaiyachati KH, Sofair AN, Schwartz JI, et al. Discharge rounds: implementation of a targeted intervention for improving patient throughput on an inpatient medical teaching service. South Med J 2016;109(5):313–7.

26. Fann JI, Moffatt-Bruce SD, DiMaio JM, et al. Human factors and human nature in cardiothoracic surgery. Ann Thorac Surg 2016;101(6):2059–66.

27. Edmondson AC. Learning from failure in health care: frequent opportunities, pervasive barriers. Qual Saf Health Care 2004;13:ii3–9.

28. Makary MA, Sexton JB, Freischlag JA, et al. Operating room teamwork among physicians and nurses: teamwork in the eye of the beholder. J Am Coll Surg 2006;202(5):746–52.

29. Yule S, Flin R, Paterson-Brown S, et al. Development of a rating system for surgeons' non-technical skills. Med Educ 2006;40(11):1098–104.

30. Flin R, Yule S, McKenzie L, et al. Attitudes to teamwork and safety in the operating theatre. Surgeon 2006;4(3):145–51.

31. Sanchez JA, Ferdinand FD, Fann JI. Patient safety science in cardiothoracic surgery: an overview. Ann Thorac Surg 2016;101(2):426–33.

32. Lamb B, Sevdalis N. How do nurses make decisions? Int J Nurs Stud 2010;48(3):281–4.

33. Vetter TR, Boudreaux AM, Jones KA, et al. The perioperative surgical home: how anaesthesiology can collaboratively achieve and leverage the triple aim in healthcare. Anesth Analg 2014;118:1131–6.

34. Taylor C, Munro AJ, Glynne-Jones R, et al. Multidisciplinary team working in cancer: what is the evidence? Br Med J 2010;340:c951.

35. Department of Health. Equity and excellence: liberating the NHS. London: Department of Health; 2010.

36. Lanceley A, Savage J, Menon U, et al. Influences on multidisciplinary team decision-making. Int J Gynecol Cancer 2008;18(2):215–22.

37. Lamb BW, Brown KF, Nagpal K, et al. Quality of care management decisions by multidisciplinary teams: a systematic review. Ann Surg Oncol 2011;18:2116–25.

Cardiothoracic Critical Care

Kevin W. Lobdell, MD[a],*, Douglas W. Haden, MD[b], Kshitij P. Mistry, MD[c]

KEYWORDS

- Critical care • Cardiothoracic surgery • Quality • Safety • Value

KEY POINTS

- High-value cardiothoracic critical care (CCC) is rapidly evolving to meet the demands of increased patient acuity and to incorporate advances in technology.
- The high-performing CCC system and culture should aim to learn quickly and continuously improve.
- CCC demands a proactive, interactive, precise, and expert team, as well as continuity.

CARDIOTHORACIC DISEASE AND THERAPY
Incidence and Prevalence

Acquired heart disease is the leading cause of death in the United States, with 611,106 deaths forecasted for 2016; it affects 11.5% of the population and is estimated to result in 3.7 million hospitalizations annually with an average stay of 4.6 days.[1] Approximately 152,000 coronary artery bypass (CAB) operations were recorded in the Society of Thoracic Surgeons-Adult Cardiac Database (STS-ACSD) in 2015, while approximately 600,000 cardiac surgical procedures were expected to be performed in 2016.[2] Congenital heart disease affects approximately 40,000 children annually in the United States, and 25% of those require surgery in their first year of life.[3]

8.5% of adults will have a diagnosis of cancer in their lifetime, and cancer was forecasted to claim 584,881 lives in 2016 (the second most common cause of death in the United States).[4] Furthermore, the American Cancer Society estimated 224,390 new cases of lung cancer in the United States for 2016 and 158,080 deaths (which accounts for approximately 25% of cancer deaths).[5,6] The American Cancer Society also forecasted 16,910 new cases and 15,690 deaths from esophageal cancer in the United States for 2016 (approximately 20% of patients survive 5 years or more after diagnosis, a four-fold improvement over the last 40 years).[7,8]

The authors have nothing to disclose.
[a] Sanger Heart and Vascular Institute, Carolinas HealthCare System, PO Box 32861, Charlotte, NC 28232, USA; [b] Carolinas HealthCare System, PO Box 32861, Charlotte, NC 28232, USA; [c] Cardiovascular Critical Care, Boston Children's Hospital, Boston, MA, USA
* Corrresponding author.
E-mail address: kevin.lobdell@carolinas.org

Surg Clin N Am 97 (2017) 811–834
http://dx.doi.org/10.1016/j.suc.2017.03.001
0039-6109/17/© 2017 Elsevier Inc. All rights reserved.

surgical.theclinics.com

Procedural Risk

CAB surgery, which accounts for 53% of acquired cardiac surgical procedures recorded in the STS-ACSD, has an average operative mortality of 2.2% and mortality and/or major morbidity in 12.3%. Major and minor complications occur in 37.5% of patients; median intensive care unit (ICU) length of stay (LOS) is 47.4 hours, with a mean of 70.9 hours. Total LOS is 8.0 days (median) and 9.3 days (mean), readmission to ICU 2.8% and 30-day readmission 10%.[9] More specifically, the average incidence of major morbidities and hospital acquired infection (HAI) includes stroke 1.3%, reoperation 3.5%, prolonged ventilation 8.2%, acute renal failure 2.1%, deep sternal wound infection 0.3%, pneumonia 2.5%, and septicemia 0.9%. Common process metrics include early extubation 49.4% (<6 hours with median initial ventilation 3.6 hours and mean 6.0 hours), reintubation 3.6%, and blood product transfusions 43%.[9] Logically, increased complexity of patient or associated procedures correlates with greater mortality, morbidity, and resource consumption. For example, left ventricular assist device implantation has been reported to have 13.2% postoperative mortality,[10] while repair of type A aortic dissection has ranged from 12% to 24%.[11]

The 2015, STS-CCSD report recorded 52,224 operations in the most recent 4-year period with an overall mortality of 3.7% (neonatal = 10.1%, infant = 3.0%, children = 0.9%, and adults = 1.7%), which increases to 16.8% for the most complex procedures (STAT Category 5).

The STS-GTSD relates a 1.3% mortality and 9.4% major morbidity for pulmonary lobectomy, 5.0% mortality and 16.0% major morbidity for pneumonectomy, and a 3.4% mortality and 33.1% major morbidity for esophagectomy.[12]

Procedure and Complication Costs

Cardiac and thoracic surgery are costly and contribute substantially to a hospital's income and profit margin.[13,14] CAB averages $73,420 in the United States,[15] while the total cost of lobectomy is estimated at $39,412,[16] and esophagectomy charges averaged $120,000 to 140,000.[17] Hospital costs for the congenital cardiac disease population are estimated at $1.9 billion.[3] Additionally, recent estimates suggest approximately 13.4% of hospital costs, 4.1% of national health expenditures, and 0.66% of the gross domestic product are attributable to critical care.[18]

The additive costs of complications are considerable, and recent estimates for CAB range from $62,773 for mediastinitis (240% greater costs than without this complication), $49,128 with renal failure, $40,704 with prolonged ventilation, $34,144 with postoperative stroke, $20,000 for reoperation for hemorrhage, to $2744 for atrial fibrillation.[19] The CAB average LOS of 7.4 days was also significantly impacted by complications (ranging from 37.8 days for mediastinitis to 9.6 days for isolated atrial fibrillation). HAIs are estimated to cost the United States $35 to 45 billion per year and are common in critical care. The clinical impact of HAIs is also enormous, since HAIs are associated with approximately 6% mortality and 17 extra days of hospitalization.[20] Improvement must include the integration of innovative tactics to mitigate the risk of HAI (eg, bioburden reduction through ultraviolet light and copper-impregnated composites).[21] Axiomatically, multiple investigations corroborate the strong correlation between poor quality and increased cost.[22,23]

HIGH-VALUE CARDIOTHORACIC CRITICAL CARE

High-value cardiothoracic critical care (CCC) must measure and manage the domains of quality (Q), safety (S), value (V), and the resources (R) applied to these efforts (V α [Q + S]/R). Global waste in health care is estimated to be approximately $4.3 trillion annually.[24] In the United States, health care consumes approximately 18% of the gross domestic product and 32% of health care expenditures are associated with hospitals.[25,26] Recently, in order to improve value and sustainability, the Center for Medicare and Medicaid Services (CMS) has proposed bundled payment models for CAB where the hospital would be accountable for the cost and quality of care during the inpatient stay and for 90 days after discharge.[27] This value-oriented payment scheme is significant, since the current reimbursement system may actually benefit hospitals with increased rate of complications. Patient-reported outcome measures are increasing and must be incorporated into the assessment of quality and value.

Quality and the High-Performance Organization

High-performance organizations (HPOs) are marked by common aspirational goals, alignment, adaptability, and accountability.[28,29] The HPO has an action bias and a strong focus on what it intends to achieve.

Safety and the High-Reliability Organization

High-reliability organizations (HROs) are characterized by their reluctance to simplify, a sensitivity to operations, a commitment to resilience, and their deference to expertise.[30,31] HROs have a firm focus on failure—and what they do not want to happen—which requires leadership commitment, a culture of safety, and effective utilization of performance improvement tools. Patient safety and the associated culture of safety are built on a foundation of trust,[32,33] transparency, and continuous improvement. The Joint Commission popularized "robust process improvement" (RPI), which is comprised of lean methodologies (which focus on elimination of waste), six-sigma (also focused on eliminating waste, but includes statistical methodology to reduce defects to nearly zero), and change management.[30]

CARDIOTHORACIC CRITICAL CARE STRUCTURE AND PROCESSES
Multidisciplinary Team Care

The focus factory approach can improve the core competencies and value proposition of a cardiovascular and thoracic service line.[34] CCC has been delivered successfully with many different models. The traditional model of cardiothoracic surgeon and/or cardiothoracic surgery residents leading CCC has been challenged by many factors, which include the limitation of resident work hours, complexity of care, and credentialing.[35–38] Currently, many high-performing cardiovascular efforts, including CCC, are multidisciplinary and include various combinations of surgeon, cardiologist, anesthesiologist, intensivist, advanced care practitioners (nurse practitioners and physician assistants), nurses, respiratory therapists, pharmacists, nutritionists, physical therapists, clinical care managers, among others.[39,40] These high-performance CCC teams must be proactive, interactive, precise, expert, and provide continuity.[41–43] Teaming is increasingly utilized in other industries and vital to the delivery of complex, high-value CCC.[44] Additionally, efforts such as TeamSTEPPS highlight the importance of effective team leadership and team training.[45,46]

Activity-based staffing has been studied for decades, and the concept of optimizing staffing for complexity is central to high-value CCC.[47,48] The authors utilize a complexity scoring methodology to quantify demands and match with resources (limiting their advanced care practitioner's (ACP's) workload to a total of 15 points) (**Table 1**).

Regularly scheduled multidisciplinary rounds, employed to engage patients and capitalize on the expertise of the health care team, may mitigate mortality risk for critically ill patients.[49–51] Organizational staffing of critical care units with closed management by

Table 1
Cardiothoracic critical care scoring

	Critical Care Complexity Scoring Worksheet			
Procedure	Simple	Complicated	Complex	Chaos
Points	1	2	3	4
Demands	Routine	Deviation from Routine	Marked Deviation from Routine	Extreme Deviation from Routine
Examples	CAB, Valve, CAB+Valve, OHT, LVAD, Lung	Temp MCS, Hemorrahge, Unstable, Tests & Travel	Initiation/ Termination MCS, Shock, Reop	—

Each patient is assigned a score (1, 2, 3, or 4) and the sum tallied. The sum is utilized to optimize matching of demand and staffing of CCC operations.

Abbreviations: CAB, coronary artery bypass surgery; CAB + Valve, coronary artery bypass surgery + valve replacement or repair; LVAD, left ventricular assist device; Lung, pulmonary resection; MCS, mechanical circulatory support; OHT, orthotopic heart transplant; Valve, valve replacement or repair.

dedicated critical care trained providers, as opposed to the open model of noncritical trained providers, has been shown to correlate with lower mortality, morbidity, and shorter LOS.[52] Nighttime intensivist staffing has not demonstrated improvement in ICU mortality in units with high-intensity daytime staffing.[53] Our patient-centered transformational redesign (PCTR) in CCC, utilizing telerounding and tele-ICU technology, mirrors that of others who have lowered mortality, morbidity, and reduced LOS.[54,55] Comprehensive, integrated innovation such as PCTR, where talent is leveraged with technology, creates value by matching demand and resources, eliminating unnecessary variation, bottlenecks, and waste, and affords the CCC team the opportunity to learn faster through more patient visits and pattern recognition.[56–58]

Human factors affecting safety and quality include adaptability, burnout, and resiliency.[59] CCC is a high-risk and high-stress endeavor, and sustainable teammate health must be a priority.

Communication Aids—Goal Sheets, Checklists, and Hand-Off Tools

Group interactions in high-risk environments, such as CCC, may be made more reliable through enhanced communication and should include vetted approaches such as read backs and Situation–Background–Assessment–Recommendation (SBAR).[60,61] Goal sheet use also positively correlates with improved communication of goals and result in shorter ICU LOS.[62] Checklists have been demonstrated to improve efficiency as well as reduce mortality and morbidity.[63–65] Similarly, hand-off tools have been utilized and shown to reduce complications and readmissions to surgical ICUs and hospitals.[66,67]

Institutional Learning and Continuous Improvement

CCC teams must share vision, goals, and mental models, and learn together.[68] In fact, learning and improving ICUs are fostered by a psychologically safe environment, evidence to support the improvement actions, and focusing on learning how (as opposed to learning what).[69]

Data-driven efforts to improve the quality, safety, and value of cardiothoracic surgical care are manifold. Mortality was reduced by 24% in the New England cardiovascular collaborative and by 20% in the Michigan surgical collaborative.[70,71] The authors' quality improvement program (QIP) demonstrated a 40% reduction in risk-adjusted mortality, improved morbidity, and process compliance, as well as improvement in leading key performance indicators such as early extubation and glycemic control.[72–75] The authors' efforts have been successfully replicated in additional facilities. Similarly, Culig and colleagues[76] started a new program and employed the Toyota Production System and found the risk-adjusted mortality was 61% less than expected, and the cost per case was also decreased by $3497 (**Fig 1**).

Critical care improvement efforts mirror the aforementioned successes in cardiac surgery QIPs.[77,78]

Avoiding complications and failure to rescue (FTR, which relates the rate of mortality after defined complications) are central to QIP efforts. Prager and colleagues[79] demonstrated that the FTR rate in cardiac surgery was significantly better in low mortality facilities for the majority of complications, but most significantly for cardiac arrest, dialysis, prolonged ventilation, and pneumonia. Novick and colleagues[80] also investigated cardiac surgery FTR and described mortality in 3.6% of patients, morbidity in 16.8%, and FTR in 19.8%. FTR in patients with acute renal failure was 48.4%, while septicemia was 42.6%. Recently, Edwards and colleagues[81] corroborated the findings in an isolated CAB population of approximately 60,400 patients, where FTR ranged from 12.1% with prolonged ventilation to 22.3% with isolated acute renal failure. Considerable variation in cost to rescue has been described without obvious outcome benefits from high-cost institutions.[82]

Risk Management and Quantified Health Care

Risk management efforts are central to high-value CCC. Risk should be quantified— through all phases of care in the periprocedural home—and modifiable risks mitigated with the aim of learning and continuously improving short- and long-term mortality, morbidity, ICU and total LOS, readmissions, cost per case, and repeat intervention.[83–88] Disruptive technologies, which include, but are not limited to wearable biosensors, biomarkers, genomics, proteomics, and artificial intelligence (AI), will be increasingly incorporated into periprocedural care to accelerate learning and improving

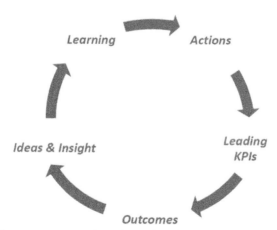

Fig. 1. Quality improvement program (QIP) flywheel. Actions link with leading keyperformance indicators (KPIs) which should be monitored in real-time. Leading KPIs link with outcomes. Ideas and insight emanate from data analysis and pattern recognition. Learning results in appropriate changes in action.

and move closer to a networked, decentralized, and personalized system of care, while simultaneously refining risk management.[89–92]

Cardiothoracic Critical Care—Clinical Systems Approach

After multiprofessional handoff from the operating room team, the cardiothoracic surgery patient is commonly managed with mechanical ventilation, inotropes, and/or vasoactive agents with varying intensity of monitoring of cardiopulmonary status, hemorrhage, urine output, and glycemic control. Initiatives to enhance recovery after surgery (ERAS) have been applied to cardiothoracic surgery with optimism, but ideal routines and results are to be determined.[93,94] Attention to modifiable risk factors and a proactive, action-oriented treatment of deviations from routine are central to high-value CCC, and a methodical, systems-based"approach is valuable for each patient and the CCC team.[95]

Neurologic System

Delirium is the most common form of neurologic dysfunction after cardiac surgery, occurring in 25% to 50% of systematically screened patients, and 92% are hypoactive.[96,97] The confusion assessment method ICU (CAM-ICU) is a simple tool for delirium assessment.[98] Risk factors for delirium after cardiac surgery include age, alcohol use, dementia, cerebrovascular disease, and the use of benzodiazepines.[96,99] In cardiac surgery patients, dexmedetomidine has been associated with less delirium, atrial fibrillation, and shorter LOS.[100,101] Current SCCM guidelines provide no recommendation for choice of sedative to prevent delirium and provide no recommendation for nonpharmacological or pharmacologic treatment for delirium, suggesting only that atypical antipsychotic medication may reduce the duration of delirium.[102]

The incidence of stroke after cardiac surgery is 1.3% for CAB (STS-NCSD) and as high as 3.9% for mitral valve plus CAB.[103–105] Considerable variation exists in stroke rates and recovery. Most strokes occur either intraoperatively or in the first 2 postoperative days.[106,107] Stroke has been associated with nine-fold increase in mortality and complications, longer LOS, and nearly doubling of costs.[19] Numerous risk factors have been identified including age, atrial fibrillation, prior stroke, and aortic atherosclerosis.[107–109]

The evaluation of neurologic deficits after cardiac surgery includes review of medical history and details of procedure and postoperative course, neurologic examination, imaging (most commonly CT, MRI, and electroencephalography [EEG]).[110] Non-focal neurologic deficits (25%–79%) are more common than focal deficits (as much as 6%). Nonenhanced CT in the first 7 postoperative days, commonly the first imaging study to be performed, has been shown to be positive in approximately 33% of patients with focal deficit, but rarely positive in patients with nonfocal deficits.[111] It is important to diagnose and appropriately treat intracerebral thromboemboli amenable to intervention and thrombolysis and intracranial hemorrhage (as well as void anticoagulants that could complicate recovery), while simultaneously avoiding excessive imaging (which is expensive, commonly requires patient transfer, and can lead to surveillance bias, which may result in more complications than the norm).

Pulmonary System

Pulmonary dysfunction is common following cardiac surgery and represents a combination of pulmonary, cardiac, and nervous system abnormalities. As aforementioned, the majority of cardiothoracic surgery patients will present to the ICU intubated after general anesthesia. While many patients, if not most, can be separated from mechanical ventilator support within hours, some will require a day or more of support.

Cardiopulmonary bypass, type and technique of operation, transfusion, anesthesia technique, and intraoperative hypothermia may all contribute to acute lung injury (ALI) and adult respiratory distress syndrome (ARDS) following cardiothoracic surgery. Aortic surgery, VAD explant-OHT, lung transplantation, and emergency procedures portend high risk for ALI and ARDS. Atelectasis, diaphragm dysfunction, and pain may also contribute to pulmonary dysfunction.[112–114]

Lung protective strategies such as low tidal volume ventilation may reduce development of postoperative ALI and ARDS, improve mortality for ARDS, and shorten LOS.[115–118] A retrospective analysis of 3434 patients recovering from cardiac surgery suggested that tidal volume greater than 10 cc/kg ideal body weight was an independent risk factor for organ failure, multiple organ failure, and prolonged stay in the ICU.[119] Also of note, restrictive fluid management in ARDS may shorten mechanical ventilation and ICU stay.[120]

Protocol-driven early extubation after cardiac surgery is a valuable practice associated with fewer pulmonary complications and use of hospital resources.[74,121–123] For those patients requiring continued ventilation, spontaneous awakening and breathing trials must be coupled with strategies to mitigate the risk of ventilator-associated pneumonia (eg, head of bed elevation or oral care).[124,125] Pulmonary complications account for approximately 55% of cardiac surgery ICU readmissions, and approximately 7% are again supported with mechanical ventilation.[126] In addition to physiotherapy and pulmonary hygiene, noninvasive ventilation has been used after cardiac surgery to prevent and treat postoperative respiratory failure. Noninvasive positive pressure ventilation (NIPPV) may be successfully employed for exacerbations of chronic obstructive lung disease and cardiogenic pulmonary edema. NIPPV has been used after cardiac surgery to both prevent and treat respiratory failure with reduced rates of reintubation, LOS, and mortality.[127–129]

High-flow nasal oxygen (HFNO) devices may provide physiologic and patient comfort advantages in comparison to NIPPV and are increasingly considered for patients with hypoxemic respiratory failure. Stéphan and colleagues[129] randomized 830 patients at high risk for respiratory failure after cardiothoracic surgery to warmed, humidified, HFNO versus NIPPV and HFNO was deemed non-inferior to NIPPV. Patients with obstructive sleep apnea were excluded, and no difference in mortality was observed. Carefully selected patients with hypoxemic respiratory failure may be successfully managed with HFNO.[130]

Risk assessment and mitigation for pulmonary complications begin preoperatively, as all patients undergoing nonemergent surgery should be encouraged to quit smoking.[131–133] Additionally, preoperative inspiratory muscle training and physical therapy appear to reduce postoperative pulmonary complications.[134–137] Patients with obstructive lung disease that is preoperatively exacerbated should receive treatment, and surgery should be delayed if feasible until they return to baseline. Postoperative deep breathing exercises or incentive spirometry after surgery may reduce pulmonary complications.[138–141] Treatment with continuous positive airway pressure may also reduce complications, particularly in patients currently unable to participate with deep breathing maneuvers.[142] Prolonged bed rest following thoracic and abdominal surgery is harmful, and early mobilization has been suggested as an integral aspect of ERAS programs.[143–145] Mobility training is commonly utilized and may reduce morbidity and cost.[146]

Cardiovascular System

Pulmonary artery catheter (PAC) use remains common in cardiac surgery, with 68% of respondents in a recent survey reporting PAC use in greater than 75% of cases.[147]

Hemodynamic data obtained from PACs may benefit cardiothoracic surgery patients with specific demands and risk profiles. Schwann and colleagues[148] suggested consideration for selective PAC placement in patients with undergoing CABG with low left ventricular ejection fraction (LVEF) (<30%), high society of thoracic surgeons (STS) score, intraortic balloon pump (IABP), congestive heart failure (CHF) (in particular with New York Heart Association [NYHA] Class IV symptoms), and those undergoing a reoperation. Other considerations include right ventricular (RV) failure, pulmonary hypertension, and those undergoing advanced heart failure surgery.[149,150] Prospective studies in well-defined populations may clarify optimal use. Common hemodynamic targets for PACs include central venous pressure (CVP) of 8 to 12 mm Hg, pulmonary wedge pressure (PCWP)/pulmonary artery diastolic pressure 10 to 14 mm Hg, confidence interval [CI] greater than 2.2 L/min/m^2, and an SvO_2 of 60% to 70%.

Noninvasive and minimally invasive hemodynamic monitoring, in particular cardiac output, are increasingly available. Various noninvasive cardiac output (CO) monitors exist employing technology that includes partial rebreathing of carbon dioxide, electrical bioimpedance, and photoplethysmography.[151–153] Proponents of this less invasive monitoring emphasize the potential to eliminate PAC-related complications.

The most commonly used minimally invasive devices employ a peripheral arterial catheter to estimate cardiac output as well as other dynamic variables such as pulse pressure and stroke volume variation. CO may be derived by pulse contour analysis alone or in conjunction with transpulmonary thermodilution or indicator dilution. Acceptable correlation of CO with PAC-derived values has been demonstrated in a variety of populations including cardiac surgery patients.[153]

Esophageal Doppler estimates CO from the velocity of descending aorta blood flow and also provides estimates of left ventricular, preload and contractility. Use of esophageal Doppler parameters has been suggested to decrease complications in select high-risk surgery populations.[151,153,154]

Transthoracic echocardiography may provide valuable information in the postoperative patient but continuous or serial examinations are impractical. Transesophageal echocardiography (TEE) is a standard intraoperative hemodynamic monitor frequently utilized to evaluate the unstable ICU patient. However, continuous monitoring has previously been impractical in the ICU until recently with the availability of miniature probes. Continuous miniature TEE has been proven feasible and safe in in the ICU. Intensive care providers can be trained to perform and interpret miniature TEE, allowing direct visualization of anatomic complications as well as biventricular function and superior vena cava filling. Relevant outcome studies are needed before widespread adoption of this promising new technology.[155,156]

The proliferation of devices allowing less invasive hemodynamic measurement parallels an increased focus on goal-directed therapy (GDT). GDT, originally popularized by Shoemaker, employs a series of actions in high-risk patients to achieve goals in an attempt to mitigate risk of untoward outcomes.[157–159] Meta-analyses of GDT in cardiac surgery patients consistently demonstrate reduced complication rates and length of stay.[160,161] Osawa and colleagues[162] reported on 126 patients randomized to cardiac output-driven algorithms utilizing intravenous fluids, inotropes, and packed red blood cell (PRBC) transfusion. CO was obtained via a lithium dilution device, and the primary outcome was a composite endpoint of 30-day mortality and major complications. There was a significant reduction in the composite endpoint along with reduced ICU and hospital LOS, reduced infection rate, and reduced occurrence of the low CO syndrome. Although the isolated 30-day mortality rate remained unchanged, the data suggest that GDT may significantly reduce complications and LOS for cardiac surgery.

Atrial fibrillation (AF), the most common dysrhythmia after cardiac surgery, ranges from 24% after CAB, 37% to 50% after valvular surgery, and as high as 60% after valvular surgery plus CAB,[103,163] and typically occurs on or after postoperative day 2. AF has been associated with a three-fold increased risk of ischemic stroke and myriad other complications including cardiac failure, pulmonary edema, need for IABP, need for pacemaker, acute kidney injury, and infections. Importantly, postoperative AF has been demonstrated to increase ICU LOS by 48 hours, add 3 days to total LOS, doubling of mortality risk, and $9000 to total hospital costs.[19] AF prophylaxis is much studied, and while definitive data are lacking, beta-blockade is commonly utilized. Amiodarone has also been suggested for AF prophylaxis and treatment.[163] AF persisting greater than 24 hours and recurrent episodes require specific treatment, and either a strategy of rate or rhythm control may be considered. Five hundred twenty-three patients with AF after cardiac surgery randomized to either rate control or rhythm control had equivalent LOS, complication rates, and persistence of AF at 60 days.[164] The benefits of anticoagulation must be weighed against the risks of bleeding and stroke. CHADS2vasc and HASBLED scores may be of value in risk assessment for anticoagulation.[163–166] Atrial flutter is less frequently observed and generally responsive to overdrive pacing or cardioversion. Should initial cardioversion fail, repeat cardioversion after intravenous amiodarone is common. As with AF, the risks and benefits of anticoagulation should be quantified and individualized.

Sustained ventricular dysrhythmias are seen in roughly 1% to 3% of patients and are associated with increased 30-day mortality. Reduced ejection fraction (<35%) is the strongest risk factor.[167,168]

Bradydysrhythmias are common following cardiac surgery and may take the form of sick sinus syndrome and varying other conduction abnormalities including atrioventricular block. As a consequence, atrial and/or ventricular epicardial pacing leads are commonly placed intraoperatively. In low-risk patients (without diabetes, preoperative arrhythmia, or need for pacing to separate from cardiopulmonary bypass), the need for postoperative pacing is as low as 2.6%, leading some centers to forgo routine placement. For the patient without epicardial leads, temporary transvenous, transesophageal, or transcutaneous pacing may be utilized. If pacing is required, most patients need it for only a short time, and only 0.8% to 3.4% of patients undergoing isolated CAB require permanent pacemaker placement. The incidence is higher in patients undergoing valvular surgery with CAB (2%–4%) and much higher in special situations such as calcific aortic stenosis, mitral valve surgery,[163] and transcatheter aortic valve replacement. Optimal timing for permanent pacemaker placement is dependent upon the clinical course but commonly occurs between postoperative day 5 to 7.[163,169] Excellent technical reviews of pacemaker selection and management can be found in the literature.[170,171]

Low CO and hypotension following cardiothoracic surgery demand immediate intervention and may be due to pneumothorax, hemorrhage, cardiac tamponade, myocardial dysfunction (right, left, or bi-ventricular), valvular dysfunction, and/or vasoplegia. Cardiac tamponade following cardiac surgery generally requires surgical exploration and can be a challenging diagnosis requiring a high index of suspicion and frequently TEE for confirmation.[172] Postoperative cardiac surgery patients may manifest shock characterized by low CO and high vascular tone. Low cardiac output syndrome (LCOS) may be defined as CI less than 2.0 L/min/m2 with systolic blood pressure (SBP) less than 90 and signs of hypoperfusion. LCOS can be related to right, left, or bi-ventricular systolic and/or diastolic dysfunction. Risk factors include age greater than 65, reduced LVEF (<50%), CAB with CPB, long CPB time, emergency surgery, diabetes mellitus with chronic kidney disease, and malnutrition.[173] The cause of LCOS must be immediately assessed and addressed directly. Optimization of ventricular function should be addressed via assessment and management of heart rate and rhythm, pre-load, afterload, and contractility.

Increased inotrope doses correlate with risk, and patients with LCOS refractory to medical support should be considered for mechanical circulatory support.[173–175] Ventricular failure may be treated with intra-aortic balloon counterpulsation (IABP), temporary ventricular assist devices inserted percutaneously or surgically implanted, total artificial hearts, or combined cardiopulmonary support. Details of choices for various populations, risks, experience, and outcomes are well described, but beyond the scope of this article.[175–181]

Vasoplegia after cardiac surgery is a state of very low vascular tone with normal to high CO leading to tissue hypoperfusion, with reported incidence varying from 2.8% in off-pump CAB to greater than 40% in patients undergoing placement of a left ventricular assist device.[182,183] Vasoplegia is a systemic inflammatory response syndrome resembling that of sepsis resulting from a complex interaction of inflammatory mediators, leukocytes, and endothelial cells.[182] Although some CCC patients will require postoperative vasopressor support, patients with vasoplegia will require large doses and frequently multiple vasopressor agents. Vasoplegia after cardiac surgery is associated with low circulating endogenous vasopressin (antidiuretic hormone) and prophylactic low-dose (<0.04 units/min) vasopressin infusion before, during, and after CPB reduces catecholamine use after separation from CPB.[183–185] Each of the catecholamine drugs has pros and cons, and the preferred agent remains a matter of debate; however, norepinephrine may be useful when both inotrope and vasomotor tone are desired.[186] Methylene blue may be administered intravenously to interfere with nitric oxide synthesis and promote increased vascular tone. Of 638 patients at a single center, 56 (8.8%) developed vasoplegia and were randomized to methylene blue or placebo. Overall mortality was 10.7% for patients with vasoplegia (vs 3.6% without vasoplegia) but was zero for those receiving methylene blue infusion. Not all studies of methylene blue have yielded positive outcomes, and the advisability and details of administration are debatable.[183]

Gastrointestinal System-Nutrition-Metabolic

Liver dysfunction increases mortality of patients undergoing cardiac surgery, where coagulopathy and hemorrhage are commonplace, and progressively increase with the severity of liver dysfunction. Liver dysfunction, in particular cirrhosis, reduces immune function, predisposing to nosocomial infection, and is associated with malnutrition and an increased risk of acute kidney injury (AKI) following cardiac surgery. The model for end-stage liver disease (MELD) score has proven useful for risk assessment and planning in the cardiac surgery population.[187,188]

Most cardiac surgery patients do not require nutritional support during their brief ICU course; however, those patients staying longer than 2 days require particular vigilance for malnutrition.[189] Malnutrition is commonly observed in cardiac surgical patients with a reported incidence ranging from 10% to 25% and it increases the risk for postoperative infection, ICU LOS, and mortality.[190] Multiple scoring systems exist to screen for malnutrition, and a recent evaluation of 4 available screening tools suggested that the MUST (malnutriton universal screening tool) might be preferable because of its ease of use and prediction of postoperative complications.[190,191] Enteral nutrition (EN) may be feasible and safe in patients requiring prolonged vasoactive support.[192] At times, EN may not meet caloric needs, and parenteral nutrition (PN) may be considered, but current guidelines recommend waiting until more than 7 days before initiation of PN. Multiple trials of EN versus PN have failed to reduce infections, mortality, or LOS.[190,193–195]

Despite extensive investigation, considerable controversy exists regarding optimal management of perioperative hyperglycemia. Hyperglycemia is linked with death, surgical site infection, and AF in some cardiac surgery patients, and various protocols have been developed to provide glycemic control.[196–201] Recent review of the authors' computerized, glucose control program included 2589 cardiothoracic surgery patients and 74,734 glucose readings; 89.77% of glucose measurements were between 70 and 149 mg%. Average time to goal (<130 mg%) was 4.02 hours, and only 11 patients (0.42%) had glucose less than 40 mg% (0.02% of readings) (Brooks N, Lobdell K, unpublished data, Presented at STS-AATS Critical Care Symposium. Quality Assurance and Improvement of a Cardiovascular Critical Care Glycemic Control Program, 2015).

Renal System

AKI occurs in as many as 40% of cardiac surgery patients depending on the definition employed. AKI increases length of stay, readmission rate, cost, and mortality in a dose-dependent fashion related to the severity of injury.[202,203] Up to 5% of patients will require renal replacement therapy (RRT), leading to a marked increase in the risk of death.

Urine output should be monitored assiduously and oliguria prevented. When oliguria occurs, it should be treated quickly by optimization of systemic blood pressure, CI, and SvO2, since oliguria is a leading indicator of AKI and other risks associated with suboptimal hemodynamics (hepatic ischemia, gut ischemia, etc).[203] Various static risk models have been developed and commonly include age, body mass index (BMI), hypertension, peripheral vascular disease, chronic pulmonary disease, serum creatinine concentration, anemia, previous cardiac surgery, emergency operation, and operation type.[204,205] A comprehensive understanding of AKI associated with cardiothoracic surgery must include all phases of care and refinement of dynamic risk models.[206]

AKI risk mitigation strategies include avoidance of nephrotoxic drugs, and more recently, high-chloride intravenous fluids have been implicated in the development of AKI. In a prospective, single-center study of 264 patients treated with usual care or GDT of stroke volume maximization, the incidence of AKI dropped from 19.9% to 6.5% with GDT.[207] In the authors' institution, routine GDT resulted in a 5-year mean incidence of acute renal failure of 1.1% (approximately50% of current STS-ACSD mean, median 1.2% and range 0.0%–2.1%) (STS-ACSD, unpublished data, 2017).

Predicting the need for renal replacement therapy (RRT) has been investigated.[208,209] Optimal timing and type of RRT remain controversial, although continuous RRT is favored in hemodynamically unstable patients compared with conventional hemodialysis.[210] RRT is resource intensive and may be associated with independent, incremental risk.[211]

Hematological System and Infections

Anemia is common and should be treated preoperatively (including autologous donation) where feasible, since it may lead to transfusion with unclear benefits.[212] In fact, according to the STS-ACSD in 2014, 43.2% of coronary artery surgery patients receive blood transfusions, while transfusion rates associated with LVAD implantation have been observed to range from 83% to 100%.[10] Twenty-five percent of all blood products transfused are in cardiac surgery patients.[213] Much has been written about the considerable variation in practice and prediction of transfusion, risks (death, complications, and cost) of this phenomenon.[214,215] The STS offers guidance through its blood conservations guidelines.[216] Investigations continue to refine understanding of the risks of anemia and transfusion and aim to optimize management of these common and vexing issues.[217–220]

Acquired coagulopathy is increasing with the use of various anticoagulants for AF, coronary and cerebrovascular disease, as well as adverse effects of nontraditional medical remedies. The CCC team must be familiar with characteristics of common drugs that affect coagulation, including half-life of effect, bridging, and reversal strategies.

The HAS-BLED bleeding risk score is useful and includes age, liver dysfunction, renal dysfunction, bleeding tendency, warfarin and antiplatelet drug use, and alcohol excess.[221]

The Society of Thoracic Surgeons provides a valuable review of antiplatelet agents for cardiac and noncardiac operations.[222]

Health care acquired infections (HAIs) are common and costly.[223] HAI after cardiac surgery is associated with approximately five-fold increase risk of death.[224] HAIs associated with CAB occur in approximately 4% to 5% of cases, with pneumonia being the most common (approximately 3%), followed by surgical site infections and septicemia.[225] Risks for HAIs commonly include smoking, diabetes mellitus, chronic lung disease, heart failure, and transfusion of blood products.[225,226] The rate of HAIs varies considerably between centers (0.9%–19.1%).[227] CCC HAI improvement programs and antibiotic stewardship efforts must focus on choice, timing, and duration of antimicrobials, chlorhexidine cleansing, bundles to prevent catheter-related blood stream infections[228] and ventilator associated events, judicious use of indwelling catheters, and an aim of early removal.

SUMMARY

High-value CCC is rapidly evolving to meet the demands of increased patient acuity and to incorporate advances in technology. The high-performing CCC system and culture should aim to learn quickly and continuously improve. CCC demands a proactive, interactive, precise, anexpert team, and continuity.

REFERENCES

1. Available at: http://www.cdc.gov/nchs/fastats/heart-disease.htm. Accessed October 5, 2016.
2. Available at: http://www.cdc.gov/nchs/fastats/inpatient-surgery.htm. Accessed October 5, 2016.
3. Available at: http://www.cdc.gov/ncbddd/heartdefects/data.html. Accessed October 5, 2016.
4. Available at: http://www.cdc.gov/nchs/fastats/cancer.htm. Accessed October 5, 2016.
5. Available at: http://www.cancer.org/cancer/lungcancer-non-smallcell/detailedguide/non-small-cell-lung-cancer-key-statistics. Accessed October 5, 2016.
6. Available at: http://www.cancer.org/cancer/lungcancer-non-smallcell/detailedguide/non-small-cell-lung-cancer-survival-rates. Accessed October 5, 2016.
7. Available at: http://www.cancer.org/cancer/esophaguscancer/detailedguide/esophagus-cancer-key-statistics. Accessed October 5, 2016.
8. Available at: http://www.cancer.org/cancer/esophaguscancer/detailedguide/esophagus-cancer-survival-rates. Accessed October 5, 2016.
9. STS-ACSD 2015. Available at: http://www.sts.org/quality-research-patient-safety/quality/quality-performance-measures. Accessed October 5, 2016.
10. Quader M, LaPar DJ, Wolfe L, et al, Investigators for the Virginia Cardiac Surgery Quality Initiative. Blood product utilization with left ventricular assist device implantation: a decade of statewide data. ASAIO J 2016;62(3):268–73.

11. Conway BD, Stamou SC, Kouchoukos NT, et al. Improved clinical outcomes and survival following repair of acute type A aortic dissection in the current era. Interact Cardiovasc Thorac Surg 2014;19(6):971–6.

12. Seder CW, Wright CD, Chang AC, et al. The society of thoracic surgeons general thoracic surgery database update on outcomes and quality. Ann Thorac Surg 2016;101(5):1646–54.

13. Resnick AS, Corrigan D, Mullen JL, et al. Surgeon contribution to hospital bottom line: not all are created equal. Ann Surg 2005;242(4):530–9.

14. Robinson JC. Variation in hospital costs, payments, and profitability for cardiac valve replacement surgery. Health Serv Res 2011;46(6 Pt 1):1928–45.

15. Available at: http://www.bloomberg.com/news/articles/2013-08-01/indias-walmart-of-heart-surgery-cuts-the-cost-by-98-percent. Accessed October 5, 2016.

16. Available at: http://jco.ascopubs.org/content/early/2014/11/20/JCO.2014.57.7155.full.pdf+html. Accessed October 5, 2016.

17. Available at: https://costprojections.cancer.gov/annual.costs.html. Accessed October 5, 2016.

18. Halpern NA, Pastores SM. Critical care medicine in the United States 2000-2005: an analysis of bed numbers, occupancy rates, payer mix, and costs. Crit Care Med 2010;38(1):65–71.

19. Speir AM, Kasirajan V, Barnett SD, et al. Additive costs of postoperative complications for isolated coronary artery bypass grafting patients in Virginia. Ann Thorac Surg 2009;88(1):40–5.

20. Savage B, Segal M, Alexander D. The cost of healthcare associated infections. Available at: https://www2.gehealthcare.com/doccart/public?guid=56c1c4429f811310VgnVCM10000024dd1403. Accessed October 18, 2016.

21. Sifri CD, Burke GH, Enfield KB. Reduced health care-associated infections in an acute care community hospital using a combination of self-disinfecting copper-impregnated composite hard surfaces and linens. Am J Infect Control 2016; 44(12):1565–71.

22. Ferraris VA, Ferraris SP, Singh A. Operative outcome and hospital cost. J Thorac Cardiovasc Surg 1998;115(3):593–602.

23. Osnabrugge RL, Speir AM, Head SJ, et al. Cost, quality, and value in coronary artery bypass grafting. J Thorac Cardiovasc Surg 2014;148(6):2729–35.

24. Available at: http://www.ahic.nihi.ca/ahic/docs/IBV%20Study%20Redefining%20the%20Value%20of%20Healthcare.pdf. Accessed October 18, 2016.

25. Available at: http://data.worldbank.org/indicator/SH.XPD.TOTL.ZS. Accessed October 5, 2016.

26. Available at: http://www.cdc.gov/nchs/fastats/health-expenditures.htm. Accessed October 5, 2016.

27. Available at: https://www.cms.gov/Newsroom/MediaReleaseDatabase/Fact-sheets/2016-Fact-sheets-items/2016-07-25.html. Accessed October 5, 2016.

28. Available at: http://www.hpocenter.com/hpo-framework/. Accessed October 5, 2016.

29. Available at: https://www.bcg.com/documents/file84953.pdf. Accessed October 5, 2016.

30. Chassin MR, Loeb JM. High-reliability health care: getting there from here. Milbank Q 2013;91(3):459–90.

31. Available at: https://archive.ahrq.gov/professionals/quality-patient-safety/quality-resources/tools/hroadvice/hroadvice.pdf. Accessed October 5, 2016.

32. Available at: http://www.chron.com/news/health/article/Journey-to-high-reliability-health-care-3985238.php. Accessed October 5, 2016.

33. Mishra AK, Mishra KE. Trust is everything: becoming the leader others will follow. Chapel (NC): Author; 2008.

34. Cook D, Thompson JE, Habermann EB, et al. From 'solution shop' model to 'focused factory' in hospital surgery: increasing care value and predictability. Health Aff (Millwood) 2014;33(5):746–55.

35. Katz NM. The emerging specialty of cardiothoracic surgical critical care: the leadership role of cardiothoracic surgeons on the multidisciplinary team. J Thorac Cardiovasc Surg 2007;134(5):1109–11.

36. Katz NM. The evolution of cardiothoracic critical care. J Thorac Cardiovasc Surg 2011;141(1):3–6.

37. Whitson BA, D'Cunha J. The thoracic surgical intensivist: the best critical care doctor for our thoracic surgical patients. Semin Thorac Cardiovasc Surg 2011;23(1):12–3.

38. Katz NM. Meeting the expanded challenges of the cardiothoracic intensive care unit. J Thorac Cardiovasc Surg 2015;150(4):777–8.

39. Lopez-Sendon J, McAreavey D, Nallamothu B, et al. Evolution of critical care cardiology: transformation of the cardiovascular intensive care unit and the emerging need for new medical staffing and training models: a scientific statement from the American Heart Association. Circulation 2012;126(11):1408–28.

40. Holmes DR Jr, Mohr F, Hamm CW, et al. Venn diagrams in cardiovascular disease: the heart team concept. Ann Thorac Surg 2013;95(2):389–91.

41. Kumar K, Zarychanski R, Bell DD, et al, Cardiovascular Health Research in Manitoba Investigator Group. Impact of 24-hour in-house intensivists on a dedicated cardiac surgery intensive care unit. Ann Thorac Surg 2009;88(4):1153–61.

42. Kumar K, Singal R, Manji RA, et al, Cardiovascular Health Research in Manitoba Investigator Group. The benefits of 24/7 in-house intensivist coverage for prolonged-stay cardiac surgery patients. J Thorac Cardiovasc Surg 2014;148(1):290–7.

43. Shake JG, Pronovost PJ, Whitman GJ. Cardiac surgical ICU care: eliminating "preventable" complications. J Card Surg 2013;28(4):406–13.

44. Available at: http://hbswk.hbs.edu/item/the-importance-of-teaming. Accessed October 5, 2016.

45. Baker D, Salas E, Barach P, et al. The relation between teamwork and patient safety. In: Carayon P, editor. Handbook of human factors and ergonomics in health care and patient safety. Taylor & Francis; 2006. p. 259–71.

46. Barach P, Weinger M. Trauma team performance. In: Wilson WC, Grande CM, Hoyt DB, editors. Trauma: emergency resuscitation and perioperative anesthesia management, vol. 1. New York: Marcel Dekker, Inc; 2007. p. 101–13.

47. Guccione A, Morena A, Pezzi A, et al. The assessment of nursing workload. Minerva Anestesiol 2004;70(5):411–6 [in Italian].

48. Available at: http://www.wsj.com/articles/hospital-icus-mine-big-data-in-push-for-better-outcomes-1435249003. Accessed October 5, 2016.

49. Kim MM, Barnato AE, Angus DC, et al. The effect of multidisciplinary care teams on intensive care unit mortality. Arch Intern Med 2010;170(4):369–76.

50. Lobdell KW, Stamou SC, Mishra AK, et al. Multidisciplinary rounds: the work, not more work. Ann Thorac Surg 2010;89(3):1010.

51. Cardarelli M, Vaidya V, Conway D, et al. Dissecting multidisciplinary cardiac surgery rounds. Ann Thorac Surg 2009;88(3):809–13.

52. Pronovost PJ, Angus DC, Dorman T, et al. Physician staffing patterns and clinical outcomes in critically ill patients: a systematic review. JAMA 2002;288(17):2151–62.

53. Wallace DJ, Angus DC, Barnato AE, et al. Nighttime intensivist staffing and mortality among critically ill patients. N Engl J Med 2012;366(22):2093–101.
54. Available at: http://sts-365.ascendeventmedia.com/sts-daily/critical-care-symposium-to-examine-role-of-tele-icus-in-improving-quality-value/. Accessed October 18, 2016.
55. Lilly CM, Zubrow MT, Kempner KM, et al, Society of Critical Care Medicine Tele-ICU Committee. Critical care telemedicine: evolution and state of the art. Crit Care Med 2014;42(11):2429–36.
56. Available at: http://mhealthintelligence.com/news/kaiser-ceo-telehealth-outpaced-in-person-visits-last-year. Accessed October 13, 2016.
57. Available at: https://www.ahcmedia.com/articles/print/86620-the-quality-cost-connection-improve-patient-flow-by-reducing-bottlenecks. Accessed October 13, 2016.
58. Rechel B, Wright S, Barlow J, et al. Hospital capacity planning: from measuring stocks to modelling flows. Bull World Health Organ 2010;88(8):632–6.
59. Fann JI, Moffatt-Bruce SD, DiMaio JM, et al. Human factors and human nature in cardiothoracic surgery. Ann Thorac Surg 2016;101(6):2059–66.
60. The better the team, the safer the world: golden rules of group interaction in high-risk environments. Evidence based suggestions for improving performance 2004. Available at: https://books.google.com/books/about/The_Better_the_Team_the_Safer_the_World.html?id=AabsGAAACAAJ.
61. Sanchez J, Lobdell K. Quality improvement: methods, principles, and role in healthcare. Nova Science Publishers, Inc.; 2013. p. 51–60.
62. Pronovost P, Berenholtz S, Dorman T, et al. Improving communication in the ICU using daily goals. J Crit Care 2003;18(2):71–5.
63. Gawande A. The checklist: if something so simple can transform intensive care, what else can it do? New Yorker 2007;86–101.
64. Haynes AB, Weiser TG, Berry WR, et al, Safe Surgery Saves Lives Study Group. A surgical safety checklist to reduce morbidity and mortality in a global population. N Engl J Med 2009;360(5):491–9.
65. Casale AS, Paulus RA, Selna MJ, et al. "ProvenCareSM": a provider-driven pay-for-performance program for acute episodic cardiac surgical care. Ann Surg 2007;246(4):613–21.
66. Toccafondi G, Albolino S, Tartaglia R, et al. The collaborative communication model for patient handover at the interface between high-acuity and low-acuity care. BMJ Qual Saf 2012;21(Suppl 1):i58–66.
67. Hesselink G, Schoonhoven L, Barach P, et al. Improving patient handovers from hospital to primary care. a systematic review. Ann Intern Med 2012;157(6): 417–28.
68. Available at: https://hbr.org/2008/07/the-competitive-imperative-of-learning. Accessed October 5, 2016.
69. Tucker AL, Nembhard IM, Edmondson AC. Implementing new practices: an empirical study of organizational learning in hospital intensive care units. Management Sci 2007;6:894–907.
70. O'Connor GT, Plume SK, Olmstead EM, et al. A regional intervention to improve the hospital mortality associated with coronary artery bypass graft surgery. The Northern New England Cardiovascular Disease Study Group. JAMA 1996; 275(11):841–6.
71. Share DA, Campbell DA, Birkmeyer N, et al. How a regional collaborative of hospitals and physicians in Michigan cut costs and improved the quality of care. Health Aff (Millwood) 2011;30(4):636–45.

72. Stamou SC, Camp SL, Stiegel RM, et al. Quality improvement program decreases mortality after cardiac surgery. J Thorac Cardiovasc Surg 2008; 136(2):494–9.

73. Stamou SC, Camp SL, Reames MK, et al. Continuous quality improvement program and major morbidity after cardiac surgery. Am J Cardiol 2008;102(6): 772–7.

74. Camp SL, Stamou SC, Stiegel RM, et al. Can timing of tracheal extubation predict improved outcomes after cardiac surgery? HSR Proc Intensive Care Cardiovasc Anesth 2009;1(2):39–47.

75. Camp SL, Stamou SC, Stiegel RM, et al. Quality improvement program increases early tracheal extubation rate and decreases pulmonary complications and resource utilization after cardiac surgery. J Card Surg 2009;24(4):414–23.

76. Culig MH, Kunkle RF, Frndak DC, et al. Improving patient care in cardiac surgery using Toyota production system based methodology. Ann Thorac Surg 2011;91(2):394–9.

77. Curtis JR, Cook DJ, Wall RJ, et al. Intensive care unit quality improvement: a "how-to" guide for the interdisciplinary team. Crit Care Med 2006;34(1):211–8.

78. Lobdell K, Camp S, Stamou S, et al. Quality improvement in cardiac critical care. HSR Proc Intensive Care Cardiovasc Anesth 2009;1(1):16–20.

79. Reddy HG, Shih T, Englesbe MJ, et al. Analyzing "failure to rescue": is this an opportunity for outcome improvement in cardiac surgery? Ann Thorac Surg 2013;95(6):1976–81.

80. Ahmed EO, Butler R, Novick RJ. Failure-to-rescue rate as a measure of quality of care in a cardiac surgery recovery unit: a five-year study. Ann Thorac Surg 2014; 97(1):147–52.

81. Edwards FH, Ferraris VA, Kurlansky PA, et al. Failure to rescue rates after coronary artery bypass grafting: an analysis from the society of thoracic surgeons adult cardiac surgery database. Ann Thorac Surg 2016;102(2):458–64.

82. Pradarelli JC, Healy MA, Osborne NH, et al. Variation in medicare expenditures for treating perioperative complications: the cost of rescue. JAMA Surg 2016; 151(12):e163340.

83. Available at: http://riskcalc.sts.org/stswebriskcalc/#/. Accessed October 5, 2016.

84. Available at: http://www.euroscore.org/calc.html. Accessed October 5, 2016.

85. Lobdell KW, Fann JI, Sanchez JA. "What's the risk?" Assessing and mitigating risk in cardiothoracic surgery. Ann Thorac Surg 2016;102(4):1052–8.

86. Hekmat K, Kroener A, Stuetzer H, et al. Daily assessment of organ dysfunction and survival in intensive care unit cardiac surgical patients. Ann Thorac Surg 2005;79(5):1555–62.

87. Doerr F, Badreldin AM, Heldwein MB, et al. A comparative study of four intensive care outcome prediction models in cardiac surgery patients. J Cardiothorac Surg 2011;6:21.

88. Exarchopoulos T, Charitidou E, Dedeilias P, et al. Scoring systems for outcome prediction in a cardiac surgical intensive care unit: a comparative study. Am J Crit Care 2015;24(4):327–34.

89. McElroy I, Sareh S, Zhu A, et al. Use of digital health kits to reduce readmission after cardiac surgery. J Surg Res 2016;204(1):1–7.

90. Deininger S, Hoenicka M, Müller-Eising K, et al. Renal function and urinary biomarkers in cardiac bypass surgery: a prospective randomized trial comparing three surgical techniques. Thorac Cardiovasc Surg 2016;64(7):561–8.

91. Available at: http://www.cbsnews.com/videos/artificial-intelligence/. Accessed October 13, 2016.
92. Available at: https://www.nih.gov/precision-medicine-initiative-cohort-program/scale-scope. Accessed October 14, 2016.
93. Fleming IO, Garratt C, Guha R, et al. Aggregation of marginal gains in cardiac surgery: feasibility of a perioperative care bundle for enhanced recovery in cardiac surgical patients. J Cardiothorac Vasc Anesth 2016;30(3):665–70.
94. Jones NL, Edmonds L, Ghosh S, et al. A review of enhanced recovery for thoracic anaesthesia and surgery. Anaesthesia 2013;68(2):179–89.
95. Ad N, Holmes SD, Shuman DJ, et al. Potential impact of modifiable clinical variables on length of stay after first-time cardiac surgery. Ann Thorac Surg 2015; 100(6):2102–7.
96. McPherson JA, Wagner CE, Boehm LM, et al. Delirium in the cardiovascular ICU: exploring modifiable risk factors. Crit Care Med 2013;41(2):405–13.
97. Kazmierski J, Kowman M, Banach M, et al, IPDACS study. Incidence and predictors of delirium after cardiac surgery: results from the IPDACS study. J Psychosom Res 2010;69(2):179–85.
98. Jackson P, Khan A. Delirium in critically ill patients. Crit Care Clin 2015;31(3): 589–603.
99. Saczynski JS, Marcantonio ER, Quach L, et al. Cognitive trajectories after postoperative delirium. N Engl J Med 2012;367(1):30–9.
100. Geng J, Qian J, Cheng H, et al. The influence of perioperative dexmedetomidine on patients undergoing cardiac surgery: a meta-analysis. PLoS One 2016;11(4): e0152829.
101. Liu X, Zhang K, Wang W, et al. Dexmedetomidine sedation reduces atrial fibrillation after cardiac surgery compared to propofol: a randomized controlled trial. Crit Care 2016;20(1):298.
102. Barr J, Fraser GL, Puntillo K, et al, American College of Critical Care Medicine. Clinical practice guidelines for the management of pain, agitation, and delirium in adult patients in the intensive care unit. Crit Care Med 2013;41(1):263–306.
103. STS-ACSD definitions. Available at: http://www.sts.org/sites/default/files/documents/STSAdultCVDataSpecificationsV2_81.pdf. Accessed October 31, 2017.
104. Shahian DM, O'Brien SM, Filardo G, et al, Society of Thoracic Surgeons Quality Measurement Task Force. The society of thoracic surgeons 2008 cardiac surgery risk models: part 1–coronary artery bypass grafting surgery. Ann Thorac Surg 2009;88(1 Suppl):S2–22.
105. Shahian DM, O'Brien SM, Filardo G, et al, Society of Thoracic Surgeons Quality Measurement Task Force. The Society of Thoracic Surgeons 2008 cardiac surgery risk models: part 3–valve plus coronary artery bypass grafting surgery. Ann Thorac Surg 2009;88(1 Suppl):S43–62.
106. Tarakji KG, Sabik JF 3rd, Bhudia SK, et al. Temporal onset, risk factors, and outcomes associated with stroke after coronary artery bypass grafting. JAMA 2011; 305(4):381–90.
107. Roach GW, Kanchuger M, Mangano CM, et al. Adverse cerebral outcomes after coronary bypass surgery. Multicenter Study of Perioperative Ischemia Research Group and the Ischemia Research and Education Foundation Investigators. N Engl J Med 1996;335(25):1857–63.
108. Lahtinen J, Biancari F, Salmela E, et al. Postoperative atrial fibrillation is a major cause of stroke after on-pump coronary artery bypass surgery. Ann Thorac Surg 2004;77(4):1241–4.

109. McKhann GM, Grega MA, Borowicz LM Jr, et al. Stroke and encephalopathy after cardiac surgery: an update. Stroke 2006;37(2):562–71.

110. Beaty CA, Arnaoutakis GJ, Grega MA, et al. The role of head computed tomography imaging in the evaluation of postoperative neurologic deficits in cardiac surgery patients. Ann Thorac Surg 2013;95(2):548–54.

111. Kunt A, Atbaş Ç, Hidiroğlu M, et al. Predictors and outcomes of minor cerebrovascular events after cardiac surgery: a multivariable analysis of 1346 patients. J Cardiovasc Surg 2013;54(4):537–43.

112. Stephens RS, Shah AS, Whitman GJ. Lung injury and acute respiratory distress syndrome after cardiac surgery. Ann Thorac Surg 2013;95(3):1122–9.

113. Apostolakis EE, Koletsis EN, Baikoussis NG, et al. Strategies to prevent intraoperative lung injury during cardiopulmonary bypass. J Cardiothorac Surg 2010;5:1.

114. Ng CS, Wan S, Yim AP, et al. Pulmonary dysfunction after cardiac surgery. Chest 2002;121(4):1269–77.

115. Fuller BM, Mohr NM, Drewry AM, et al. Lower tidal volume at initiation of mechanical ventilation may reduce progression to acute respiratory distress syndrome: a systematic review. Crit Care 2013;17(1):R11.

116. Serpa Neto A, Cardoso SO, Manetta JA, et al. Association between use of lung-protective ventilation with lower tidal volumes and clinical outcomes among patients without acute respiratory distress syndrome: a meta-analysis. JAMA 2012; 308(16):1651–9.

117. Ventilation with lower tidal volumes as compared with traditional tidal volumes for acute lung injury and the acute respiratory distress syndrome. The acute respiratory distress syndrome network. N Engl J Med 2000;342(18):1301–8.

118. Futier E, Constantin JM, Paugam-Burtz C, et al, IMPROVE Study Group. A trial of intraoperative low-tidal-volume ventilation in abdominal surgery. N Engl J Med 2013;369(5):428–37.

119. Lellouche F, Dionne S, Simard S, et al. High tidal volumes in mechanically ventilated patients increase organ dysfunction after cardiac surgery. Anesthesiology 2012;116(5):1072–82.

120. National Heart, Lung, and Blood Institute Acute Respiratory Distress Syndrome (ARDS) Clinical Trials Network, Wiedemann HP, Wheeler AP, Bernard GR, et al. Comparison of two fluid-management strategies in acute lung injury. N Engl J Med 2006;354(24):2564–75.

121. Fitch ZW, Debesa O, Ohkuma R, et al. A protocol-driven approach to early extubation after heart surgery. J Thorac Cardiovasc Surg 2014;147(4):1344–50.

122. Meade MO, Guyatt G, Butler R, et al. Trials comparing early vs late extubation following cardiovascular surgery. Chest 2001;120(6 Suppl):445S–53S.

123. Rashid A, Sattar KA, Dar MI, et al. Analyzing the outcome of early versus prolonged extubation following cardiac surgery. Ann Thorac Cardiovasc Surg 2008;14(4):218–23.

124. Girard TD, Kress JP, Fuchs BD, et al. Efficacy and safety of a paired sedation and ventilator weaning protocol for mechanically ventilated patients in intensive care (Awakening and Breathing Controlled trial): a randomised controlled trial. Lancet 2008;371(9607):126–34.

125. Nair GB, Niederman MS. Ventilator-associated pneumonia: present understanding and ongoing debates. Intensive Care Med 2015;41(1):34–48.

126. Vohra HA, Goldsmith IR, Rosin MD, et al. The predictors and outcome of recidivism in cardiac ICUs. Eur J Cardiothorac Surg 2005;27(3):508–11.

127. De Santo LS, Bancone C, Santarpino G, et al. Noninvasive positive-pressure ventilation for extubation failure after cardiac surgery: pilot safety evaluation. J Thorac Cardiovasc Surg 2009;137(2):342–6.

128. Olper L, Corbetta D, Cabrini L, et al. Effects of non-invasive ventilation on reintubation rate: a systematic review and meta-analysis of randomised studies of patients undergoing cardiothoracic surgery. Crit Care Resusc 2013;15(3):220–7.

129. Stéphan F, Barrucand B, Petit P, et al, BiPOP Study Group. High-flow nasal oxygen vs noninvasive positive airway pressure in hypoxemic patients after cardiothoracic surgery: a randomized clinical trial. JAMA 2015;313(23):2331–9.

130. Zochios V, Klein AA, Jones N, et al. Effect of high-flow nasal oxygen on pulmonary complications and outcomes after adult cardiothoracic surgery: a qualitative review. J Cardiothorac Vasc Anesth 2016;30(5):1379–85.

131. Warner MA, Offord KP, Warner ME, et al. Role of preoperative cessation of smoking and other factors in postoperative pulmonary complications: a blinded prospective study of coronary artery bypass patients. Mayo Clin Proc 1989;64(6):609–16.

132. Schmid M, Sood A, Campbell L, et al. Impact of smoking on perioperative outcomes after major surgery. Am J Surg 2015;210(2):221–9.

133. Mills E, Eyawo O, Lockhart I, et al. Smoking cessation reduces postoperative complications: a systematic review and meta-analysis. Am J Med 2011;124(2):144–54.

134. Hulzebos EH, Smit Y, Helders PP, et al. Preoperative physical therapy for elective cardiac surgery patients. Cochrane Database Syst Rev 2012;(11):CD010118.

135. Katsura M, Kuriyama A, Takeshima T, et al. Preoperative inspiratory muscle training for postoperative pulmonary complications in adults undergoing cardiac and major abdominal surgery. Cochrane Database Syst Rev 2015;(10):CD010356.

136. Starobin D, Kramer MR, Garty M, et al. Morbidity associated with systemic corticosteroid preparation for coronary artery bypass grafting in patients with chronic obstructive pulmonary disease: a case control study. J Cardiothorac Surg 2007;2:25.

137. Lee HW, Lee JK, Oh SH, et al. Effect of perioperative systemic steroid treatment on patients with obstructive lung disease undergoing elective abdominal surgery. Clin Respir J 2016. [Epub ahead of print].

138. Westerdahl E, Lindmark B, Eriksson T, et al. Deep-breathing exercises reduce atelectasis and improve pulmonary function after coronary artery bypass surgery. Chest 2005;128(5):3482–8.

139. Freitas ER, Soares BG, Cardoso JR, et al. Incentive spirometry for preventing pulmonary complications after coronary artery bypass graft. Cochrane Database Syst Rev 2012;(9):CD004466.

140. Cassidy MR, Rosenkranz P, McCabe K, et al. reducing postoperative pulmonary complications with a multidisciplinary patient care program. JAMA Surg 2013;148(8):740–5.

141. Haeffener MP, Ferreira GM, Barreto SS, et al. Incentive spirometry with expiratory positive airway pressure reduces pulmonary complications, improves pulmonary function and 6-minute walk distance in patients undergoing coronary artery bypass graft surgery. Am Heart J 2008;156(5):900.e1-8.

142. Zarbock A, Mueller E, Netzer S, et al. Prophylactic nasal continuous positive airway pressure following cardiac surgery protects from postoperative pulmonary complications: a prospective, randomized, controlled trial in 500 patients. Chest 2009;135(5):1252–9.

143. van der Leeden M, Huijsmans R, Geleijn E, et al. Early enforced mobilisation following surgery for gastrointestinal cancer: feasibility and outcomes. Physiotherapy 2016;102(1):103–10.

144. Haines KJ, Skinner EH, Berney S, Austin Health POST Study Investigators. Association of postoperative pulmonary complications with delayed mobilisation following major abdominal surgery: an observational cohort study. Physiotherapy 2013;99(2):119–25.

145. Castelino T, Fiore JF Jr, Niculiseanu P, et al. The effect of early mobilization protocols on postoperative outcomes following abdominal and thoracic surgery: a systematic review. Surgery 2016;159(4):991–1003.

146. Takahashi T, Kumamaru M, Jenkins S, et al. In-patient step count predicts rehospitalization after cardiac surgery. J Cardiol 2015;66(4):286–91.

147. Judge O, Ji F, Fleming N, et al. Current use of the pulmonary artery catheter in cardiac surgery: a survey study. J Cardiothorac Vasc Anesth 2015;29(1):69–75.

148. Schwann NM, Hillel Z, Hoeft A, et al. Lack of effectiveness of the pulmonary artery catheter in cardiac surgery. Anesth Analg 2011;113(5):994–1002.

149. Schwann TA, Zacharias A, Riordan CJ, et al. Safe, highly selective use of pulmonary artery catheters in coronary artery bypass grafting: an objective patient selection method. Ann Thorac Surg 2002;73(5):1394–401.

150. Ranucci M. Which cardiac surgical patients can benefit from placement of a pulmonary artery catheter? Crit Care 2006;10(Suppl 3):S6.

151. Thiele RH, Bartels K, Gan TJ. Cardiac output monitoring: a contemporary assessment and review. Crit Care Med 2015;43(1):177–85.

152. Saugel B, Cecconi M, Wagner JY, et al. Noninvasive continuous cardiac output monitoring in perioperative and intensive care medicine. Br J Anaesth 2015;114(4):562–75.

153. Kenaan M, Gajera M, Goonewardena SN. Hemodynamic assessment in the contemporary intensive care unit: a review of circulatory monitoring devices. Crit Care Clin 2014;30(3):413–45.

154. Marik PE. Noninvasive cardiac output monitors: a state-of the-art review. J Cardiothorac Vasc Anesth 2013;27(1):121–34.

155. Sarosiek K, Kang CY, Johnson CM, et al. Perioperative use of the imacor hemodynamic transesophageal echocardiography probe in cardiac surgery patients: initial experience. ASAIO J 2014;60(5):553–8.

156. Treskatsch S, Balzer F, Knebel F, et al. Feasibility and influence of hTEE monitoring on postoperative management in cardiac surgery patients. Int J Cardiovasc Imaging 2015;31(7):1327–35.

157. Shoemaker WC. Cardiorespiratory patterns of surviving and nonsurviving postoperative patients. Surg Gynecol Obstet 1972;134(5):810–4.

158. Shoemaker WC, Appel PL, Kram HB, et al. Prospective trial of supranormal values of survivors as therapeutic goals in high-risk surgical patients. Chest 1988;94(6):1176–86.

159. Shoemaker WC, Patil R, Appel PL, et al. Hemodynamic and oxygen transport patterns for outcome prediction, therapeutic goals, and clinical algorithms to improve outcome. Feasibility of artificial intelligence to customize algorithms. Chest 1992;102(5 Suppl 2):617S–25S.

160. Giglio M, Dalfino L, Puntillo F, et al. Haemodynamic goal-directed therapy in cardiac and vascular surgery. A systematic review and meta-analysis. Interact Cardiovasc Thorac Surg 2012;15(5):878–87.

161. Aya HD, Cecconi M, Hamilton M, et al. Goal-directed therapy in cardiac surgery: a systematic review and meta-analysis. Br J Anaesth 2013;110(4):510–7.

162. Osawa EA, Rhodes A, Landoni G, et al. Effect of perioperative goal-directed hemodynamic resuscitation therapy on outcomes following cardiac surgery: a randomized clinical trial and systematic review. Crit Care Med 2016;44(4):724–33.

163. Peretto G, Durante A, Limite LR, et al. Postoperative arrhythmias after cardiac surgery: incidence, risk factors, and therapeutic management. Cardiol Res Pract 2014;2014:615987.

164. Gillinov AM, Bagiella E, Moskowitz AJ, et al. Rate control versus rhythm control for atrial fibrillation after cardiac surgery. N Engl J Med 2016;374(20):1911–21.

165. Chua SK, Shyu KG, Lu MJ, et al. Clinical utility of CHADS2 and CHA2DS2-VASc scoring systems for predicting postoperative atrial fibrillation after cardiac surgery. J Thorac Cardiovasc Surg 2013;146(4):919–26.

166. Lip GY, Lane DA. Stroke prevention in atrial fibrillation: a systematic review. JAMA 2015;313(19):1950–62.

167. Steinberg JS, Gaur A, Sciacca R, et al. New-onset sustained ventricular tachycardia after cardiac surgery. Circulation 1999;99(7):903–8.

168. Yeung-Lai-Wah JA, Qi A, McNeill E, et al. New-onset sustained ventricular tachycardia and fibrillation early after cardiac operations. Ann Thorac Surg 2004; 77(6):2083–8.

169. Steyers CM 3rd, Khera R, Bhave P. Pacemaker dependency after cardiac surgery: a systematic review of current evidence. PLoS One 2015;10(10): e0140340.

170. Reade MC. Temporary epicardial pacing after cardiac surgery: a practical review: part 1: general considerations in the management of epicardial pacing. Anaesthesia 2007;62(3):264–71.

171. Reade MC. Temporary epicardial pacing after cardiac surgery: a practical review. Part 2: Selection of epicardial pacing modes and troubleshooting. Anaesthesia 2007;62(4):364–73.

172. Price S, Prout J, Jaggar SI, et al. 'Tamponade' following cardiac surgery: terminology and echocardiography may both mislead. Eur J Cardiothorac Surg 2004; 26(6):1156–60.

173. Lomivorotov VV, Efremov SM, Kirov MY, et al. Low-cardiac-output syndrome after cardiac surgery. J Cardiothorac Vasc Anesth 2017;31(1):291–308.

174. Samuels LE, Darzé ES. Management of acute cardiogenic shock. Cardiol Clin 2003;21(1):43–9.

175. Werdan K, Gielen S, Ebelt H, et al. Mechanical circulatory support in cardiogenic shock. Eur Heart J 2014;35(3):156–67.

176. Ranucci M, Ballotta A, Castelvecchio S, et al, Surgical and Clinical Outcome REsearch (SCORE) Group. Perioperative heart failure in coronary surgery and timing of intra-aortic balloon pump insertion. Acta Anaesthesiol Scand 2010; 54(7):878–84.

177. Deschka H, Holthaus AJ, Sindermann JR, et al. Can perioperative right ventricular support prevent postoperative right heart failure in patients with biventricular dysfunction undergoing left ventricular assist device implantation? J Cardiothorac Vasc Anesth 2016;30(3):619–26.

178. Aissaoui N, Morshuis M, Schoenbrodt M, et al. Temporary right ventricular mechanical circulatory support for the management of right ventricular failure in critically ill patients. J Thorac Cardiovasc Surg 2013;146(1):186–91.

179. Adachi I, Khan MS, Guzmán-Pruneda FA, et al. Evolution and impact of ventricular assist device program on children awaiting heart transplantation. Ann Thorac Surg 2015;99(2):635–40.

180. Kirsch ME, Nguyen A, Mastroianni C, et al. SynCardia temporary total artificial heart as bridge to transplantation: current results at la pitié hospital. Ann Thorac Surg 2013;95(5):1640–6.
181. Acheampong B, Johnson JN, Stulak JM, et al. Postcardiotomy ECMO support after high-risk operations in adult congenital heart disease. Congenit Heart Dis 2016;11(6):751–5.
182. Argenziano M, Chen JM, Choudhri AF, et al. Management of vasodilatory shock after cardiac surgery: identification of predisposing factors and use of a novel pressor agent. J Thorac Cardiovasc Surg 1998;116(6):973–80.
183. Omar S, Zedan A, Nugent K. Cardiac vasoplegia syndrome: pathophysiology, risk factors and treatment. Am J Med Sci 2015;349(1):80–8.
184. Morales DL, Garrido MJ, Madigan JD, et al. A double-blind randomized trial: prophylactic vasopressin reduces hypotension after cardiopulmonary bypass. Ann Thorac Surg 2003;75(3):926–30.
185. Papadopoulos G, Sintou E, Siminelakis S, et al. Perioperative infusion of low-dose of vasopressin for prevention and management of vasodilatory vasoplegic syndrome in patients undergoing coronary artery bypass grafting-A double-blind randomized study. J Cardiothorac Surg 2010;5:17.
186. Egi M, Bellomo R, Langenberg C, et al. Selecting a vasopressor drug for vaso-plegic shock after adult cardiac surgery: a systematic literature review. Ann Thorac Surg 2007;83(2):715–23.
187. Lopez-Delgado JC, Esteve F, Javierre C, et al. Influence of cirrhosis in cardiac surgery outcomes. World J Hepatol 2015;7(5):753–60.
188. Thielmann M, Mechmet A, Neuhäuser M, et al. Risk prediction and outcomes in patients with liver cirrhosis undergoing open-heart surgery. Eur J Cardiothorac Surg 2010;38(5):592–9.
189. Rahman A, Agarwala R, Martin C, et al. Nutrition therapy in critically ill patients following cardiac surgery: defining and improving practice. JPEN J Parenter Enteral Nutr 2016. [Epub ahead of print].
190. Evans AS, Hosseinian L, Mohabir T, et al. Nutrition and the cardiac surgery intensive care unit patient–an update. J Cardiothorac Vasc Anesth 2015;29(4):1044–50.
191. Lomivorotov VV, Efremov SM, Boboshko VA, et al. Prognostic value of nutritional screening tools for patients scheduled for cardiac surgery. Interact Cardiovasc Thorac Surg 2013;16(5):612–8.
192. Berger MM, Revelly JP, Cayeux MC, et al. Enteral nutrition in critically ill patients with severe hemodynamic failure after cardiopulmonary bypass. Clin Nutr 2005;24(1):124–32.
193. Taylor BE, McClave SA, Martindale RG, et al. Guidelines for the provision and assessment of nutrition support therapy in the adult critically ill patient: society of critical care medicine (SCCM) and American Society for Parenteral and Enteral Nutrition (A.S.P.E.N.). Crit Care Med 2016;44(2):390–438.
194. Harvey SE, Parrott F, Harrison DA, et al, CALORIES Trial Investigators. Trial of the route of early nutritional support in critically ill adults. N Engl J Med 2014;371(18):1673–84.
195. Casaer MP, Mesotten D, Hermans G, et al. Early versus late parenteral nutrition in critically ill adults. N Engl J Med 2011;365(6):506–17.
196. Available at: http://www.sts.org/education-meetings/sts-webinar-series. Accessed October 31, 2017.
197. McDonnell ME, Alexanian SM, White L, et al. A primer for achieving glycemic control in the cardiac surgical patient. J Card Surg 2012;27(4):470–7.

198. Pezzella AT, Holmes SD, Pritchard G, et al. Impact of perioperative glycemic control strategy on patient survival after coronary bypass surgery. Ann Thorac Surg 2014;98(4):1281–5.

199. Ad N, Tran HA, Halpin L, et al. Practice changes in blood glucose management following open heart surgery: from a prospective randomized study to everyday practice. Eur J Cardiothorac Surg 2015;47(4):733–9.

200. Lobdell KW. Computerized euglycemia in cardiovascular and thoracic surgery. Ann Thorac Surg 2009;88(3):1048–9.

201. Stamou SC, Nussbaum M, Carew JD, et al. Hypoglycemia with intensive insulin therapy after cardiac surgery: predisposing factors and association with mortality. J Thorac Cardiovasc Surg 2011;142(1):166–73.

202. Brown JR, Hisey WM, Marshall EJ, et al. Acute kidney injury severity and long-term readmission and mortality after cardiac surgery. Ann Thorac Surg 2016; 102(5):1482–9.

203. Engoren M, Maile MD, Heung M, et al. The association between urine output, creatinine elevation, and death. Ann Thorac Surg 2016. http://dx.doi.org/10.1016/j.athoracsur.2016.07.036.

204. Thakar CV, Arrigain S, Worley S, et al. A clinical score to predict acute renal failure after cardiac surgery. J Am Soc Nephrol 2005;16:162–8.

205. Mehta RH, Grab JD, O'Brien SM, et al, Society of Thoracic Surgeons National Cardiac Surgery Database Investigators. Bedside tool for predicting the risk of postoperative dialysis in patients undergoing cardiac surgery. Circulation 2006;114:2208–16.

206. Jiang W, Teng J, Xu J, et al. Dynamic predictive scores for cardiac surgery-associated acute kidney injury. J Am Heart Assoc 2016;5(8). pii: e003754.

207. Thomson R, Meeran H, Valencia O, et al. Goal-directed therapy after cardiac surgery and the incidence of acute kidney injury. J Crit Care 2014;29(6): 997–1000.

208. Chen J, Zhang G, Wang C, et al. Predicting renal replacement therapy after cardiac valve surgery: external validation and comparison of two clinical scores. Interact Cardiovasc Thorac Surg 2016;23(6):869–975.

209. Pannu N, Graham M, Klarenbach S, et al, APPROACH Investigators and the Alberta Kidney Disease Network. A new model to predict acute kidney injury requiring renal replacement therapy after cardiac surgery. CMAJ 2016; 188(15):1076–83.

210. Liu Y, Davari-Farid S, Arora P, et al. Early versus late initiation of renal replacement therapy in critically ill patients with acute kidney injury after cardiac surgery: a systematic review and meta-analysis. J Cardiothorac Vasc Anesth 2014;28(3):557–63.

211. Elseviers MM, Lins RL, Van der Niepen P, et al, SHARF Investigators. Renal replacement therapy is an independent risk factor for mortality in critically ill patients with acute kidney injury. Crit Care 2010;14(6):R221.

212. Schwann TA, Habib JR, Khalifeh JM, et al. Effects of blood transfusion on cause-specific late mortality after coronary artery bypass grafting-less is more. Ann Thorac Surg 2016;102(2):465–73.

213. US Department of Health and Human Services. The 2007 Nationwide Blood Collection and Utilization Survey Report. 2007. Available at: https://wayback.archive-it.org/3919/20140402175908/http://www.hhs.gov/ash/bloodsafety/2007nbcus_survey.pdf. Accessed October 28, 2016.

214. Likosky DS, Paugh TA, Harrington SD, et al, Michigan Society of Thoracic and Cardiovascular Surgeons Quality Collaborative. Prediction of transfusions after

isolated coronary artery bypass grafting surgical procedures. Ann Thorac Surg 2017;103(3):764–72.

215. Horvath KA, Acker MA, Chang H, et al. Blood transfusion and infection after cardiac surgery. Ann Thorac Surg 2013;95(6):2194–201.

216. Society of Thoracic Surgeons Blood Conservation Guideline Task Force, Ferraris VA, Brown JR, et al. 2011 update to the Society of Thoracic Surgeons and the Society of cardiovascular anesthesiologists blood conservation clinical practice guidelines. Ann Thorac Surg 2011;91(3):944–82.

217. LaPar DJ, Crosby IK, Ailawadi G, et al, Investigators for the Virginia cardiac surgery quality initiative. Blood product conservation is associated with improved outcomes and reduced costs after cardiac surgery. J Thorac Cardiovasc Surg 2013;145(3):796–803.

218. Paone G, Brewer R, Likosky DS, et al, Membership of the Michigan society of thoracic and cardiovascular Surgeons. Transfusion rate as a quality metric: is blood conservation a learnable skill? Ann Thorac Surg 2013;96(4):1279–86.

219. Beattie WS, Karkouti K, Wijeysundera DN, et al. Risk associated with preoperative anemia in noncardiac surgery: a single-center cohort study. Anesthesiology 2009;110(3):574–81.

220. von Heymann C, Kaufner L, Sander M, et al. Does the severity of preoperative anemia or blood transfusion have a stronger impact on long-term survival after cardiac surgery? J Thorac Cardiovasc Surg 2016;152(5):1412–20.

221. Available at: http://www.uptodate.com/contents/anticoagulation-in-older-adults #H10666069. Accessed October 31, 2017.

222. Ferraris VA, Saha SP, Oestreich JH, et al, Society of Thoracic Surgeons. 2012 update to the Society of Thoracic Surgeons guideline on use of antiplatelet drugs in patients having cardiac and noncardiac operations. Ann Thorac Surg 2012;94(5):1761–81.

223. Lobdell KW, Stamou S, Sanchez JA. Hospital-acquired infections. Surg Clin North Am 2012;92(1):65–77.

224. Fowler VG Jr, O'Brien SM, Muhlbaier LH, et al. Clinical predictors of major infections after cardiac surgery. Circulation 2005;112(9 Suppl):I358–65.

225. Likosky DS, Wallace AS, Prager RL, et al. Sources of variation in hospital-level infection rates after coronary artery bypass grafting: an analysis of the society of thoracic surgeons adult heart surgery database. Ann Thorac Surg 2015; 100(5):1570–5.

226. Strobel RJ, Liang Q, Zhang M, et al, Michigan Society of Thoracic and Cardiovascular Surgeons Quality Collaborative. A preoperative risk model for postoperative pneumonia after coronary artery bypass grafting. Ann Thorac Surg 2016; 102(4):1213–9.

227. Shih T, Zhang M, Kommareddi M, et al, Michigan Society of Thoracic and Cardiovascular Surgeons Quality Collaborative. Center-level variation in infection rates after coronary artery bypass grafting. Circ Cardiovasc Qual Outcomes 2014;7(4):567–73.

228. Pronovost P, Needham D, Berenholtz S, et al. An intervention to decrease catheter-related bloodstream infections in the ICU. N Engl J Med 2006;355: 2725–32.

The Surgical Treatment of Coronary Artery Occlusive Disease

Modern Treatment Strategies for an Age Old Problem

Thomas A. Schwann, MD, MBA

KEYWORDS

- Coronary artery bypass grafting • Multiple arterial grafts
- Percutaneous coronary intervention • Practice guidelines

KEY POINTS

- Coronary artery disease remains a formidable challenge to clinicians and both percutaneous interventions and surgical techniques for myocardial revascularization continue to improve.
- In light of emerging data, multiple practice guidelines have been published to assist clinicians in their therapeutic decisions.
- The multidisciplinary Heart Team concept needs to be embraced by all cardiovascular providers to optimize patient outcomes.

THE HISTORICAL EVOLUTION OF CORONARY ARTERY BYPASS GRAFTING

Coronary artery disease (CAD) remains a significant public health problem in the United States and the Western world, accounting for substantial morbidity and mortality. Each year, 370,000 people die of CAD and 735,000 people suffer a myocardial infarction.[1] Coronary atherosclerosis has afflicted humanity throughout the ages and indeed was noted to be present in Egyptian mummies.[2] Surgical treatment of CAD began at the beginning of the 20th century with pioneering work of the Alexis Carrel, who first demonstrated a possible surgical option by performing the first descending aorta to coronary artery interposition graft using the carotid artery in a canine model.[3] Carrel went on to receive a Nobel Prize in Physiology and Medicine, partially based on this seminal contribution. Early surgical strategies in humans to

No conflict of interest to disclose.
Department of Surgery, University of Toledo College of Medicine & Life Sciences, 3000 Arlington Avenue, Toledo, OH 43614, USA
E-mail address: Thomas.Schwann@utoledo.edu

Surg Clin N Am 97 (2017) 835–865
http://dx.doi.org/10.1016/j.suc.2017.03.007
0039-6109/17/© 2017 Elsevier Inc. All rights reserved.

relieve angina included thoracic sympathectomy,[4] aorta to coronary sinus grafting,[5] and ligation of the distal left internal thoracic artery (LITA) with the hope that this maneuver will increase myocardial perfusion by shunting blood into the coronary circulation and away from the chest wall via the pericardiophrenic branch of the LITA.[6] Arthur Vineberg advanced the field of cardiac surgery by implanting the LITA into the left ventricular (LV) anterior wall in an effort to directly improve myocardial blood supply and relieve angina. Vineberg hypothesized that the implanted LITA would arborize and establish microcirculatory connections to the native coronary circulation and thus create a "third coronary artery."[7] After the development of coronary angiography in 1958 by Sones and Shirley,[8] a remarkably high LITA patency rate of 92% and a communication rate of 54% between the LITA and the coronary circulation was documented by investigators from the Cleveland Clinic in a report in the late 1960s.[9]

After the development of coronary angiography, direct coronary artery revascularization via coronary artery bypass grafting (CABG) became the dominant treatment of choice for coronary occlusive disease. Sabiston reported the first aortocoronary artery bypass in 1962[10] and, shortly thereafter, Kolessov and Potashov[11] described the first LITA to left anterior descending coronary artery bypass graft. Favalaro[12] popularized saphenous vein graft (SVG)-based CABG at the Cleveland Clinic as routine therapy for CAD, whereas Green[13] was an avid advocate of the routine use of LITA in CABG. Multiple studies in the early 1980s established the specific role and efficacy of CABG and more clearly defined its indications: Coronary Artery Surgery Study (CASS), the European Coronary Artery Bypass Trial, and the Veterans Administration Coronary Artery Bypass Trial.[14–16]

Percutaneous coronary angioplasty was introduced in 1977[17] and was found to have a relatively reasonable safety profile.[18] Percutaneous coronary angioplasty rapidly grew in popularity, eventually supplanting CABG as the dominant form of coronary revascularization. The percutaneous approach to CAD underwent multiple iterations, with the development of bare metal stenting, which was followed shortly thereafter by the introduction of drug-eluting stents into routine clinical practice. Thus, percutaneous coronary angioplasty (PTCA) was replaced by percutaneous coronary intervention (PCI). These improvements decreased target vessel restenosis rates, but at the cost of catastrophic stent thrombosis despite dual antiplatelet therapy.

Comparison of outcomes of CABG versus PCI was extensively studied in the late 1990's and early 2000's. Multiple randomized, prospective studies were published and the results consistently showed equipoise between the two revascularization modalities.[19–27] Uniformly, these analyses were underpowered to detect differences in outcomes, enrolled a highly selected study groups (frequently <5% of those screened were included in the study populations) and excluded higher risk patients (those with diabetes mellitus, multivessel coronary disease, and impaired ventricular function) in whom the benefits of CABG were well-defined. The documented equivalent outcomes between PCI and CABG in these highly selected study cohorts were inappropriately generalized across all patient demographics and this, in part, underpinned the rapid growth of PCI techniques. Recently, additional retrospective as well as prospective analyses reflective of more real-life coronary revascularization practice patterns, such as the SYNTAX (Synergy Between Percutaneous Coronary Intervention With TAXUS and Cardiac Surgery) Trial,[28,29] the FREEDOM (Future Revascularization Evaluation in Patients with Diabetes Mellitus: Optimal Management of Multi Vessel Disease) Trial,[30] CARDia (Coronary Artery Revascularization in Diabetes) Study[31] and the ASCERT (ACCF and STS Database Collaboration on the Comparative Effectiveness of Revascularization Strategies) Trial[32] have been instrumental in elucidating the patient subcohorts that derive best long-term outcomes with either CABG or PCI. In contradistinction with the older studies, the more recent trials have found a consistent, improved long-term survival in higher risk patients with CAD of CABG compared with PCI. Based in part on these data, multiple practice guidelines have been formulated with the specific intent of informing practitioners regarding the optimal revascularization options for patients based on preoperative patient characteristics and complexity of their CAD.[33–36] Currently, CABG and PCI are appropriately viewed as complimentary rather than competitive therapeutic alternatives.

In an effort to improve patient-centered outcomes after CABG, a transition from all saphenous vein coronary grafting to increased reliance on arterial grafts as conduits for myocardial revascularization has taken place over the last 3 decades. This modification was initially based on the seminal work of Loop and associates[37] and subsequently corroborated by Edwards and colleagues,[38] using data from the emerging Society of Thoracic Surgery Adult Cardiac Surgery Database, and other investigators reporting similarly superior outcomes with the use of a single arterial graft in the form of the LITA with supplemental SVG.[39–42] These studies uniformly identified a decreased perioperative mortality and a long-term survival advantage of adding the LITA to SVG and the conclusions were compelling enough to establish the use of LITA in CABG surgery as a benchmark of quality by the Society of Thoracic Surgeons (STS). The adoption of the LITA into standard practice was relatively slow, with significant regional differences, such that only 75.6% to 88.6% of Medicare patients[43] and 92.4% of all patients[44] underwent CABG with a single LITA in the first decade of the 21st century. More recent advances in CABG surgery focused on the incremental survival benefits of multiple arterial grafts in the form of bilateral internal thoracic artery (BITA) grafting[45–51] or in the form of radial artery (RA) as the second arterial graft in conjunction with LITA,[52–58] with or without additional supplemental SVG. Indeed, multiple arterial CABG (MABG) has been shown to be a superior grafting strategy compared with single arterial CABG (SABG) or PCI.[59]

CURRENT EVIDENCE-BASED CORONARY ARTERY BYPASS GRAFTING BEST PRACTICE GUIDELINES

Optimal outcomes of CABG are predicated on the following factors: (1) judicious patient selection designed to optimize long-term benefits of myocardial revascularization (CABG vs PCI) while minimizing perioperative morbidity and mortality and (2) appropriate grafting strategy with preferential use of arterial over venous conduits facilitating a complete versus incomplete myocardial revascularization.

Optimal Patient Selection for Coronary Artery Bypass Grafting Versus Percutaneous Coronary Intervention in Stable Ischemic Heart Disease

There has been considerable debate about the best treatment modality for patients with stable ischemic heart disease (SIHD) with 10 observational studies comparing CABG with PCI using drug-eluting stents, which constitutes the best percutaneous technology.[32,60–68] Most of these involved a relatively short follow-up period and reported conflicting results. In a meta analysis of more than 24,000 patients with severe triple vessel CAD, the rate of death or myocardial infarction was equivalent, albeit with a significantly higher reintervention rate among PCI patients.[69] Recently, the following large comparative outcome studies defined specific patient populations that benefit most from CABG.

The SYNTAX (Synergy Between Percutaneous Coronary Intervention With TAXUS and Cardiac Surgery) Trial
The SYNTAX score is a tool that allows for a reproducible quantitative assessment of the degree and complexity of coronary atherosclerosis and is a useful tool for

therapeutic decision making between surgical and percutaneous revascularization options.[29] The SYNTAX study was a multi institutional, prospective, randomized study of patients who were candidates for either CABG or PCI using drug-eluting stents. In this study, 1800 patients were randomized and their degree of CAD was calculated by the SYNTAX score, which incorporated among other factors, the degree of coronary stenosis, its complexity and its location. A web-based application enabled the calculation of the SYNTAX Score (**Table 1**). The patients were divided into terciles based on their SYNTAX scores: low tercile was a score of less than 22, intermediate tercile was a score between 22 and 33, and high tercile was a score of greater than 33. At 5 years, CABG was associated with a significantly lower rate of major adverse cardiac and cardiovascular events (MACCE; 26.9% in the CABG group and 37.3% in the PCI group; P<.0001). The rate of myocardial infarctions (3.8% in the CABG group vs 9.7% in the PCI group; P<.0001) and repeat revascularizations (13.7% in the CABG group and 25.9% in the PCI group; P<.0001) were significantly higher with PCI. In patients with intermediate and high SYNTAX scores, MACCE was significantly higher in the PCI group versus the CABG group (intermediate SYNTAX score, 25.8% in the CABG group and 36.0% in the PCI group [P = .008], high SYNTAX score, 26.8% in the CABG group and 44.0% in the PCI group [P<.0001]). The occurrence of MACCE correlated with the SYNTAX score in PCI patients only and there was no such correlation with CABG. The differences in MACCE between those treated with PCI and CABG increased with an increasing SYNTAX scores. A clear overall survival benefit was noted in the CABG group in patients with high SYNTAX scores (11.4% mortality rate in the CABG group and a 19.2% mortality rate in the PCI group; P = .005]). Thus, in patients with mild CAD, PCI is a reasonable therapeutic option, whereas in patients with moderate or severe CAD, CABG is the optimal treatment if the operative risk is not prohibitive.

ASCERT (ACCF and STS Database Collaboration on the Comparative Effectiveness of Revascularization Strategies) Trial

The ASCERT Trial was a collaborative outcomes study linking the American College of Cardiology Foundation National Cardiovascular Data Registry (CathPCI Registry) and the Society of Thoracic Surgeons Adult Cardiac Surgery Database to the claims data from the Centers of Medicare and Medicaid Services for the years between 2004 and 2008. Long-term outcomes between CABG and PCI were compared in Medicare patients older than 65 using inverse probability weighting based on propensity scores as a risk adjustment methodology. The patient records were matched using probabilistic matching techniques (based on the patients date of birth, sex, hospital identification number, admission date, and discharge date) obviating the need for specific patient identifiers. The study cohort included patients with double and triple vessel CAD. Patients with an acute myocardial infarction were excluded. A total of 86,244 CABG patients were matched with 103,549 PCI patients. The median follow-up was 2.67 years. Patients undergoing PCI received drug-eluting stents in 78% of cases, bare metal stents in 16% of cases, and 6% received no stents. At the 1-year follow-up, there were no differences in adjusted mortality rates (6.24% for CABG patients and 6.55% for the PCI group; risk ratio, 0.95; 95% confidence interval, 0.90–1.00). At the 4-year follow-up, the CABG group showed a statistically significant lower mortality compared with the PCI group (16.4% vs 20.8%; risk ratio, 0.79; 95% confidence interval, 0.76–0.82). Importantly, this CABG-associated survival advantage was seen across multiple CABG subgroups based on sex, age, presence or absence of diabetes, body mass index, presence or absence of chronic lung disease, ejection fraction, and glomerular filtration rate, and in both high-risk and low-risk surgical groups. Thus, this large observational study, reflecting the real life treatment patterns from national datasets, with a relatively short follow-up period documents a clear survival advantage of CABG over PCI. Other important endpoints, such as MACCE, including reintervention rates and costs were not available.

CARDia (Coronary Artery Revascularization in Diabetes) Study

The CARDia study was a randomized, prospective, 24-center trial from the United Kingdom PCI versus CABG non-inferiority outcome study in 510 diabetic patients with symptomatic multivessel CAD. At the relatively short 1-year follow-up, there was a nonsignificantly higher rate of composite outcomes of death, myocardial infarction, and stroke (driven principally by a higher rate of myocardial infarction) and a significantly higher rates of repeat revascularization in the PCI group. The prespecified noninferiority margin for PCI was met. The mortality rates in both treatment groups were equivalent and the stroke risk was nonsignificantly lower in the PCI group.

The indications for surgical myocardial revascularization continue to evolve as both surgical techniques and percutaneous techniques evolve and improve. There has been significant progress in the development of multiple practice guideline defining specific patient cohorts, based on patient demographics and degree as well as complexity of coronary atherosclerotic lesions, that are best treated with either CABG or PCI.[33–36]

What frequently in the past was a unilateral therapeutic decision by either the cardiologist or the cardiac surgeon, has now been delegated to a multidisciplinary Heart Team as the best mechanism for directing the optimal therapy for each individual patient.[35,70] The Heart Team, composed of both an interventional cardiologist, a cardiac surgeon and other providers is tasked with reviewing the patient's pertinent medical history including the coronary anatomy and based on these, selecting the optimal therapeutic alternative and together articulating that recommendation to the patient. In addition, recent emphasis on shared decision making between patients and providers has been articulated, with physicians serving as content experts while the patient deciding what outcome is of primary importance to them. The concept of the Heart Team has been incorporated into multiple recent comparative outcomes studies, including the SYNTAX and FREEDOM trials.[29,30] The Heart Team must critically assess the expected benefits of an intervention (enhanced survival, improved quality of life, or relief of symptomatology) and weight these against the periprocedural and long-term risks (death, myocardial infarctions, strokes, repeat revascularizations, infections, bleeding, etc) while also considering such region-specific factors as operator and institutional experience and outcomes. The Heart Team maybe aided by objective, empirically derived, and well-validated risk stratification tools such as the Society of Thoracic Surgery Peri-operative Risk Model[71] and the EuroScore II Model[72] to assess perioperative risk of mortality and morbidity, the SYNTAX Score[73] to assess the complexity and severity of coronary lesions, and the National Cardiovascular Database Registry (NCDR CathPCI) Risk Score[74] to predict risk in PCI patients. Although helpful in establishing an objective level of risk associated with an intervention, these tools remain underused in clinical practice because they are complex and somewhat cumbersome, and have not been unified into a universally accepted single tool. Attempts at refining their usefulness are progressing with the development of the SYNTAX II Score incorporating patient demographics and coronary lesion characteristics into a single tool.[75] It must be remembered that no model will be able to predict outcomes for any single individual, but only for a group of patients. In addition, as more data points become available in the increasingly comprehensive and complex registries, additional elements will need to be entered into the decision making matrix such as patient frailty, for example. To present patients with a full assessment of the impact of a given intervention,

Table 1
SYNTAX score calculator

Steps	Variable Assessed	Description
Step 1	Dominance	The weight of individual coronary segments varies according to coronary artery dominance (right or left). Codominance does not exist as an option in the SYNTAX score.
Step 2	Coronary segment	The diseased coronary segment directly affects the score as each coronary segment is assigned a weight, depending on its location, ranging from 0.5 (ie, posterolateral branch) to 6 (ie, left main in case of left dominance)

Step 3	Diameter stenosis	The score of each diseased coronary segment is multiplied by 2 in case of a stenosis 50%–99% and by 5 in case of total occlusion.
		In case of total occlusion, additional points will be added as follows:
		Age >3 mo or unknown +1
		Blunt stump +1
		Bridging +1
		First segment visible distally +1 per nonvisible segment
		Side branch at the occlusion +1 if <1.5 mm diameter
		+1 if both <1.5 and ≥1.5 mm diameter
		+0 if ≥1.5 mm diameter (ie, bifurcation lesion)
Step 4	Trifurcation lesion	The presence of a trifurcation lesion adds additional points based on the number of diseased segments:
		1 segment +3
		2 segments +4
		3 segments +5
		4 segments +6
Step 5	Bifurcation lesion	The presence of a bifurcation lesion adds additional points based on the type of bifurcation according to the Medina classification.[29]
		Medina 1,0,0 or 0,1,0 or 1,1,0: add 1 additional point
		Medina 1,1,1 or 0,0,1 or 1,0,1 or 0,1,1: add 2 additional points
		Additionally, the presence of a bifurcation angle <70° adds 1 additional point
Step 6	Aortoostial lesion	The presence of aortoostial lesion segments adds 1 additional point.
Step 7	Severe tortuosity	The presence of severe tortuosity proximal of the diseased segment adds 2 additional points.
Step 8	Lesion length	Lesion length >20 mm adds 1 additional point.
Step 9	Calcification	The presence of heavy calcification adds 2 additional points.
Step 10	Thrombus	The presence of thrombus adds 1 additional point.
Step 11	Diffuse disease/small vessels	The presence of diffusely diseased and narrowed segments distal to the lesion (ie, when at least 75% of the length of the segment distal to the lesion has a vessel diameter of <2 mm) adds 1 point per segment number.

Data from Windecker S, Kolh P, Alfonso F, et al. 2014 ESC/EACTS guidelines on myocardial revascularization. Eur Heart J 2014;35:2541–619.

the risks of the associated underlying pathologic condition without treatment must also be considered. Unfortunately, our understanding of this is rather rudimentary at best; currently, there are no clinically based registries designed to gather these data, and administrative databases pose significant and well-described limitations. Perhaps large datasets embedded in the evolving transition into electronic medical records may yield valuable information through artificial intelligence tools such as IBM's Watson. Increased attention to patient reported outcomes are also likely to impact future refinements of currently available practice guidelines. Unfortunately until the risk models for interventions as well as the natural history of non surgically or percutaneously treated SIHD are further refined and integrated and until more robust patient self reported outcomes become available, the Heart Team of today will need to continue to relay principally on subjective factors in choosing the optimal therapeutic option for patients using clinical judgment and robust inter-disciplinary dialogue as the central basis for decision making in the face of ambiguity. The degree to which the Heart Team concept is incorporated into clinical practice patterns across the United States remains a subject of considerable debate with ongoing considerations of novel reimbursement systems rewarding a greater reliance on the Heart team for clinical decision making.

A decision tree for optimal therapy for patients with multi-vessel SIHD is provided in **Fig. 1**. A summary of latest best practice guidelines of multiple professional societies for patients with SIHD is summarized in **Table 2**.

UNPROTECTED LEFT MAIN CORONARY ARTERY STENOSIS

Traditionally, patients with significant left main (LM) coronary artery lesions were advised to undergo CABG, but recent emerging data suggest equipoise between CABG and PCI in selected patients with LM coronary artery lesions with equivalent clinically relevant outcome data up to 5 years after the intervention. Significant LM luminal stenosis have been identified in 4% of patients undergoing angiographic evaluation and 80% of these patients have additional 3-vessel atherosclerotic burden.[76] In the SYNTAX Trial, in patients with LM lesions, the outcomes with PCI compared with CABG were noninferior. The clinical endpoints were equivalent in patients with isolated LM lesions or in patients with LM lesions and uncomplicated CAD as evidenced by a SYNTAX score of less than 22. Because the overall primary endpoint of the SYNTAX Trail was not met (noninferiority of PCI vs CABG) any subcohort analysis must, however, be interpreted with caution. In addition, 45% of screened patients with LM lesions had such severity and complexity of coronary disease that they were unable to be randomized and 89% of them underwent CABG. In contradistinction, 705 patients with LM lesions of the 1800 overall patient study cohort were able to be randomized between CABG and PCI. Most LM lesion patients with a low SYNTAX score had single vessel CAD or isolated LM disease. Those with an intermediate SYNTAX score had 2-vessel CAD, and those with a high SYNTAX score had triple vessel CAD. At the 5-year follow-up, there was little difference in outcomes between CABG and PCI in low or intermediate SYNTAX scores. In high SYNTAX score LM lesion patients, a significantly higher rate of MACCE was documented in the PCI cohort versus the CABG cohorts, 46.5% and 29.7%, respectively ($P = .003$).[29] Other, smaller, randomized, prospective trials reported similar outcomes, albeit only on shorter term follow-up.[77,78] In the LE MANS (Study of Unprotected Left Main Stenting vs Bypass Surgery) Trial involving 105 patients randomized between surgery and PCI, there were no appreciable differences between the 2 study groups at either 30 days or 2 years. Importantly only 35% of patients in the PCI group received optimal therapy with drug-eluting stents and only 72% of the CABG cohort received even 1 internal thoracic artery graft. In the PRECOMBAT

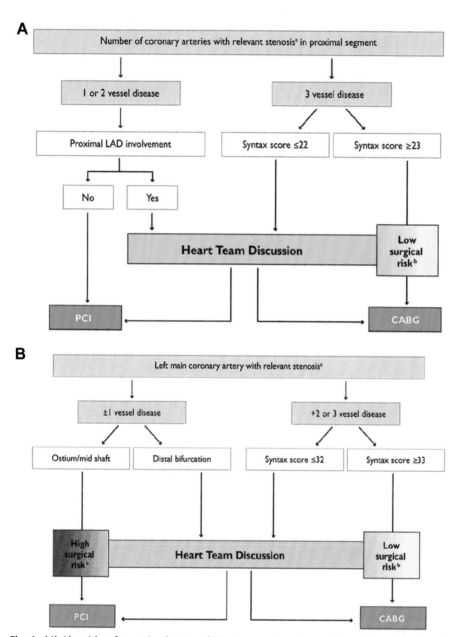

Fig. 1. (*A*) Algorithm for optimal revascularization strategy in patients with stable ischemic heart disease without left main coronary involvement. (*B*) Algorithm for optimal revascularization strategy in patients with stable ischemic heart disease with left main coronary involvement. [a] Greater than 50% stenosis and proof of ischemia, greater than 90% stenosis in 2 angiographic views or fractional flow reserve of less than 0.080. [b] Coronary artery bypass grafting (CABG) is the preferred option in most patients unless patients' comorbidities or specificities deserve discussion by the Heart Team. LAD, left anterior descending artery; PCI, percutaneous coronary intervention. (*From* Kolh P, Kurlansky P, Cremer J, et al. Transatlantic Editorial: a comparison between European and North American guidelines on myocardial revascularization. Eur J Cardiothorac Surg 2016;49:1307–17; with permission.)

Table 2
ACCF/AHA and ESC/EACTS guidelines on myocardial revascularization

	ACCF/AHA 2011 (Hillis et al[34])	ACC/AHA 2014 Focused Update (Fihn et al[70])	ESC/EACTS 2014 (Windecker et al[35])
Unprotected LM or complex CAD	Class I, LOE C: Heart Team. Class IIa, LOE B: SYNTAX score.		Multidisciplinary decision making required for multivessel stable CAD. Class I, LOE C: Institutional protocols are developed by the Heart Team to implement appropriate revascularization strategy in accordance with guidelines.
Unprotected LM	Class I, LOE B: CABG. Class IIa, LOE B: PCI when both: low risk PCI procedural complications with high likelihood of good long-term outcome (SYNTAX score <22, ostial or mid segment LM) and clinical characteristics predict significantly increased surgical risk (STS predicted operative mortality >5%). Class IIB, LOE B: PCI when both anatomic conditions associated with low or intermediate risk PCI procedure complications and intermediate to high likelihood of good long-term outcome (SYNTAX score <33, bifurcation LM disease) and clinical characteristics that predict increased risk of adverse surgical outcomes (moderate to severe COPD, disability from previous stroke, prior cardiac surgery, STS predicted operative mortality >2%). Class III, LOE B: harm when PCI chosen in patients with unfavorable anatomy for PCI and who are good candidates for CABG.		SYNTAX Score <22: class I, LOE B for CABG, class I, LOE B for PCI. SYNTAX Score 23–32: class I, LOE B for CABG, class IIA, LOE B for PCI. SYNTAX score >32: class I, LOE B for CABG, class III, LOE B for PCI.

Condition		
Three-vessel CAD with or without proximal LAD disease	Class I, LOE B for CABG. Class IIa, LOE B: CABG reasonable over PCI with complex 3-vessel CAD (SYNTAX score >22) who are good candidates for CABG. Class IIb, LOE B: PCI of uncertain benefit.	SYNTAX score <22: class I, LOE A for CABG; class I, LOE B for PCI. SYNTAX score 23–32: class I, LOE A for CABG, class III, LOE B for PCI (HARM for PCI). SYNTAX score >32: class I, LOE A for CABG, class III, LOE B for PCI (HARM for PCI).
Two-vessel CAD with proximal LAD disease	Class I, LOE B for CABG. Class IIb, LOE B: PCI of uncertain benefit.	Class I, LOE B for CABG. Class I, LOE C for PCI.
Two-vessel CAD without proximal LAD disease	Class IIa, LOE B for CABG if extensive ischemia is present. Class IIb, LOE C: CABG of uncertain benefit without extensive ischemia is present. Class IIb, LOE B: PCI of uncertain benefit.	Class I, LOA C: PCI. Class IIb, LOE C: CABG.
One-vessel with proximal LAD disease	Class IIa, LOE B for CABG with LIMA for long-term benefit. Class IIb, LOE B: PCI of uncertain benefit.	Class I, LOA A: PCI. Class I, LOA A: CABG.
One vessel without proximal LAD disease	Class III, LOE B; CABG (HARM CABG). Class III, LOE B; PCI (HARM PCI).	Class IIb, LOE C: CABG. Class I, LOE C: PCI.

(continued on next page)

Table 2
(continued)

	ACCF/AHA 2011 (Hillis et al[34])	ACC/AHA 2014 Focused Update (Fihn et al[70])	ESC/EACTS 2014 (Windecker et al[35])
Diabetic patients	Class IIa, LOE B: CABG reasonable over PCI to improve survival in patients with multivessel CAD and DM, particularly if LIMA used to the LAD.	Class I, LOE B: CABG is generally preferred vs PCI to improve survival in patients with DM and multivessel CAD for which revascularization is likely to improve survival (3-vessel CAD or complex 2-vessel CAD involving the proximal LAD), particularly if LIMA can be anastomosed to LAD, provided that patient is a good candidate for surgery. Class I, LOE C: a Heart Team approach to revascularization is recommended in patients with DM and complex multivessel CAD.	Class I, LOE A: patients with multivessel CAD and acceptable surgical risk: CABG recommended over PCI. Class IIa, LOE B patients with multivessel CAD and SYNTAX score <22: PCI should be considered as alternative to CABG.

Abbreviations: ACC, American College of Cardiology; ACCF, American College of Cardiology Foundation; AHA, American Heart Association; CABG, coronary artery bypass grafting; CAD, coronary artery disease; COPD, chronic obstructive pulmonary disease; DM, diabetes mellitus; EACTS, European Association for Cardio-Thoracic Surgery; ESC, European Society of Cardiology; LAD, left anterior descending artery; LM, left main; LOE, level of evidence; PCI, percutaneous coronary intervention; STS, Society of Thoracic Surgeons.
Data from Refs.[34,35,70]

(Premier of Randomized Comparison of Bypass Surgery vs Angioplasty Using Sirolimus-Eluting Stents in Patients With Left Main Coronary Artery Disease) study, 600 patients were randomized between surgical and percutaneous techniques. The 2-year MACCE rates were uniformly excellent with either technique: 4.4% with drug-eluting stents and 4.7% with CABG, but repeat revascularization rates were significantly higher in PCI patients compared with CABG patients, at 9.0% and 4.2%, respectively ($P = .02$). The authors conclude that PCI was noninferior to CABG; however, given the wide noninferiority margin, the results should not be considered clinically directive. Equipoise between CABG and PCI was also noted in observational studies.[79] In a metaanalysis of 3773 patients from observational studies and randomized trials,[80] MACCE rates were equivalent at 1, 2, and 3 years of follow-up. The revascularization rates were significantly higher in PCI patients than in CABG patients: 1-year odds ratio of 4.36, 2-year odds ratio of 4.20, and 3-year odds ratio of 3.30. Cumulatively, these data suggest, but do not definitively prove, that PCI and CABG result in equivalent outcomes in selected patients with uncomplicated LM CAD and have been incorporated into practice guidelines specifying PCI as a reasonable therapeutic choice, especially in patients with an unfavorable acute perioperative risk profile for CABG (see **Table 2**).

Patients with Diabetes Mellitus

Diabetic patients with CAD have a higher risk of adverse cardiovascular outcomes than patients without diabetes[54] and there is growing body of data with most, but not all, studies supporting CABG as the optimal revascularization strategy in this demographic. The pivotal FREEDOM trial randomized 1900 patients to drug-eluting stents PCI or CABG.[30] The 5-year composite endpoint of death, nonfatal myocardial infarction, and nonfatal stroke was significantly better with CABG than PCI at 18.7% and 26.6%, respectively ($P = .005$). The CABG benefit was driven both by a reduction in the rate of myocardial infarction (6.0% vs 13.9%; $P<.001$) and death (10.9% vs 16.3%; $P = .049$). The risk of stroke was higher in the CABG group with the 5 year rate of 2.4% in the PCI group and 5.2% in the CABG group ($P = .03$).

Other studies also support superior outcomes of CABG versus PCI in diabetics including the BARI (Bypass Angioplasty Revascularization Investigation) study[81] and the BARI-2D (BARI in Type 2 Diabetes) study.[82] In a collaborative analysis of 10 randomized studies comparing CABG against PCI,[83] CABG was found to favorably impact the survival of diabetic patients with a hazard ratio of 0.70 and a 95% confidence interval of 0.56 to 0.87. CABG was also found to be superior to PCI in a meta-analysis of 8 randomized trials comprising 3131 patients, with CABG decreasing long-term mortality by one-third.[84] Other studies, however, have found no surgical therapeutic advantage compared with CABG. The 5-year results of a diabetic subcohort of the SYNTAX trial showed equivalent mortality with CABG and PCI, at 12.9% and 19.5%, respectively ($P = .065$).[85] Similarly, a meta analysis of 4 trials[86] showed equivalent mortality with either modality (CABG 7.9%, PCI 12.4%; $P = .09$).

In summary, the preponderance of data supports the superiority of CABG over PCI in diabetic patients with stable CAD and has been given a class I recommendation in the 2014 American College of Cardiology/American Heart Association/American Association for Thoracic Surgery/Preventive Cardiovascular Nurses Association/Society for Cardiovascular Angiography and Interventions/STS Focused Update of the Guidelines for Patients with Stable Ischemic Heart Disease[70] as well as the European Association for Cardio-Thoracic Surgery and the European Society of Cardiology 2014 Guidelines on Myocardial Revascularization.[87] The European guidelines set a class IIa recommendation for PCI in diabetics with a low SYNTAX score.

Patients with Left Ventricular Dysfunction

LV dysfunction is a frequently encountered problem by cardiac surgeons. Despite the increased perioperative risk and diminished long-term survival associated with LV dysfunction,[71,88,89] CABG remains a viable option in many patients,[90–94] because patients with more advanced LV dysfunction derive the most benefit from CABG.[95,96] CABG has been found to be superior to medical therapy[90,93,95,96] in part owing to the finding that up to 30% of sudden cardiac deaths in patients with LV dysfunction are attributed to acute coronary events,[97] an outcome likely mitigated by CABG. CABG has also been shown to improve the 1, 5, 10, and 15-year survival rates compared with PCI in patients with LV dysfunction.[98] Surgical revascularization in patients with ischemic cardiomyopathy can be accomplished with acceptable perioperative mortality and a concomitant improvement in the patients' functional status and cardiac function.[91–94,96] Improvements in perioperative techniques have decreased early CABG mortality even in patients with a LV ejection fraction of less than 30% from as high as 5.3% to 6.9%[91,99] to 2.3% in a recent analysis from the STS database.[94] Topkara and colleagues[100] reported an in-hospital mortality rate of 6.5% in patients with an LV ejection fraction of less than 20% versus 1.4% in patients with an LV ejection fraction of greater than 40%. Despite these findings, the STITCH (Surgical Treatment for Ischemic Heart Failure) trial,[101] which compared CABG with medical therapy, did not show improved long-term all-cause mortality with surgical therapy (36% vs 41%; $P = .12$). Importantly, however, CABG did positively effect a number of secondary endpoints, such as cardiovascular mortality (28% vs 33%; $P = .05$) and cardiovascular rehospitalization (58% vs 68%; $P<.001$). In addition, in an as-treated analysis[93] that controlled for patient crossover between therapeutic modality, CABG resulted in a reduction in all-cause mortality (33% vs 44%; $P<.001$). A 10-year follow-up report[102] found that CABG was associated with reduced all cause mortality (58.9% vs 66.1%; $P = .02$) and cardiovascular mortality (40.5% vs 49.3%; $P = .006$), as well as the composite outcome of death and cardiovascular rehospitalization (76.6% vs 87.0%; $P<.001$). As in the general CABG population, the use of multiple arterial grafts in patients with diminished LV ejection fraction also results in improved survival and has been noted with the BITA grafting strategy[45] or with the use of the RA as a second arterial conduit in conjunction with the LITA.[103]

CORONARY REVASCULARIZATION IN PATIENTS WITH ACUTE CORONARY SYNDROMES

The recommendations and indications for CABG in patients with stable coronary disease are frequently extended to patient with either non–ST-segment elevation myocardial infarction (NSTEMI) or ST-segment elevation (STEMI) myocardial infarction, although the data supporting them are lacking. Indeed, 60% of CABG operations are performed in the setting of an acute hospitalization for unstable symptoms and a full 29% are performed in the immediate postinfarct period (STS Research Center, http://www.STS.org/documents, personal communication, 2016). Although PCI remains the principal therapeutic modality in the vast majority of patients with unstable coronary syndromes, CABG nevertheless is an important fall back strategy in the event that the coronary anatomy is not suitable for PCI, those with a complication of PCI, or in those patients who, in addition to myocardial revascularization, require surgical intervention for a mechanical complication of an ischemic myocardial insult, such as a ventricular septal defect or rupture of ventricular free wall, or those who develop acute mitral regurgitation secondary to papillary muscle rupture.

Optimal Coronary Artery Bypass Grafting Strategy

Multiple arterial grafts: More is better

LITA-based CABG with supplemental SVG has been the gold standard for surgical myocardial revascularization since the early 1990s when the STS leadership chose LITA grafting as a benchmark of clinical excellence and third party payers tied more favorable reimbursement to LITA based single arterial CABG (SABG) compared to using saphenous vein grafts exclusively. The observed long-term improved survival[37,40] and decreased perioperative mortality[40] associated with SABG has been attributed to the superior patency of arterial grafts compared with venous grafts.[104–110] Over the past 2 decades, there has emerged remarkably consistent data that MABG improves long-term survival compared with SABG. The two most common conduits used in conjunction with the gold standard LITA to achieve MABG are the right internal thoracic artery (RITA) resulting in BITA configuration (BITA-MABG) and the RA (RA-MABG). The gastroepiploic artery is used rarely in the United States, but more liberally in Asia. Importantly, compared with SABG, there have been no reports of adverse impact on survival of patients undergoing MABG. The published practice guidelines support the use of MABG. The 2011 American College of Cardiology Foundation/American Heart Association Guideline for Coronary Artery Bypass Graft Surgery (class IIb recommendation, level of evidence [LOE] B for RA; class IIa recommendation, LOE B for BITA), the European Society of Cardiology/European Association for Cardio-Thoracic Surgery Guidelines on Myocardial Revascularization (class I recommendation, LOE B for RA; class IIa recommendation, LOE B for BITA) and the Society of Thoracic Surgeons Clinical Practice Guidelines on Arterial Conduits for Coronary Artery Bypass Grafting (class IIa, LOE B for RA; class IIa recommendation, LOE B for BITA) uniformly recommend MABG.[34–36] Indeed, the data are compelling enough for some surgical experts to call for MABG to be considered the new benchmark of quality.[111] Despite these data, the surgical community has been slow to adopt this grafting technique into their armamentarium and its penetration into clinical practice is currently mediocre at best. In the United States, more than 90% of CABG patients still undergo SABG (STS Research Center, http://www.STS.org/documents, personal communication, 2016). Similarly, only 12% of patients in one Canadian province received more than 1 arterial graft,[112] and only 15% of patients in the Society for Cardiothoracic Surgery in Great Britain and Ireland received more than one arterial graft while 5% received 3 or more.[113] These data reflecting the overall general practice patterns of cardiac surgeons stand in stark contrast with other clinicians with an interest in MABG, who report substantially higher BITA MABG rates. Puskas and colleagues[47] reported a BITA MABG use rate of 23% and Kurlansky and colleagues[46] reported a BITA use rate of 48%. Locker and colleagues[48] reported a MABG use rate of 13.8% in Mayo Clinic patients. American RA enthusiasts have reported RA use rates of between 60% and 80%,[114,115] with excellent long-term clinical outcomes and no increased acute perioperative morbidity or mortality.

The principal obstacle against the wider adoption of MABG techniques into clinical practice stem from the lack of supportive prospective, randomized studies and questions regarding the generalizability to the general CABG population of observational data from institutions that have a dedication to and an expertise in MABG. In addition, although the increased technical complexity of MABG and concerns regarding the well-described sternal wound complications in case of BITA grafting,[51,116] a "never event" designated by the Center for Medicare & Medicaid Services, may be compelling factors in preventing a more extensive adoption of MABG into routine practice, in face of the documented patient survival benefits, the discrepancy between evidence-based literature and practice is difficult to reconcile. Thus, arguably, a significant number of CABG patients maybe deprived of optimal therapy. Tranbaugh and colleagues[114] estimated that, compared with the current low use of MABG in the general American CABG population a more robust MABG use rate might well result in 10,000 fewer deaths and an additional 64,000 person-years of life over the course of a decade. It should be remembered that the transition from all SVG CABG to the current gold standard of single arterial, LITA-based, CABG occurred without prospective, randomized data. The ART (Arterial Revascularization Trial) study is currently enrolling patients with the aim of comparing long-term survival outcomes between BITA-MABG and SABG in a randomized, prospective study methodology, but those outcomes will not be forthcoming for several more years. As Barlow[117] argues, there will likely be no other "silver bullet" prospective, randomized data to settle the MABG versus SABG debate and that this controversy will need to be adjudicated with the existing retrospective studies available today for the patients of today and the foreseeable future.

MABG has also been shown to extend the CABG versus PCI survival advantage in selected patients.[59,118]

Bilateral internal thoracic artery–multiple arterial coronary artery bypass grafting versus single arterial coronary artery bypass grafting

The internal thoracic arteries are the best conduits available for surgical myocardial reconstruction and have proven long-term durability with a 10-year patency of greater than 90%.[119] The long-term durability of ITA grafts stems from their unique morphologic structure. The ITA has a discontinuous internal elastic lamina and is principally an elastic artery with minimal muscular elements in its media,[120] which is quite thin, and this likely contributes to relatively rare clinically evident vasospasm. The ITA is also remarkably resistant to atherosclerosis and generates multiple vasoactive mediators including anti inflammatory agents and vasodilators such as nitric oxide[121] **Fig. 2.**

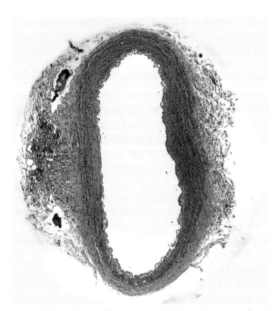

Fig. 2. Photomicrograph of section of left internal thoracic artery (stain: hematoxylin and eosin stain; original magnification, ×4). (*From* Rehman SM, Yi G, Taggart DP. The radial artery: current concepts on its use in coronary revascularization. Ann Thorac Surg 2013;96:1901; with permission.)

The patency rates of ITA grafts are target dependent, with the greatest durability observed when the ITA is placed to the left anterior descending coronary artery and has worst durability when placed to the right coronary artery system.[119] Despite this finding, the survival advantage of BITA-MABG compared with SABG is preserved regardless of whether the second ITA is placed to the right or left coronary systems.[122,123] There is consistency of superior outcomes with the BITA-MABG configuration compared with SABG in retrospective observational studies[45–48,99,124–129] as well as in meta analyses.[49,50] The only randomized, controlled trial (the ART Trial) evaluating the differences in outcomes between BITA-MABG and SABG will not be available for a number of years, but the short-term, 1-year data reported equally excellent outcomes between the two grafting techniques. It is likely that the equivalent outcomes stem from too short a follow-up time to allow for any meaningful graft patency-mediated clinical outcome differences.

A significant hurdle to the wider adoption of the BITA-MABG grafting strategy is the increased complexity of this operation requiring consecutive rather than concurrent graft harvesting and an increased risk of deep sternal wound infections (DSWI) and wound healing complications.[51,116,130] Although most data do point to the increased risk of DSWI with BITA-MABG, some investigators find no such association,[46,47,124,125,127] especially if the ITA grafts are harvested in a skeletonized fashion. The reported risk factors for DSWI are, among others, diabetes mellitus, female gender, obesity, prolonged surgery, mediastinal reexploration, and smoking, and the risks seem to be additive.[131,132] In a meta analysis of 32 studies, Dai and coworkers[116] found a 60% increased risk of DSWI with BITA versus SABG. The contradictory findings maybe attributable to a lack of consistent definitions, lack of power to discriminate differences in relatively rare postoperative events such as DSWI, and differing surgical techniques used in these studies. Specifically, it has been hypothesized that BITA grafting devascularizes the anterior chest wall to a greater extent than single LITA harvesting in SABG and that this physiologic effect can be ameliorated by skeletonizing the both ITA grafts as opposed to harvesting them as pedicled grafts.[133] Such physiologic effects of skeletonization of BITA grafts are associated with a decrease in the risk of DSWI.[116,131,134,135] Importantly, DSWI has been reported to increase hospital mortality and costs.[132]

Radial artery multiple arterial coronary artery bypass grafting versus single arterial coronary artery bypass grafting

The RA is the second most commonly used arterial graft in CABG surgery behind the LITA. Its ease of harvest, its ability to reach all target vessels, and its documented superior patency without an appreciable concern for increased risk of DSWI account for its popularity. Its use however remains low and well below 10% in contemporary CABG series (STS Research Center, http://www.STS.org/documents, personal communication, 2016), despite the fact that this conduit has been perhaps the most studied graft used in CABG. Multiple randomized, controlled studies,[55–57,136,137] meta analyses,[138–140] and observational studies[48,52–54,103,115,141–143] have documented excellent RA durability and improved long-term survival when the RA is used in conjunction with the LITA, compared with SABG. Indeed in all studies with a follow-up of longer than 2 years, RA has been shown to have better patency than SVG. The RA morphology (**Fig. 3**) makes it a less ideal graft than the LITA and its particularly pronounced muscular media component predisposes it to troublesome vasospasm and makes this graft more sensitive to competitive flow issues.[120] Although the incidence of atherosclerotic changes and intimal hyperplasia is higher in the RA than it is in the LITA, the RA is nevertheless relatively resistant to atherosclerosis. Recently, Gaudino and colleagues[144] reported that the RA undergoes remodeling after

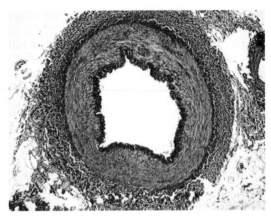

Fig. 3. Photomicrograph of radial artery (stain: elastic-Van Gieson; original magnification, ×100). (*From* Rehman SM, Yi G, Taggart DP. The radial artery: current concepts on its use in coronary revascularization. Ann Thorac Surg 2013;96:1901; with permission.)

implantation into the coronary circulation leading to significant anatomic and vasoreactive modification such that the RA is transformed from a muscular conduit to an elastomuscular conduit akin to the ITA, the undisputed best coronary conduit. In addition, the RA maintains superior physiologic function compared with SVG as evidenced by preservation of its flow-mediated vasodilatation properties.[145]

Given the muscular elements in the media of the RA, the patency of the RA is more dependent on the underlying target vessel stenosis than other conduits and this graft is more susceptible to premature failure owing to competitive flow through the native coronary artery target. Thus, a number of investigators have suggested that, to ensure optimal results, RA use should be restricted to target vessels with a high degree of stenosis, either greater than 70% or even greater than 90%[55,146] in the case of the right coronary artery. This right coronary artery specific observation may be owing to its relatively larger caliber compared with branches of the circumflex and left anterior descending arteries, thus increasing the chances for competitive flow-mediated negative effects. The recommendation for RA use simply on the degree of target vessel stenosis may be an oversimplification, if the concern is driven by competitive flow. A more sophisticated, albeit complex, guide for RA use will likely include the minimal luminal cross sectional area of the target vessel versus the cross-sectional area of the RA graft and thus the size of both the target vessel and RA graft will need to be considered in addition to the maximal degree of target vessel stenosis.

There is debate about whether the RA or the RITA is the second best coronary bypass graft to use with the LITA. The randomized, controlled RAPCO (Radial Artery Patency and Clinical Outcomes) trial compared the patency of the RA and RITA and found no difference in the durability of RA, RITA, and SVG at the 5-year follow-up with no detectable differences in clinical outcomes.[57,147] Nasso and colleagues,[148] in another randomized trial, also reported equipoise between these grafting strategies. Observational studies, however, are contradictory with some noting clinical outcomes that are equivalent between RA-MABG and RITA-MABG,[149–151] others reporting superior RA-MABG,[152] and still others noting superior RITA-MABG outcomes.[153,154] The results of these relatively small, retrospective analyses must be interpreted with caution owing to significant methodologic issues and the final adjudication between RA and RITA superiority will need further scrutiny. Until further definitive data become available, it is reasonable to principally use the RA in favor over the RITA in patients with a high risk of sternal complications, including diabetics, the obese, those with altered immune status, and those with chronic pulmonary disease. Indeed RA-MABG may be particularly advantageous in diabetic patients requiring CABG (**Fig. 4**).[58]

How many arterial grafts are enough?
The value of more than 2 arterial grafts in CABG remains unclear with the very limited available data offering conflicting conclusions.[112,155–157] CABG with three or more arterial grafts is rare, but there have been reports of successful all-arterial coronary revascularization.[48,158,159] The rationale for this approach rests on the excellent durability of arterial grafts and the recently reported decreased down stream disease progression distal to arterial versus venous grafts.[160] The specific role of this grafting strategy requires further analysis.

Complete myocardial revascularization
Despite 40 years of CABG experience, the precise and uniformly accepted definition of incomplete myocardial revascularization and complete myocardial revascularization is lacking and, thus, not surprisingly, the impact of incomplete myocardial revascularization on survival is not well-defined. Traditionally, incomplete myocardial revascularization has been defined by the lack of a graft placed to 1 or more of the 3 principal epicardial coronary systems with at least a 50% stenosis: the so-called anatomic incomplete myocardial revascularization.[161] Alternatively, a so-called functional incomplete myocardial revascularization results from the lack of a graft placed to each diseased coronary artery target.[162] Still others have defined incomplete myocardial revascularization based on the residual postprocedural myocardial jeopardy index,[163] a decremental deviation from an ab initio grafting strategy as formulated in the SYNTAX Trial[164] or a residual post-operative Syntax score of greater than

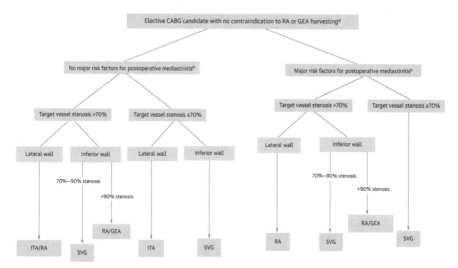

Fig. 4. Algorithm for optimal graft selection in LITA based CABG. Composite and elongated grafts are not considered. [a] In the case of contraindications to RA or GEA harvesting, SVG should be used. [b] Defined as obesity, diabetes, and severe chronic lung disease, especially in combination. CABG, coronary artery bypass graft; GEA, gastroepiploic artery; ITA, internal thoracic artery; LITA, left internal thoracic artery; RA, radial artery; SVG, saphenous vein graft. (*From* Gaudino M, Taggart D, Suma H, et al. The choice of conduits in coronary artery bypass surgery. J Am Coll Cardiol 2015;66(15):1734; with permission.)

zero.[165] In addition to the variable definitions of incomplete myocardial revascularization, the lack of consistent incorporation of data on the coronary target size or its percent stenosis in studies dealing with this subject further complicates matters and obfuscates study conclusions. Given this lack of standardization in defining incomplete myocardial revascularization, it should not be surprising that the reported rates of incomplete myocardial revascularization in CABG vary widely: from 5% reported by Ngaage and colleagues,[166] to 36.8% in the SYNTAX Trial,[164] to as high as 69% in the BARI trial.[163]

Given the traditionally universal commitment to avoiding incomplete myocardial revascularization, no surgeon enters the operating room with an a priori plan to conclude the procedure with an incomplete myocardial revascularization. Not infrequently, however, patient-specific circumstances dictate intraoperative decision making that necessarily results in incomplete myocardial revascularization. This may be owing to such factors as unacceptably small target vessels, diffuse malignant atherosclerosis, lack of conduits, the presence of a porcelain aorta precluding proximal anastomosis placement, or the conscious decision to forego a graft placement to a coronary artery supplying nonviable myocardium. Other possible reasons for incomplete myocardial revascularization is an inability to identify the target vessel intraoperatively or accepting incomplete myocardial revascularization in an effort to minimize operative time. The reported impact of incomplete myocardial revascularization on clinically relevant outcomes is inconsistent.[167–173] The explanation for the possible association of diminished long-term survival and incomplete myocardial revascularization is likely multi factorial. Farooq and colleagues,[165] analyzing the SYNTAX database, report an association of incomplete myocardial revascularization with a greater burden and complexity of anatomic coronary disease as well as clinical comorbidities, both known to adversely affect survival. Rastan and colleagues[171] made a similar observation between incomplete myocardial revascularization and complexity of coronary lesions. Thus, it is likely that the long-term adverse outcomes associated with incomplete myocardial revascularization may be due to both the persistent residual myocardial ischemic burden from too few grafts as well as from factors difficult to control for in risk adjustment methodologies, such as poor quality of coronary targets, for example, given the necessity for subjective judgment to define them. Confronting such a challenge, the surgeon must balance mutually contradictory priorities. By proceeding with a technically challenging and time-consuming process of grafting poor coronary targets in the quest to avoid incomplete myocardial revascularization and its long-term negative association with survival, the surgeon must necessarily accept the risks of acute graft failure and the acute negative sequela of a possibly longer operative time. Ngaage and colleagues[166] studied the challenge of the optimal approach to small coronary artery targets. In a series of 5171 CABG patients, these investigators note that grafting small coronary arteries did not increase the acute perioperative risk of adverse outcomes. Importantly, the incomplete myocardial revascularization resulting from not grafting these small vessels did increase acute major adverse cardiac events, suggesting that a complete revascularization even in the face of poor coronary targets should be pursued.

A number of preoperative patient factors have been found to be predictive of incomplete myocardial revascularization, including older age, diabetes, and peripheral vascular disease.[165] Interestingly, MABG may mitigate the negative effects of incomplete myocardial revascularization. Kieser and colleagues[168] reported no adverse long-term outcomes associated with incomplete myocardial revascularization in patients younger than 80 years in a CABG cohort with a 98% MABG rate. Rastan and colleagues,[171] in a large CABG series with a 21% rate of all arterial grafting, found no difference in survival up to 5 years postoperatively between patients with incomplete myocardial revascularization and complete myocardial revascularization.

SUMMARY

Coronary artery bypass surgery remains, more than 50 years after its introduction into clinical practice, the most studied surgical procedure and an important element of our therapeutic armamentarium for patients with CAD. Both PCI and CABG are best viewed as complimentary and are best deployed in a collaborative multi disciplinary Heart Team–based setting. The indications for its use continue to evolve and paradoxically its value is most apparent in high risk patient groups. With emerging data supporting the incremental survival benefits of multiple arterial grafting in coronary revascularization, MABG should be encouraged.

REFERENCES

1. Allam AH, Thompson RC, Wann S, et al. Atherosclerosis in ancient Egyptian mummies. The Horus Study. JACC Cardiovasc Imaging 2011;4(4):315–27.
2. Mozaffarian D, Benjamin EJ, Go AS, et al. Heart disease and stroke statistics - 2015 update; a report from the American Heart Association. Circulation 2015; 131:e20–322.
3. Carrel A. On the experimental surgery of the thoracic aorta and the heart. Ann Surg 1910;52:83.
4. Jonnesco T. Angine de poitrine guerie par la resection du sympathique cervico-thoracique. Bull Acad Med 1920;84:93–102.
5. Marks C. A history of coronary artery surgery. South Med J 1973;66:249–53.
6. Fieschi. Quoted by Battezzati M, Tagliaferro A, De Marchi G. The ligature of the internal mammary arteries in disorders of vascularization of the myocardium. Minerva Med 1958;46:1173.
7. Vineberg A. Development of an anastomosis between the coronary vessels and a transplanted internal mammary artery. Can Med Assoc J 1946;55:117–9.
8. Sones FM Jr, Shirey EK, Proudfit WL, et al. Cine-coronary angiography. Circulation 1959;20:773–4.
9. Ferguson DJ, Shirey EK, Sheldon WC, et al. Left internal mammary artery implant – postoperative assessment. Circulation 1968;38:II24–6.
10. Mueller RL, Rosengart TK, Isom OW. The history of surgery for ischemic heart disease. Ann Thorac Surg 1997;63:869–78.
11. Kolessov V, Potashov L. Surgery of coronary arteries. Eksp Khir Anesteziol 1965; 10:3.
12. Favaloro RG. Saphenous vein graft in the surgical treatment of coronary artery disease; operative technique. J Thorac Cardiovasc Surg 1969;58:178.
13. Green GE, Spencer FC, Tice DA, et al. Arterial and venous microsurgical bypass grafts for coronary artery disease. J Thorac Cardiovasc Surg 1970;60: 491–503.
14. Coronary Artery Surgery Study (CASS). A randomized trial of coronary artery bypass surgery. Survival data. Circulation 1983;68:939–50.
15. Varnauskas E. Twelve year follow up of survival in the randomized European coronary surgery study. N Engl J Med 1988;319:332–7.
16. Eleven-year survival in the veterans administration randomized trial of coronary bypass surgery for stable angina. The veterans administration coronary artery bypass surgery cooperative study group. N Engl J Med 1984;311:1333–9.
17. Gruntzig A. Transluminal dilatation of coronary stenosis. Lancet 1978;1:263.

18. Dorros G, Cowley MJ, Simpson J, et al. Percutaneous transluminal coronary angioplasty: report of complications from the National Heart, Lung and Blood Institute PTCA Registry. Circulation 1983;67:723–30.

19. Coronary angioplasty versus coronary artery bypass surgery: the randomized intervention treatment of angina (RITA) trial. Lancet 1993;341:573–80.

20. First year results of the CABRI (Coronary Angioplasty versus Bypass Revascularization Investigation). CABRI trial participants. Lancet 1995;346:1179–84.

21. Hueb WA, Bellotti G, de Oliveria SA, et al. The medicine, angioplasty or surgery study (MASS): a prospective randomized trial of medical therapy, balloon angioplasty or bypass surgery for single proximal left anterior descending artery stenosis. J Am Coll Cardiol 1995;26:1600–5.

22. King SB 3rd, Lembo NJ, Weintraub WS, et al. A randomized trial comparing coronary angioplasty with coronary bypass surgery. Emory Angioplasty versus Surgery Trial (EAST). N Engl J Med 1994;331:1044–50.

23. Rodriguez A, Boullon F, Perez-Baliano N, et al. Argentine randomized trial of percutaneous transluminal coronary angioplasty versus coronary artery bypass surgery in multiple vessel disease (ERACI): in-hospital and 1 year follow up. ERACI group. J Am Coll Cardiol 1993;22:1060–7.

24. Rodriguez A, Bernardi V, Navia J, et al. Argentine randomized study: coronary angioplasty with stenting versus coronary bypass surgery in patients with multiple vessel disease (ERACI II): 30 day and one year follow up results. ERACI II investigators. J Am Coll Cardiol 2001;37:51–8.

25. Sedlis SP, Morrison DA, Lorin JD, et al, Investigators od the Dept. of Veterans Affairs Cooperative Study AWESOME. Percutaneous coronary intervention versus coronary artery bypass graft surgery for diabetic patient with unstable angina and risk factors for adverse outcomes with bypass: outcome of diabetic patients in the AWESOME randomized registry. J Am Coll Cardiol 2002;40:1555–6.

26. So SI. Coronary artery bypass surgery versus percutaneous coronary intervention with stent implantation in patients with multi vessel coronary artery disease (the sent or surgery trial): a randomised controlled trial. Lancet 2002;360:965–70.

27. Serruys PW, Unger F, Sousa JE, et al, Arterial revascularization Therapies Study Group. Comparison of coronary artery bypass surgery with stenting for treatment of multi vessel disease. N Engl J Med 2001;344:1117–24.

28. Serruys PW, Morice MC, Kappetein AP, et al. Percutaneous coronary intervention versus coronary artery bypass grafting for severe coronary artery disease. N Engl J Med 2009;360:961–72.

29. Mohr FW, Marice MC, Kappatein AP, et al. Coronary artery bypass graft surgery versus percutaneous coronary intervention in patients with three- vessel disease and left main coronary disease: 5-year follow up of the randomized, clinical SYNTAX trial. Lancet 2013;381:629–38.

30. Farkouh ME, Domanski M, Sleeper LA, et al. Strategies for multivessel revascularization in patients with diabetes. N Engl J Med 2012;367:2375–84.

31. Kapur A, Hall RJ, Malik IS, et al. Randomized comparison od percutaneous coronary intervention with coronary artery bypass grafting in diabetic patients. 1-year results of the CARDIa (Coronary Artery Revascularization in Diabetes) trial. J Am Coll Cardiol 2010;55:432–40.

32. Weintraub WS, Grau-Sepulveda MV, Weiss JM, et al. Comparative effectiveness of revascularization strategies. N Engl J Med 2012;366:1467–76.

33. Eagle KA, Guyton RA, Davidoff R, et al. ACC/AHA 2004 guideline update for coronary artery bypass graft surgery. Circulation 2004;110:1168–76.
34. Hillis DL, Smith PK, Anderson JL, et al. 2011 ACCF/AHA guideline for coronary artery bypass surgery: executive summary: a report of the American College of Cardiology Foundation/American Heart Association Task Force on Practice Guidelines. Circulation 2011;124:2610–42.
35. Windecker S, Kolh P, Alfonso F, et al. 2014 ESC/EACTS guidelines on myocardial revascularization. Eur Heart J 2014;35:2541–619.
36. Aldea GS, Bakaeen FG, Pal J, et al. The Society of Thoracic Surgeons clinical practice guidelines on arterial conduits for coronary artery bypass grafting. Ann Thorac Surg 2016;101:801–9.
37. Loop FD, Lytle BD, Cosgrove DM, et al. Influence of the internal mammary artery graft on 10-year survival and other cardiac events. N Engl J Med 1986;314:1–6.
38. Edwards FH, Clark RE, Schwartz M. Impact of internal mammary artery conduits on operative mortality in coronary revascularization. Ann Thorac Surg 1994;57:27–32.
39. Grover FL, Johnson RR, Marshall G, et al. Impact of mammary grafts on coronary bypass operative mortality and morbidity: Department of Veterans Affairs Cardiac Surgeons. Ann Thorac Surg 1994;57:559–68.
40. Gardner TJ, Greene PS, Rykiel MF, et al. Routine use of the left internal mammary artery graft in the elderly. Ann Thorac Surg 1990;49:188–94.
41. Cameron AAC, Davis KB, Green GE, et al. Coronary bypass surgery with internal-thoracic-artery grafts: effects on survival over a 15-year period. N Engl J Med 1996;334:216–9.
42. Leavitt BJ, O'Connor GT, Olmstead EM, et al. Use of the internal mammary artery graft and in-hospital mortality and other adverse outcomes associated with coronary artery bypass surgery. Circulation 2001;103:507–12.
43. McNeely C, Markwell S, Vassileva C. Trends in patient characteristics and outcomes of coronary artery bypass grafting in 2000 to 2012 Medicare population. Ann Thorac Surg 2016;102:132–8.
44. Tabata M, Grab JD, Khalpey Z, et al. Prevalence and variability of internal mammary artery graft use in contemporary multivessel coronary artery bypass graft surgery. Analysis of the Society of Thoracic Surgeons national cardiac database. Circulation 2009;120:935–40.
45. Lytle BW, Blackstone EH, Sabik JF, et al. The effect of bilateral internal thoracic artery grafting on survival during 20 postoperative years. Ann Thorac Surg 2004;78(6):2005–12.
46. Kurlansky PA, Traad EA, Dorman MJ, et al. Thirty-year follow-up defines survival benefit for second internal mammary artery in propensity-matched groups. Ann Thorac Surg 2010;90:101–8.
47. Puskas JD, Sadiq A, Vassiliades TA, et al. Bilateral internal thoracic artery grafting is associated with significantly improved long-term survival, even among diabetics. Ann Thorac Surg 2012;94:710–6.
48. Locker C, Schaff HV, Dearani JA, et al. Multiple arterial grafts improve late survival of patients undergoing coronary artery bypass surgery: analysis of 8622 patients with multivessel disease. Circulation 2012;126:1023–30.
49. Weiss AJ, Zhao S, Tian DH, et al. A meta-analysis comparing internal mammary artery with left internal mammary artery for coronary artery bypass grafting. Ann Cardiothorac Surg 2013;2:390–400.
50. Yi GY, Shine B, Rehman SM, et al. Effect of bilateral internal mammary artery grafts on long term survival. Circulation 2014;130:539–45.

51. Taggart DP, Altman DG, Gray AM, et al, on behalf of the ART Investigators. Randomized trial to compare bilateral vs single internal mammary artery coronary bypass grafting: 1 year results of the Arterial Revascularization Trial. Eur Heart J 2010;31:2470–81.

52. Zacharias A, Habib RH, Schwann T, et al. Improved survival with radial artery versus vein conduits in coronary bypass surgery with left internal thoracic artery to left anterior descending artery grafting. Circulation 2004;109:1489–96.

53. Tranbaugh RF, Dimitrova KR, Friedmann P, et al. Radial artery conduits improve long-term survival after coronary artery bypass grafting. Ann Thorac Surg 2010; 90:1165–72.

54. Schwann TA, Al-Shaar L, Engoren M, et al. Late effects of radial artery vs saphenous vein grafting for multivessel coronary bypass surgery in diabetics: a propensity-matched analysis. Eur J Cardiothorac Surg 2013;44:701–10.

55. Deb S, Cohen EA, Singh SK, et al, for the RAPS Investigators. Radial artery and saphenous vein patency more than 5 years after coronary artery bypass surgery: results from RAPS (Radial Artery Patency Study). J Am Coll Cardiol 2012;60:28–35.

56. Collins P, Webb CM, Chong CF, et al, for the RSVP Trial Investigators. Radial artery versus saphenous vein patency randomized trial: five year angiograpjic follow up. Circulation 2008;117:2859–64.

57. Hayward PA, Buxton BF. Mid-term results of the radial artery patency and clinical outcomes randomized trial. Ann Cardiothorac Surg 2013;2:458–66.

58. Deb S, Singh SK, Moussa F, et al, on behalf of the Radial Artery Patency Study Investigators. The long-term impact of diabetes on graft patency after coronary artery bypass grafting surgery: a sub-study of the multi center Radial Artery Patency Study. J Thorac Cardiovasc Surg 2014;148:1246–53.

59. Habib RH, Dimitrova KR, Badour SA, et al. CABG vs PCI: greater benefit in long-term outcomes with multiple arterial bypass grafting. J Am Coll Cardiol 2015;66: 1417–27.

60. Hannan EL, Wu C, Walfor G, et al. Drug eluting stents vs. coronary artery bypass grafting in multivessel disease. N Engl J Med 2005;352:2174–83.

61. Briguori C, Condorelli G, Airoldi, et al. Comparison of coronary drug eluting stents versus coronary artery bypass grafting in patients with diabetes mellitus. Am J Cardiol 2007;99:779–84.

62. Javaid A, Steinberg DH, Buch AN, et al. Outcomes of coronary artery bypass grafting versus percutaneous coronary intervention with drug eluting stents for patients with multivessel coronary artery disease. Circulation 2007;116:1200–6.

63. Lee MS, Jamal F, Kedia G, et al. Comparison of bypass surgery with drug eluting stents for diabetic patients with multivessel disease. Int J Cardiol 2007;123:34–42.

64. Park DW, Yun SC, Lee SW, et al. Long term mortality after percutaneous coronary intervention with drug eluting stent implantation versus coronary artery bypass surgery for treatment of multivessel coronary artery disease. Circulation 2008;117:2079–86.

65. Tarantini G, Ramondo A, Napodano M, et al. PCI versus CABG for multivessel coronary disease in diabetics. Catheter Cardiovasc Interv 2009;73:50–8.

66. Varani E, Bulducelli M, Vecchi G, et al. Comparison of multiple drug eluting stent percutaneous coronary intervention and surgical revascularization in patients with multivessel coronary disease: one year clinical results and total treatment costs. J Invasive Cardiol 2007;19:469–75.

67. Yang JH, Gwon HC, Cho SJ, et al. Comparison of coronary artery bypass grafting with drug eluting stent implantation for the treatment of multivessel coronary artery disease. Ann Thorac Surg 2008;85:665–70.

68. Yang ZK, Shen WF, Zhang RY, et al. Coronary artery bypass surgery versus percutaneous coronary intervention with drug eluting stent implantation in patients with multivessel coronary disease. J Interv Cardiol 2007;20:10–6.

69. Benedetto U, Melina G, Angeloni E, et al. Coronary artery bypass grafting versus drug eluting stents in multivessel coronary disease. A meta-analysis on 24,268 patients. Eur J Cardiothorac Surg 2009;36:611–5.

70. Fihn SD, Blankenship JC, Alexander KP, et al. 2014 ACC/AHA/AATS/PCNA/SCAI/STS focused update of the guidelines for the diagnosis and management of patients with stable ischemic heart disease. Circulation 2014;130:1749–67.

71. Shahian DM, O'Brien SM, Filardo G, et al. The Society of Thoracic Surgeons 2008 cardiac surgery risk models; part 1: coronary artery bypass grafting surgery. Ann Thorac Surg 2009;88(Suppl 1):S2–22.

72. Nashef SA, Roques F, Aharples LD, et al. EuroSCORE II. Eur J Cardiothorac Surg 2012;41:734–44.

73. Papadopoulou SL, Girasis C, Dharampal A, et al. CT-SYNTAX score: a feasibility and reproducibility study. JACC Cardiovasc Imaging 2013;6:413–5.

74. Peterson ED, Dai D, DeLong ER, et al. Contemporary mortality risk prediction for percutaneous coronary intervention: results from 588,398 procedures in the National Cardiovascular Data registry. J Am Coll Cardiol 2010;55:1923–32.

75. Farooq V, van Klaveren D, Steyerberg EW, et al. Anatomical and clinical characteristics to guide decision making between coronary artery bypass surgery and percutaneous coronary intervention for individual patients: development and validation of SYNTAX score II. Lancet 2013;381:639–50.

76. Ragasta M, Dee S, Sarembock IJ, et al. Prevalence of unfavorable angiographic characteristics for percutaneous intervention in patients with unprotected left main coronary artery disease. Catheter Cardiovasc Interv 2006;68:357–62.

77. Buszman PE, Kiesz SR, Bochenek A, et al. Acute and late outcomes of unprotected left main stenting in comparison with surgical revascularization. J Am Coll Cardiol 2008;51:538–45.

78. Park SJ, Kim YH, Park DW, et al. Randomized trial of stents versus bypass surgery for left main coronary artery disease. N Engl J Med 2011;364:1718–27.

79. Chieffo A, Meliga E, Latib A, et al. Drug eluting stent for left main coronary artery disease: the DELTA registry: a multi center registry evaluating percutaneous coronary intervention versus coronary artery bypass grafting for left main treatment. JACC Cardiovasc Interv 2012;5:718–27.

80. Naik H, White AJ, Chakravarty T, et al. A meta-analysis of 3,773 patients treated with percutaneous coronary intervention or surgery for unprotected left main coronary artery stenosis. JACC Cardiovasc Interv 2009;2:739–47.

81. BARI Investigators. The final 10-year follow-up results from the BARI randomized trial. J Am Coll Cardiol 2007;49:1600–6.

82. The BARI 2D Study Group. A randomized trial of therapies for type 2 diabetes and coronary artery disease. N Engl J Med 2009;360:2503–15.

83. Hlatky MA, Boothroyd DB, Bravata DM, et al. Coronary artery bypass surgery compared with percutaneous coronary interventions for multi vessel disease: a collaborative analysis of individual patient data from ten randomized trials. Lancet 2009;373:1190–7.

84. Verma S, Farkouh ME, Yanagawa B. Comparison of coronary artery bypass surgery and percutaneous coronary intervention in patients with diabetes: a meta-analysis of randomized controlled trial. Lancet Diabetes Endocrinol 2013;1:317–28.

85. Kappetein AP, Head SJ, Morice MC, et al. Treatment of complex coronary artery disease in patients with diabetes: 5-year results comparing outcomes of bypass surgery and percutaneous coronary intervention in the SYNTAX trial. Eur J Cardiothorac Surg 2013;43:1006–13.

86. Daemen J, Boersma E, Flather M, et al. long term safety and efficacy of percutaneous coronary intervention with stenting and coronary artery bypass surgery for multi-vessel coronary artery disease: a meta-analysis with r year patient level data from the ARTS, ERACI-II, MASSII, and SoS trials. Circulation 2008;118: 1146–54.

87. Kohl P, Windecker S, Alfanso F, et al. 2014 ESC/EACTS guidelines on myocardial revascularization of the European Society of Cardiology (ESC) and the European Association for Cardio-Thoracic Surgery (EACTS). Developed with the special contribution from the European Association of Percutaneous Cardiovascular Interventions (EAPCI). Eur J Cardiothorac Surg 2014;46:517–92.

88. Shahian DM, O'Brien SM, Sheng S, et al. Predictors of long term survival after coronary artery bypass surgery. Results from the Society of Thoracic Surgeons Adult Cardiac Surgery Database (The ASCERT Study). Circulation 2012;125: 1491–500.

89. Puskas JD, Kilgo PD, Thourani VH, et al. The Society of Thoracic Surgeons 30 day predicted risk of mortality score also predicts long term survival. Ann Thorac Surg 2012;93:26–35.

90. Alderman EL, Fisher LD, Litwin P, et al. Results of coronary artery surgery in patients with poor left ventricular function (CASS). Circulation 1983;68:785–95.

91. Elefteriades JA, Morales DLS, Gradel C, et al. Results of coronary artery bypass grafting by a single surgeon in patients with left ventricular ejection fractions < 30%. Am J Cardiol 1997;79:1573–8.

92. Nardi P, Pellegrino A, Scafuri A, et al. Long term outcome of coronary artery bypass grafting in patients with left ventricular dysfunction. Ann Thorac Surg 2009;87:1401–8.

93. Velazquez EJ, Lee KL, Deja MA, et al. Coronary artery bypass in patients with left ventricular dysfunction. N Engl J Med 2011;364:1607–16.

94. Keeling WB, Williams ML, Slaughter MS, et al. Off pump and on pump coronary revascularization in patients with low ejection fraction: a report from the Society of Thoracic Surgeons National Database. Ann Thorac Surg 2013;96:83–9.

95. Allman KC, Shaw LJ, Hachamovitch R, et al. Myocardial viability testing and impact of revascularization on prognosis in patients with coronary artery disease and left ventricular dysfunction: a meta-analysis. J Am Coll Cardiol 2002;39: 1151–8.

96. Panza JA, Velazquez EJ, She L, et al. Extent of coronary and myocardial disease and benefit from surgical revascularization in LV dysfunction. J Am Coll Cardiol 2014;64:553–61.

97. Urtesky BF, Thygesen K, Armstrong PW, et al. Acute coronary findings at autopsy in heart failure patients with sudden death. Results from the Assessment of Treatment with Lisinopril and Survival (ATLAS) Trial. Circulation 2000;102: 611–6.

98. Nagendran J, Norris CM, Graham MM, for the APPROACH Investigators. Ann Thorac Surg 2013;96:2038–44.

99. Galbut D, Kurlansky PA, Traad EA, et al. Bilateral internal thoracic artery grafting improves long term survival in patients with reduced ejection fraction: a propensity matched study with 30 year follow-up. J Thorac Cardiovasc Surg 2012;143: 844–53.

100. Topkara VK, Cheema FH, Kasavaramanujam S, et al. Coronary artery bypass grafting in patients with low ejection fraction. Circulation 2005;112(Suppl 9): I344–50.

101. Velazquez EJ, Lee KL, O'Connor CM, et al. The rationale and design of the Surgical Treatment for Ischemic Heart Failure (STITCH) trial. J Thorac Cardiovasc Surg 2007;134:1540–7.

102. Velazquez EJ, Lee KL, Jones RH, et al. Coronary artery bypass surgery in patients with ischemic cardiomyopathy. N Engl J Med 2016;374:1511–20.

103. Schwann TA, Al-Shaar L, Tranbaugh RF, et al. Multi versus single coronary artery bypass surgery across the ejection fraction spectrum. Ann Thorac Surg 2015; 100:810–7.

104. Lytle BW, Loop FD, Cosgrove DM, et al. Long-term (5-12 years) serial studies of internal mammary artery and saphenous vein coronary artery bypass grafts. J Thorac Cardiovasc Surg 1985;89:248–58.

105. Sabik JF, Lytle BW, Blackstone EH, et al. Does competitive flow reduce internal thoracic artery graft patency? Ann Thorac Surg 2003;76(5):1490–6.

106. Yoshizumi T, Ito T, Maekawa A, et al. Is the mid-term outcome of free right internal thoracic artery with a proximal anastomosis modification inferior to in situ right internal thoracic artery graft to the left anterior descending artery? Gen Thorac Cardiovasc Surg 2012;60:480–8.

107. Al-Ruzzeh S, George S, Bustami M, et al. Early clinical and angiographic outcome of pedicled right internal thoracic artery graft to the left anterior descending artery. Ann Thorac Surg 2002;73:1431–5.

108. Tatoulis J, Buxton BF, Fuller JA, et al. The right internal thoracic artery: the forgotten conduit – 5,766 patients and 991 angiograms. Ann Thorac Surg 2011;92:9–15.

109. Ura M, Sakata R, Nakayamay, et al. Analysis by early angiography of right internal thoracic artery grafting via the transverse sinus: predictors of graft failure. Circulation 2000;101:640–6.

110. Ura M, Sakata R, Nakayama Y, et al. Technical aspects and outcome of in situ right internal thoracic artery grafting to the major branches of the circumflex artery via the transverse sinus. Ann Thorac Surg 2001;71:1485–90.

111. Puskas JD, Yanagawa B, Taggart DP. Advancing the state of the art in surgical coronary revascularization. Ann Thorac Surg 2016;101:419–21.

112. Guru V, Fremes SE, Tu JV. How many arterial grafts are enough? A population based study of midterm outcomes. J Thorac Cardiovasc Surg 2006;131:1021–8.

113. Rehman SM, Yi G, Taggart DP. The radial artery: current concepts on its use in coronary revascularization. Ann Thorac Surg 2013;96:1900–9.

114. Tranbaugh RF, Lucido DJ, Dimitrova KR, et al. Multiple arterial bypass grafting should be routine. J Thorac Cardiovasc Surg 2015;150:1537–45.

115. Schwann TA, Zacharias A, Riordan CJ, et al. Does radial use as a second arterial conduit for coronary artery bypass grafting improve long-term survival in diabetics? Eur J Cardiothorac Surg 2008;33:914–23.

116. Dai C, Lu Z, Zhu H, et al. Bilateral internal mammary artery grafting and risk of sternal wound infection: evidence from observational studies. Ann Thorac Surg 2013;95:1938–45.

117. Barlow CW. What is the best second conduit for coronary artery bypass grafting? With no silver bullet study we should not ignore good regular bullets when we got them. J Thorac Cardiovasc Surg 2015;150:1535–6.

118. Locker C, Shaff HV, Daly RC, et al. Multiple arterial grafts improve survival with coronary bypass surgery versus conventional coronary artery bypass grafting compared to percutaneous interventions. J Thorac Cardiovasc Surg 2016; 152:369–79.

119. Tatoulis J, Buxton BF, Fuller JA, et al. The right internal thoracic artery: is it underutilized? Curr Opin Cardiol 2011;26:528–35.

120. Ruengsakulrach P, Sinclair R, Komedo M, et al. Comparative histopathology of radial artery versus internal thoracic artery and risk factors for development of internal hyperplasia and atherosclerosis. Circulation 1999;100(Suppl 19): II139–44.

121. Otsuka F, Yahagi K, Sakalura K, et al. Why is the mammary artery so special and what protects it from atherosclerosis. Ann Cardiothorac Surg 2013;2:519–26.

122. Sabik JF, Stockins A, Nowicki ER, et al. Does the location of the second internal thoracic artery graft influence outcome of coronary artery bypass grafting? Circulation 2008;118(Suppl 1):S210–5.

123. Kurlansky PA, Traad EA, Dorman MJ, et al. Location of the second internal mammary artery graft does not influence outcome of coronary artery bypass grafting. Ann Thorac Surg 2011;91:1378–84.

124. Shi WY, Hayward PA, Tatoulis J, et al. Are all forms of total arterial revasculariation equal? A comparison of single versus bilateral internal thoracic artery grafting strategies. J Thorac Cardiovasc Surg 2015;150:1526–34.

125. Stevens LM, Carrier M, Perrault LP, et al. Single versus bilateral internal thoracic artery grafts with concomitant saphenous vein grafts for multivessel coronary artery bypass grafting: Effects on mortality and event –free survival. J Thorac Cardiovasc Surg 2004;127:1408–15.

126. Rankin JS, Tuttle RH, Wechsler AS, et al. Techniques and benefits of multiple internal mammary artery bypass at 20 years of follow-up. Ann Thorac Surg 2007; 83:1008–15.

127. LaPar DJ, Crosby IK, Rich JB, et al, and Investigators for the Virginia Surgery Quality Initiative. Bilateral internal mammary artery use for coronary artery bypass grafting remains underutilized: a propensity-matched multi-institutional analysis. Ann Thorac Surg 2015;100:8–15.

128. Grau JB, Ferrari G, Mak AWC, et al. Propensity matched analysis of bilateral internal mammary artery versus single internal mammary artery grafting at 17-year follow-up: validation of a contemporary surgical experience. Eur J Cardiothorac Surg 2012;41:770–6.

129. Benedetto U, Montecalvo A, Kattach H, et al. Impact of the second intern thoracic artery on short- and long-term outcomes in obese patients: a propensity score matched analysis. J Thorac Cardiovasc Surg 2015;149:841–7.

130. Raza S, Sabik JF, Masabni K, et al. Surgical revascularization techniques that minimize risk and maximize late survival after coronary artery bypass grafting in patients with diabetes. J Thorac Cardiovasc Surg 2014;148:1257–66.

131. Benedetto U, Altman DG, Gerry S, et al, on Behalf of the Arterial Revascularization Trial Investigators. Pedicled and skeletonized single and bilateral internal thoracic artery grafts and the incidence of sternal wound complications: insights from the Arterial Revascualarization Trial. J Thorac Cardiovasc Surg 2016;152: 270–6.

132. El Oakley RM, Wright JE. Post operative mediastinitis: classification and management. Ann Thorac Surg 1996;61:1030–6.
133. Cohen AJ, Lockman J, Lorberboym M, et al. Assessment of sternal vascularity with single photon emission computed tomography after harvesting of the internal thoracic artery. J Thorac Cardiovasc Surg 1999;118:496–502.
134. Toumpoulis IK, Theakos N, Dunning J. Does bilateral internal thoracic artery harvest increase the risk of mediastinitis? Interact Cardiovasc Thorac Surg 2007;6:787–92.
135. De Paulis R, de Notaris S, Scaffia R, et al. The effect of bilateral internal thoracic artery harvesting on superficial and deep sternal infection: the role of skeletonization. J Thorac Cardiovasc Surg 2005;129:536–43.
136. Desai ND, Cohen EA, Naylor CD, et al, Radial Artery Patency Study Investigators. A randomized comparison of radial-artery and saphenous-vein coronary bypass grafts. N Engl J Med 2004;351:2302–9.
137. Goldman S, Sethi GK, Holman W, et al. Radial artery grafts vs saphenous vein grafts in coronary artery bypass surgery: a randomized trial. JAMA 2011;305:167–74.
138. Benedetto U, Angeloni E, Refice S, et al. Radial artery versus saphenous vein graft patency: meta-analysis of randomized controlled trials. J Thorac Cardiovasc Surg 2010;139:229–31.
139. Athenasiou T, Saso S, Rao C, et al. Radial artery versus saphenous vein conduits for coronary artery bypass surgery: forty years of competition – which conduit offers better patency? A systematic review and meta-analysis. Eur J Cardiothorac Surg 2011;40:208–20.
140. Cao C, Manganas C, Horton M, et al. Angiographic outcomes of radial artery versus saphenous vein in coronary artery bypass graft surgery: a meta-analysis of randomized controlled studies. J Thorac Cardiovasc Surg 2012;146:255–61.
141. Schwann TA, Tranbaugh RF, Dimitrova KR, et al. Time-varying (0-15 years) survival benefit of radial artery versus saphenous vein grafting: a multi-institutional analysis of 9852 patients. Ann Thorac Surg 2014;97:1328–34.
142. Schwann TA, Habib RH. The effect of patient sex on survival in patients undergoing isolated coronary artery bypass surgery receiving a radial artery. Eur J Cardiothorac Surg 2014;47:331–2.
143. Habib RH, Schwann TA, Engoren M. Late effects of radial artery versus saphenous vein grafting in patients 70 years or older. Ann Thorac Surg 2012;94:1478–84.
144. Gaudino M, Prati F, Caradonna E, et al. Implantation in coronary circulation induces morphofunctional transformation of radial grafts from muscular to elastomuscular. Circulation 2005;112:I208–11.
145. Webb CM, Moat NE, Chong CF, et al. Vascular reactivity and flow characteristics of radial artery and long saphenous vein coronary bypass grafts. A 5-year follow-up. Circulation 2010;122:861–7.
146. Gaudino M, Alessandrini F, Pragliola C, et al. Effect of target artery location and severity of stenosis on mid-term patency of aorta-anastomosed vs internal thoracic artery anastomosed radial artery grafts. Eur J Cardiothorac Surg 2014;25:424–8.
147. Hayward PAR, Gordon IR, Hare DL, et al. Comparable patencies of radial artery and right internal thoracic artery or saphenous vein beyond 5 years: results from the Radial Artery Patency and Clinical Outcomes trial. J Thorac Cardiovasc Surg 2010;139:60–7.

148. Nasso G, Coppola R, Bonifazi R, et al. Arterial revascularization in primary coronary artery bypass grafting; Direct comparison of 4 strategies –Results of the Stand in Y Mammary Study. J Thorac Cardiovasc Surg 2009;137:1093–100.

149. Tranbaugh RF, Dimitrova KR, Lucido DJ, et al. The second best arterial graft: a propensity analysis of the radial artery versus the free right internal thoracic artery to bypass the circumflex artery. J Thorac Cardiovasc Surg 2014;147: 133–42.

150. Califiore AM, DiMAuro M, D'Allessandro S, et al. Revascularization of the lateral wall: long term angiographic and clinical results of radial artery versus right internal thoracic artery. J Thorac Cardiovasc Surg 2002;123:225–31.

151. Schwann TA, Hashim SW, Badour S, et al. Equipoise between radial artery and right internal thoracic artery as the second arterial conduit in left internal thoracic artery based coronary artery bypass graft surgery; a multi institutional study. Eur J Cardiothorac Surg 2016;49:188–95.

152. Caputo M, Reeves B, Marchetto G, et al. Radial versus right internal thoracic artery as a second arterial conduit for coronary surgery: early and intermediate outcomes. J Thorac Cardiovasc Surg 2003;126:39–47.

153. Kelly R, Buth KJ, Legare JF. Bilateral internal thoracic artery grafting is superior to other forms of multiple arterial grafting in providing survival benefit after coronary bypass surgery. J Thorac Cardiovasc Surg 2012;144:1408–15.

154. Ruttmann E, Fischler N, Sakic A, et al. Second internal thoracic artery versus radial artery in coronary artery bypass grafting. A long term, propensity score matched follow up study. Circulation 2011;124:1321–9.

155. Glineur D, D'hoore W, Price, et al. Survival benefit of multiple arterial grafting in a 25-year single-institutional experience: the importance of the third arterial graft. Eur J Cardiothorac Surg 2012;42(2):284–90 [discussion: 290–1].

156. Lev-Ran O, Mohr R, Uretzky G, et al. Graft of choice to right coronary system in left-sided bilateral internal thoracic artery grafting. Ann Thorac Surg 2003;75(1): 88–92.

157. Di Mauro M, Contini M, Iaco AL, et al. Bilateral internal thoracic artery on the left side: a propensity score-matched study of impact of the third conduit on the right side. J Thorac Cardiovasc Surg 2009;137(4):869–74.

158. Buxton BF, Shi WY, Tatoulis J, et al. Total arterial revascularization with internal thoracic and radial artery grafts in triple-vessel coronary artery disease is associated with improved survival. J Thorac Cardiovasc Surg 2014;148:1238–43.

159. Zacharias A, Schwann TA, Riordan CJ, et al. Late results of conventional versus all arterial revascularization based on internal thoracic and radial artery grafting. Ann Thorac Surg 2009;87:19–26.

160. Dimitrova KR, Hoffman DM, Geller CM, et al. Arterial grafts protect the native coronary vessels from atherosclerotic disease progression. Ann Thorac Surg 2012;94:475–81.

161. McNeer JF, Conley MJ, Starmer CF, et al. Complete and incomplete revascularization at aortocoronary bypass surgery: experience with 392 consecutive patients. Am Heart J 1974;88(2):176–82.

162. Vander Salm TJ, Kip KE, Jones RH, et al. What constitutes optimal surgical revascularization? Answers from the Bypass Angioplasty Revascularization Investigation (BARI). J Am Coll Cardiol 2002;39(4):565–657.

163. Schwartz L, Bertolet M, Feit F, et al. Impact of completeness of revascularization on long-term cardiovascular outcomes in patients with type 2 diabetes mellitus: results from the Bypass Angioplasty Revascularization Investigation 2 Diabetes (BARI 2D). Circ Cardiovasc Interv 2012;5(2):166–73.

164. Head SJ, Mack MJ, Holmes DR Jr, et al. Incidence, predictors and outcomes of incomplete revascularization after percutaneous coronary intervention and coronary artery bypass grafting: a subgroup analysis of 3-year SYNTAX data. Eur J Cardiothorac Surg 2012;41(3):535–41.

165. Farooq V, Serruys PW, Bourantas CV, et al. Quantification of incomplete revascularization and its association with five-year mortality in the Synergy Between Percutaneous Coronary Intervention With Taxus and Cardiac Surgery (SYNTAX) trial validation of the residual SYNTAX score. Circulation 2013;128(2):141–51.

166. Ngaage DL, Hashmi I, Griffin S, et al. To graft or not to graft? Do coronary artery characteristics influence early outcomes of coronary artery bypass surgery? Analysis of coronary anastomoses of 5171 patients. J Thorac Cardiovasc Surg 2010;140(1):66–72, 72.e1.

167. Kleisli T, Cheng W, Jacobs MJ, et al. In the current era, complete revascularization improves survival after coronary artery bypass surgery. J Thorac Cardiovasc Surg 2005;129(6):1283–91.

168. Kieser TM, Curran HJ, Rose MS, et al. Arterial grafts balance survival between incomplete and complete revascularization: a series of 1000 consecutive coronary artery bypass graft patients with 98% arterial grafts. J Thorac Cardiovasc Surg 2014;147(1):75–83.

169. Moon MR, Sundt TM 3rd, Pasque MK, et al. Influence of internal mammary artery grafting and completeness of revascularization on long-term outcome in octogenarians. Ann Thorac Surg 2001;72(6):2003–7.

170. Lytle BW, Loop FD, Taylor PC, et al. The effect of coronary reoperation on the survival of patients with stenoses in saphenous vein bypass grafts to coronary arteries. J Thorac Cardiovasc Surg 1993;105(4):605–12 [discussion: 612–4].

171. Rastan AJ, Walther T, Falk V, et al. Does reasonable incomplete surgical revascularization affect early or long-term survival in patients with multivessel coronary artery disease receiving left internal mammary artery bypass to left anterior descending artery? Circulation 2009;120(Suppl 11):S70–7.

172. Kozower BD, Moon MR, Barner HB, et al. Impact of complete revascularization on long-term survival after coronary artery bypass grafting in octogenarians. Ann Thorac Surg 2005;80(1):112–6 [discussion: 116–7].

173. Scott R, Blackstone EH, McCarthy PM, et al. Isolated bypass grafting of the left internal thoracic artery to the left anterior descending coronary artery: late consequences of incomplete revascularization. J Thorac Cardiovasc Surg 2000; 120(1):173–84.

Mitral Valve Repair
The French Correction Versus the American Correction

 CrossMark

Sarah A. Schubert, MD[a],*, James H. Mehaffey, MD[b],
Eric J. Charles, MD[b], Irving L. Kron, MD[a]

KEYWORDS

- Mitral valve repair • French correction • American correction
- Degenerative mitral valve disease

KEY POINTS

- Mitral valve repair is associated with better short- and long-term outcomes, fewer thromboembolic complications, and improved survival compared with mitral valve replacement.
- Carpentier's "French correction" of degenerative mitral valve pathology aims to restore normal valve anatomy through leaflet resection, chordal manipulation, and rigid annuloplasty.
- The "American correction" of degenerative mitral valve pathology intends to restore normal valve function through use of artificial chordae, minimal leaflet resection, and flexible annuloplasty.

Degenerative mitral valve disease is found in 2% to 3% of adults in the United States, making it the most common organic mitral valve pathology.[1] Although degenerative mitral valve pathology does not always progress to clinically significant mitral regurgitation (MR), patients who develop symptoms attributable to MR have a worse prognosis with mortality rates of 34% annually.[2,3]

With surgery essentially unavoidable in these patients, mitral valve repair has demonstrated superior short-[4–6] and long-term[7–9] outcomes in a wide variety of patients with degenerative[5,8,10,11] or functional[9,12–15] mitral valve disease.[6,16] Valve replacement, however, may be considered in patients with combined degenerative and ischemic MR, MR caused by papillary muscle rupture, or those undergoing reoperation following prior failed repair.[17] Nevertheless, mitral valve repair for either

The authors have nothing to disclose.
[a] Division of Thoracic and Cardiovascular Surgery, Department of Surgery, University of Virginia, 1215 Lee Street, Box 800679, Charlottesville, VA 22908, USA; [b] Department of Surgery, University of Virginia, Box 800709, Charlottesville, VA 22908, USA
* Corresponding author.
E-mail address: ss9kw@virginia.edu

Surg Clin N Am 97 (2017) 867–888
http://dx.doi.org/10.1016/j.suc.2017.03.009
surgical.theclinics.com

degenerative or ischemic MR has been consistently associated with lower risk of thromboembolism and improved survival.[6]

Not surprisingly, as the outcomes with mitral valve repair have surpassed those of mitral valve replacement, the methods of mitral valve repair have evolved and improved. The optimal methods for surgical repair of MR have varied over time and even across continents. Beginning with suture annuloplasty,[18] then commissural fusion with suture,[19] and open leaflet plication,[20] techniques of mitral valve repair have continued to multiply and progress.

Alain Carpentier's method of leaflet repair with quadrangular resection and rigid annuloplasty to correct annular dilatation emerged as the most successful and reproducible means of correcting MR.[21–25] Developed through autopsy and pathology studies of the mitral valve, Carpentier's method of mitral valve repair aimed to restore normal dimensions to the mitral valve and apparatus,[22] a so-called anatomic approach that has come to be known as the "French correction."[25]

Yet, as imaging techniques have improved and knowledge of the dynamic structure and function of the mitral valve has grown, Lawrie and colleagues[26] turned to a functional correction of MR, which he referred to as the "American correction."[27,28] The primary tenet of this repair is colloquially "respect, not resect," in reference to the mitral valve leaflets and chordae, which are generally spared with this approach. Furthermore, Lawrie's method relies on a flexible annuloplasty ring to correct annular dilatation and Gore-Tex (WL Gore and Associates, Inc, Newark, DE) artificial chordae to repair prolapse and realign leaflets.[28,29]

Although these techniques are traditionally compared in opposition with one another, in reality, these methods of mitral valve repair simply reflect an evolution in principles as operative techniques are enhanced and as more is discovered about the mitral valve's dynamic structure and functions.

MITRAL VALVE ANATOMY

Located between the left atrium and left ventricle, the mitral valve apparatus is comprised of the mitral annulus, anterior and posterior leaflets, chordae tendinae, and the papillary muscles. The valvular apparatus works in concert with the subvalvular apparatus, namely the chordae tendinae and papillary muscles, to permit normal blood flow from the left atrium to the left ventricle during diastole and prevent reversal of flow during systole (**Fig. 1**).

The mitral annulus is an ovoid ring of fibrous tissue that is continuous with the fibrous skeleton of the heart. The right fibrous trigone is formed from the confluence of the mitral and tricuspid annuli to which the noncoronary leaflet of the aortic valve and the membranous interventricular septum are attached. The left fibrous trigone is formed from the fibrous continuity between the aortic and mitral valves. With the anterolateral and posteromedial commissures located at the lowest point in the mitral annulus, the normal configuration of the valvular annulus is in the shape of a saddle (**Fig. 2**). The mitral valve annulus is thinnest at the insertion of the posterior leaflet, thus making it the most mobile portion of the valve and consequently most vulnerable to dilatation.[1,30]

The anterior leaflet of the mitral valve comprises approximately two-thirds of the area of the valvular orifice but only one-third for the annular circumference, whereas the posterior leaflet comprises the other two-thirds of the annular circumference (**Fig. 3**). A normal line of coaptation exists between the leaflets, ranging from 7 mm to 9 mm, thus allowing for valve competency with a variety of physiologic systolic pressures and volumes. Of note, the commissures do not extend into the annulus,

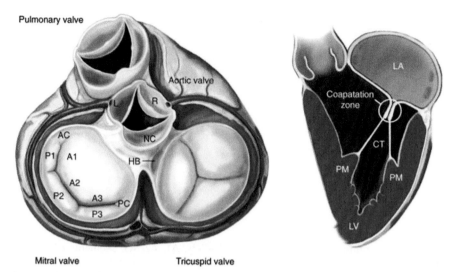

Pulmonary valve

Mitral valve   Tricuspid valve

Fig. 1. Anatomy of the mitral valve and mitral apparatus. (*Left*) Anatomic view of the cardiac valves in systole with the left and right atrium cropped away and the great vessels transected. The mitral valve apparatus consists of the mitral leaflets, mitral annulus, chordae tendineae, the papillary muscles, and the left ventricle. (*Right*) Normal function of the mitral apparatus brings both leaflets together in systole and creates the coaptation zone. A1, A2, A3, segments of the anterior leaflet; AC, anterior commissure; CT, chordae tendineae; HB, His bundle; L, left coronary cusp; LA, left atrium; LV, left ventricle; NC, noncoronary cusp; P1, P2, P3, segments of the posterior leaflet; PC, posterior commissure; PM, papillary muscle; R, right coronary cusp. (*From* Castillo JG, Adams DH. Mitral valve repair and replacement. In: Otto C, editor. Valvular heart disease: a companion to Braunwald's heart disease. 4th edition. Philadelphia: Elsevier Saunders; 2014. p. 327; with permission.)

leaving so-called commissural leaflets that must be respected during commissurotomy to prevent subsequent leaflet tearing and valvular regurgitation.[30]

The posterior leaflet is divided into three segments: P1, P2, and P3 based on normal indentations along the leaflet free edge, with corresponding segments A1, A2, and A3 in the anterior leaflet, albeit without visible anatomic delineations as those in the posterior leaflet (see **Fig. 3**). The posterior leaflet, also known as the mural leaflet, is attached to the ventricular free wall, thus directly subjecting it to the repeated stresses of ventricular contractions and making it more vulnerable to prolapse, particularly within the P2 leaflet.[30]

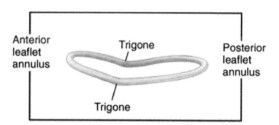

Fig. 2. Schematic configuration of the mitral annulus. (*From* Carpentier A, Adams DH, Filsoufi F. Surgical anatomy and physiology. In: Carpentier A, editor. Carpentier's reconstructive valve surgery: from valve analysis to valve reconstruction. Philadelphia: Elsevier Saunders; 2010. p. 30; with permission.)

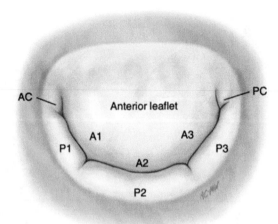

Fig. 3. Normal configuration of mitral valve leaflets. A1, A2, A3, segments of anterior leaflet; AC, anterior commisure; P1, P2, P3, segments of posterior leaflet; PC, posterior commissure. (*From* Carpentier A, Adams DH, Filsoufi F. Surgical anatomy and physiology. In: Carpentier A, editor. Carpentier's reconstructive valve surgery: from valve analysis to valve reconstruction. Philadelphia: Elsevier Saunders; 2010. p. 33; with permission.)

The subvalvular apparatus consists of the chordae tendinae, collagenous connections between the papillary muscles and the ventricular leaflet surface, and papillary muscles, which are part of the muscular ventricular wall (**Fig. 4**). Primary or marginal chordae attach to the free edge of the leaflet, thus preventing leaflet prolapse. Secondary or intermediary chordae attach to the ventricular leaflet surface and act to

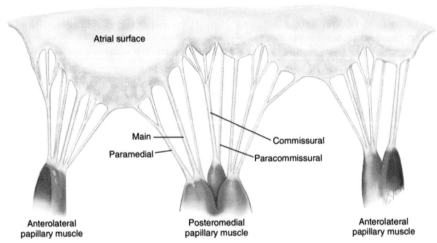

Fig. 4. Mitral subvalvular apparatus. The chordae tendinae attach the valve leaflets to the papillary muscles, with the main chordae originating from the middle of the leaflet free edge and others identified according to their position relative to the commissures and to the leaflet free edge. There is wide variability in chordal branching and attachments. (*From* Carpentier A, Adams DH, Filsoufi F. Surgical anatomy and physiology. In: Carpentier A, editor. Carpentier's reconstructive valve surgery: from valve analysis to valve reconstruction. Philadelphia: Elsevier Saunders; 2010. p. 37; with permission.)

reduce leaflet tension. Tertiary chordae (basal chordae), which are only present on the posterior leaflet, attach the leaflet base to the annulus and myocardium.[1]

Two papillary muscles originate from the left ventricular myocardium: the anterolateral papillary muscle and the posteromedial papillary muscle (**Fig. 5**). Each papillary muscle anchors chordae from both leaflets, and the configurations of chordal attachments to each papillary muscle, and even to the ventricular wall, can widely vary.[30] Working in concert, all of these components of the mitral valve apparatus serve to maintain valvular competence and direct proper blood flow from the left atrium to the left ventricle.

THE FRENCH CORRECTION

Alain Carpentier was the first to systematically describe regurgitant mitral valve pathology and standardize the myriad of methods for repairing the mitral valve.[25,31] He divided mitral valve pathology into three primary types based on leaflet motion (**Table 1**). Type I MR describes MR with normal leaflet motion. This type of MR develops from annular dilation, leaflet tear, leaflet perforation, or vegetation. These structural deficiencies are usually the result of ischemic or dilated cardiomyopathy, long-standing atrial fibrillation, trauma, or endocarditis (**Fig. 6**). Type II describes a valve with leaflet prolapse, which results from chordal rupture, papillary muscle rupture, chordal elongation, or papillary muscle elongation. Leaflet prolapse is usually secondary to degenerative processes, such as fibroelastic deficiency, Barlow disease, or Marfan syndrome, but it can also develop as a result of endocarditis, trauma, or ischemic cardiomyopathy (**Fig. 7**). Type III describes a valve with restricted leaflet motion. Type IIIa refers to restricted leaflet opening primarily during diastole, usually the result of rheumatic disease causing commissure fusion, chordae thickening, and chordae fusion. Type IIIb refers to restricted leaflet opening primarily during systole, resulting from leaflet tethering caused by papillary muscle displacement from localized ventricular dyskinesia or global ventricular dilatation from later stages of various cardiomyopathies (**Fig. 8**).[1,25] Because the cause of valvular dysfunction determines prognosis and treatment strategy depends on this cause, Carpentier's classification scheme aids selection of appropriate surgical repair techniques.

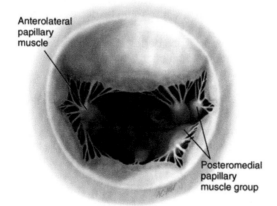

Fig. 5. View of the anterolateral and posteromedial papillary muscles through the mitral valve orifice. (*From* Carpentier A, Adams DH, Filsoufi F. Surgical anatomy and physiology. In: Carpentier A, editor. Carpentier's reconstructive valve surgery: from valve analysis to valve reconstruction. Philadelphia: Elsevier Saunders; 2010. p. 35; with permission.)

Table 1
Carpentier's functional classification of mitral regurgitation

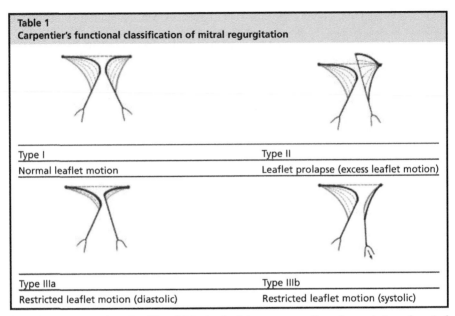

Type I	Type II
Normal leaflet motion	Leaflet prolapse (excess leaflet motion)
Type IIIa	Type IIIb
Restricted leaflet motion (diastolic)	Restricted leaflet motion (systolic)

From Carpentier A, Adams DH, Filsoufi F. Pathophysiology, preoperative valve analysis, and surgical indications. In: Carpentier A, editor. Carpentier's reconstructive valve surgery: from valve analysis to valve reconstruction. Philadelphia: Elsevier Saunders; 2010. p. 45; with permission.

The rationale behind Carpentier's French correction of a regurgitant mitral valve is restoration of the normal anatomic relationships within the valve apparatus, and the first step toward that restoration is a careful examination of the diseased valve. The atrium is examined for jet lesions indicative of prolapse of an opposing leaflet, and the annulus diameter is assessed for degree of dilatation. All leaflets are unfurled with a nerve hook and examined for thickening, tethering, or prolapse, and the chordae are inspected for rupture or elongation.

Repair of the valve proceeds with a quadrangular resection of the prolapsed portion of the posterior leaflet with corresponding annular plication, followed by suture reapproximation of the free leaflet edges (**Fig. 9**).

Correcting anterior leaflet prolapse depends on the causative lesion, whether it is chordal rupture or elongation. When chordal rupture has occurred, the free edge of the prolapsed leaflet is fixed to intact secondary chordae or chordae from the mural leaflet are transposed to the free edge of the prolapsed anterior leaflet, which requires sufficient mobilization of the corresponding papillary muscle (**Fig. 10**).

When anterior leaflet prolapse is the result of chordal elongation, the excess chordal length can essentially be tucked into an invagination created within the attached papillary muscle and then suturing each side of the divided papillary muscle back together around the extra chordal length (**Fig. 11**). Another method of mending chordal elongation is shortening of the papillary muscle (**Fig. 12**).

Restricted leaflet motion is another source of MR, and it is the result of four different lesions: (1) leaflet thickening, (2) chordal thickening, (3) commissural fusion, and (4) chordal fusion. Commisurotomy is done to correct commissural fusion. Chordal thickening, which occurs with the secondary chordae, is alleviated with resection of the thickened chordae or fenestration of thickened marginal chordae.

Type I - Normal Leaflet Motion

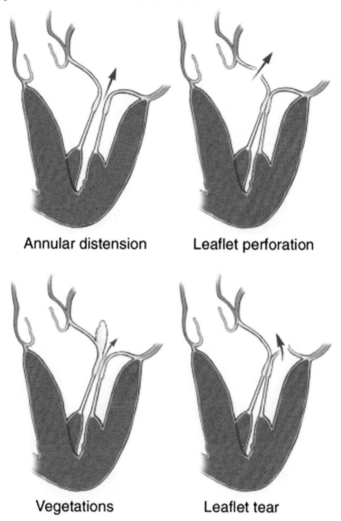

Annular distension	Leaflet perforation
Vegetations	Leaflet tear

Fig. 6. Type I functional MR according to Carpentier's classification. Type I describes MR with normal leaflet motion, usually arising from annular dilatation, leaflet perforation, vegetation, or leaflet tear. (*From* Carpentier A, Adams DH, Filsoufi F. Pathophysiology, preoperative valve analysis, and surgical indications. In: Carpentier A, editor. Carpentier's reconstructive valve surgery: from valve analysis to valve reconstruction. Philadelphia: Elsevier Saunders; 2010. p. 47; with permission.)

Finally, to correct the annular dilatation that accompanies essentially all cases of mitral insufficiency, Carpentier pioneered the development of a rigid prosthetic annuloplasty ring. The ring is intended to restore the normal systolic size and shape of the annulus, thus also restoring leaflet coaptation and preventing further deformation of the annulus (**Fig. 13**).

Since first describing the use of a rigid annuloplasty ring, Carpentier has developed three different types of annuloplasty rings to refine repair according to the anatomic

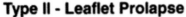

Type II - Leaflet Prolapse

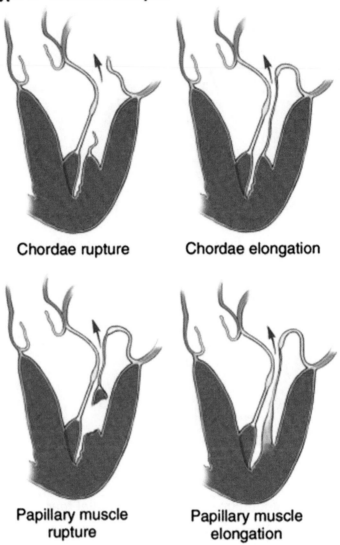

Chordae rupture   Chordae elongation

Papillary muscle   Papillary muscle
rupture   elongation

Fig. 7. Type II functional MR according to Carpentier's classification. Type II describes MR from leaflet prolapse, usually the result of chordal or papillary muscle rupture or elongation. (*From* Carpentier A, Adams DH, Filsoufi F. Pathophysiology, preoperative valve analysis, and surgical indications. In: Carpentier A, editor. Carpentier's reconstructive valve surgery: from valve analysis to valve reconstruction. Philadelphia: Elsevier Saunders; 2010. p. 47; with permission.)

deformation: (1) the Carpentier-Edwards Classic Ring, (2) the Carpentier-Edwards Physio Ring, and (3) the Carpentier-McCarthy-Adams Etiologix IMR Ring for ischemic MR (Edwards LifeSciences Corp, Irvine, CA). The Physio ring is designed for degenerative MR, with a large anteroposterior diameter and a slight saddle shape to restore normal systolic contour to the valvular annulus.[32] Sizing of the annuloplasty ring is

Type III Restricted Leaflet Motion

Type IIIa - Diastolic

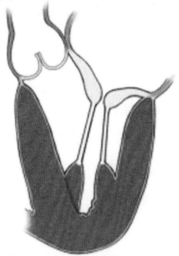

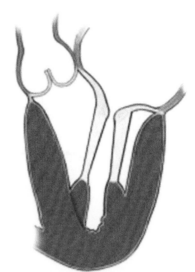

**Commissure fusion/
leaflet thickening**

**Chordae thickening/
fusion**

Type IIIb - Systolic

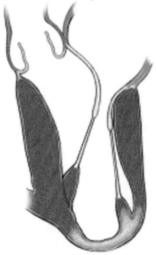

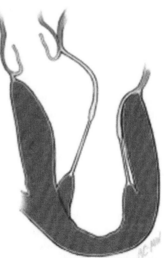

Myocardial infarction

Ventricular dilatation

Fig. 8. Type IIIa and IIIb functional MR according to Carpentier's classification. Type IIIa describes MR from restricted leaflet motion during diastole and type IIIb describes MR from restricted leaflet motion during systole. (*From* Carpentier A, Adams DH, Filsoufi F. Pathophysiology, preoperative valve analysis, and surgical indications. In: Carpentier A, editor. Carpentier's reconstructive valve surgery: from valve analysis to valve reconstruction. Philadelphia: Elsevier Saunders; 2010. p. 48; with permission.)

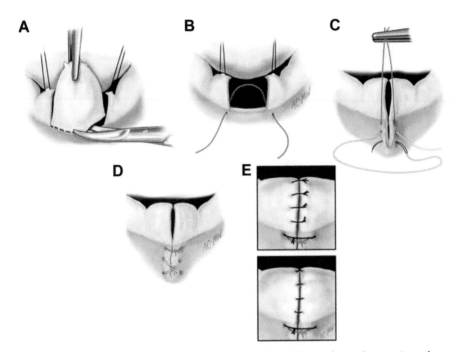

Fig. 9. Quadrangular resection of prolapsed P2 leaflet. (*A*) Quadrangular portion of prolapsed P2 leaflet is excised. (*B*) An interrupted mattress suture is placed through the annulus at the limits of the resected area. (*C*) A figure-of-eight suture is placed through the annulus to plicate the annulus. (*D*) Completed annular plication. (*E*) Interrupted sutures are placed to reapproximate the resected leaflet edges, with knots inverted or everted. (*From* Carpentier A, Adams DH, Filsoufi F. Techniques in type II posterior leaflet prolapse. In: Carpentier A, editor. Carpentier's reconstructive valve surgery: from valve analysis to valve reconstruction. Philadelphia: Elsevier Saunders; 2010. p. 118; with permission.)

based on precise measurement of the anterior leaflet surface area by unfurling the leaflet, thus approximating the size and shape of the mitral orifice.[25]

Following correction of these annular and leaflet abnormalities, systolic anterior motion (SAM) of the mitral valve can result if there is a residual discrepancy between the annular area and the remaining leaflet tissue. SAM occurs when the anterior mitral valve leaflet prolapses into the left ventricular outflow tract (LVOT) during systole (**Fig. 14**).[33] The primary risk factors for the development of SAM following mitral valve repair are an undersized annuloplasty ring and/or excess leaflet tissue.[34,35] Consequences of this pathologic leaflet motion include residual MR and LVOT obstruction, both of which are observed on intraoperative transesophageal echocardiography. If SAM is observed intraoperatively following mitral valve repair, most instances are corrected with optimization of ventricular filling via increasing preload and afterload, improving atrioventricular synchrony through atrioventricular pacing, and stopping pharmacologic inotropic support to reduce ventricular hypercontractility. These maneuvers are also effective postoperatively and are supplemented with β-blocker administration. SAM that appears with provocative testing (dynamic SAM) usually resolves within a few weeks after surgery through LVOT remodeling.[36]

Instances of SAM that are irreversible, persist following surgery, or produce significant hemodynamic derangement must be surgically corrected. If the unfurled anterior

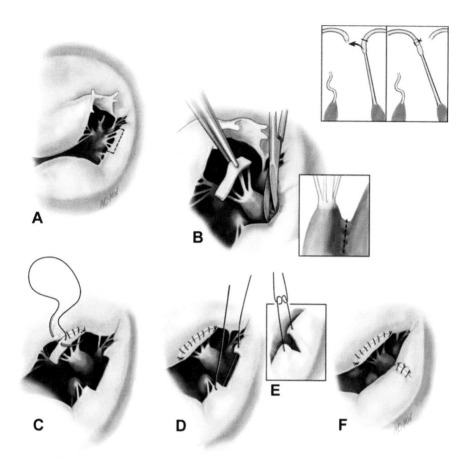

Fig. 10. Chordal transposition to correct chordal rupture. (*A*) Posterior leaflet adjacent to the area of prolapsed leaflet is identified. (*B*) Posterior leaflet tissue is mobilized with attached chordae, with mobilization of papillary muscle as necessary. (*C*) Reattachment of posterior chordae to prolapsed anterior leaflet. (*D, E*) Reapproximation of posterior leaflet edges. (*F*) Completed chordal transposition. (*From* Carpentier A, Adams DH, Filsoufi F. Techniques in type II anterior leaflet prolapse. In: Carpentier A, editor. Carpentier's reconstructive valve surgery: from valve analysis to valve reconstruction. Philadelphia: Elsevier Saunders; 2010. p. 101; with permission.)

leaflet is much larger than the annulus, the annuloplasty ring should be replaced with a ring of larger diameter[37] or the posterior leaflet height should be reduced. Carpentier advocated for a sliding annuloplasty to decrease the height of the posterior leaflet, which includes resection of a portion of the leaflet and annular plication with reapproximation of the resected leaflet edges (**Fig. 15**).[36,38]

Since developing these methods of mitral valve repair, outcomes with these particular techniques have varied. Although the repair techniques demonstrate excellent short-term results with low rates of persistent MR and even lower mortality rates, durability with Carpentier's repair techniques declines over time.[39–42] David and colleagues[39] report freedom from MR at 12 years ranging from 65% to 80%, depending on which leaflet is prolapsed. Flameng and colleagues[41] cite a constant recurrence rate of regurgitation of 2% to 3% per year, with a freedom from MR of

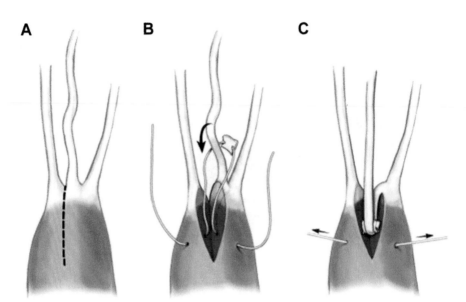

Fig. 11. Chordal shortening technique. (*A*) Papillary muscle is divided. (*B*) Pledgeted suture is passed around excess chord. (*C*) Pledgeted suture around excess chord is invaginated into divided papillary muscle, which is subsequently reapproximated. (*From* Carpentier A, Adams DH, Filsoufi F. Techniques in type II anterior leaflet prolapse. In: Carpentier A, editor. Carpentier's reconstructive valve surgery: from valve analysis to valve reconstruction. Philadelphia: Elsevier Saunders; 2010. p. 106; with permission.)

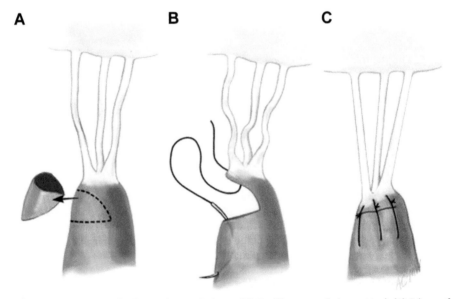

Fig. 12. Papillary muscle shortening technique. (*A*) Papillary muscle is resected. (*B*) Edges of resected papillary muscle are reapproximated. (*C*) Completed shortened papillary muscle. (*From* Carpentier A, Adams DH, Filsoufi F. Techniques in type II anterior leaflet prolapse. In: Carpentier A, editor. Carpentier's reconstructive valve surgery: from valve analysis to valve reconstruction. Philadelphia: Elsevier Saunders; 2010. p. 107; with permission.)

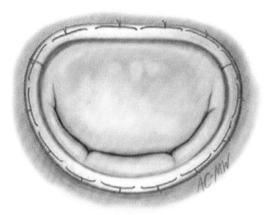

Fig. 13. Completed annuloplasty to correct annular dilatation. (*From* Carpentier A, Adams DH, Filsoufi F. Valve exposure, intraoperative valve analysis, and reconstruction. In: Carpentier A, editor. Carpentier's reconstructive valve surgery: from valve analysis to valve reconstruction. Philadelphia: Elsevier Saunders; 2010. p. 60; with permission.)

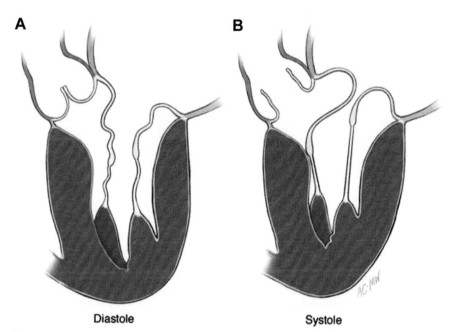

Fig. 14. SAM of the mitral valve. (*A*) Redundant chordal and leaflet tissue during diastole. (*B*) Left ventricular outflow tract obstruction from redundant chordal and leaflet tissue during systole. (*From* Carpentier A, Adams DH, Filsoufi F. Techniques in systolic anterior leaflet motion (SAM). In: Carpentier A, editor. Carpentier's reconstructive valve surgery: from valve analysis to valve reconstruction. Philadelphia: Elsevier Saunders; 2010. p. 157; with permission.)

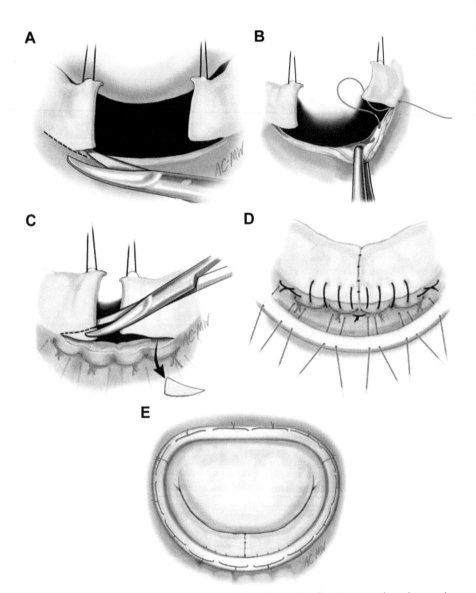

Fig. 15. Sliding leaflet annuloplasty. (*A*) Excess prolapsed leaflet is resected, and secondary chordae are resected as necessary. (*B*) Sutures are then passed successively through the annulus to reduce its diameter. (*C*) Annular sutures are tied to compress, not plicate, the annulus. (*D*) Completed sliding leaflet reconstruction with annuloplasty ring placement. (*E*) Completed sliding annuloplasty. (*From* Carpentier A, Adams DH, Filsoufi F. Techniques in type II posterior leaflet prolapse. In: Carpentier A, editor. Carpentier's reconstructive valve surgery: from valve analysis to valve reconstruction. Philadelphia: Elsevier Saunders; 2010. p. 120–2; with permission.)

65% at 10 years. In patients with Barlow disease, Jouan and colleagues[31] describe a recurrence rate of 9.8% of moderate or greater MR. Although there are varying estimates of the recurrence of MR and the subsequent need for reoperation in these patients, repairs of this type may be permanent, albeit with recurrent MR possibly remaining clinically silent. As experience with Carpentier's repair techniques began to accumulate and advanced imaging techniques that allow better comprehension of the structural dynamics of the mitral valve became available, new ideas regarding the optimal means of repairing the mitral valve began to emerge. These new ideas of mitral valve repair eventually coalesced into what is known as the "American correction."

THE AMERICAN CORRECTION

In contrast to Carpentier's French correction of degenerative MR, Gerald Lawrie developed the so-called American correction as a means of functional restoration, as opposed to anatomic restoration, of the mitral valve. Primary tenets of this American correction consist of a flexible annuloplasty ring and maintenance of the entire mitral valve leaflets with artificial chordae used to correct areas of prolapse.[26,27,29]

This idea of restoration of function developed over time as knowledge of the dynamic structure of the mitral valve throughout the cardiac cycle was elucidated. Enhanced imaging techniques, such as three-dimensional echocardiography, drove these developments. Visualization of the mitral valve in vivo, as opposed to autopsy examination, led to the understanding that movement of the entire valve apparatus determines its degree of proper function. Thus, a functional correction of the mitral valve became a more salient objective.

Valvular competency is based on leaflet coaptation, which is derived from the mitral annulus. A normally functioning mitral annulus varies in shape throughout the course of the cardiac cycle. The annulus is attached to the left ventricular myocardium posterolaterally, the aortic root anteriorly, and the left atrium superiorly, creating a saddle-shape. The commissural junction of the anterior and posterior leaflets is angulated, which becomes more acute during systole as the ventricle contracts and the aortic root and sinuses of Valsalva expand. These systolic changes displace the anterior annulus and leaflet, posteriorly, thus promoting leaflet apposition during systole.[29,43,44]

The mitral valve annulus in patients with degenerative MR, however, can double in size, with significant flattening of the valvular orifice and diminished leaflet edge apposition.[29,45,46] Without sufficient leaflet coaptation, additional stress is added to the leaflet bodies and marginal chordae during systole, thus predisposing these components to further dysfunction and future failure.[47–49]

As experience with Carpentier's techniques of rigid annuloplasty repair and leaflet resection began to accumulate, durability of the repair techniques was questioned, in light of a reoperation rate for recurrent MR of 43%.[50] Furthermore, additional investigation into mechanisms of mitral valve competence revealed that rigid annuloplasty rings induce high levels of leaflet and annular strain, thus predisposing the valvular repair to early mechanical failure.[48]

In response to these high rates of reoperation, the American correction was devised to maintain normal three-dimensional geometry and permit normal movement of the valvular apparatus throughout the cardiac cycle. First and foremost, this American correction is a nonresectional or limited resection approach, characterized by maintaining an intact annulus and leaflets. This approach is thought to more closely mimic the function and movement of a normal mitral valve, with a similar distribution of stress throughout the leaflets and annulus.[51]

Similar to Carpentier's technique, the American correction begins with a detailed examination of the valve apparatus to determine the sources of valvular insufficiency. Transition zones along the leaflet coaptation edge are marked to determine the normal points of leaflet coaptation, traction sutures are placed in the annulus, and the valve is tested with a bulb syringe (**Fig. 16**).

To correct areas of leaflet prolapse, artificial Gore-Tex cords are placed through the papillary muscle in two places and then each end of suture is brought up to the leaflet edge as a pair of chordae and secured with a double pass through the edge of the valve leaflet (**Fig. 17**). When the necessary sutures have been placed to correct the areas of prolapse, each chord length is adjusted according to intermittent examinations of leaflet coaptation. Of note, overshortening of the chordae can create a narrow regurgitant jet after weaning from bypass. This results in the papillary muscles and the leaflet edges being pulled into the ventricular lumen more than what is simulated with bulb syringe insufflation. After the chordae have been appropriately sized, the sutures are then tied, and the knots are tacked to the ventricular leaflet surfaces.[28]

A limited resection technique can also be used with a triangular leaflet resection to correct leaflet prolapse (**Fig. 18**). This simplified technique is used to reduce the height of the posterior leaflet, with a reduced incidence of postoperative SAM. Furthermore, a limited resection reduces excessively redundant leaflet tissue, as occurs with Barlow disease, in the repair compared with the use of artificial chordae. Combining a triangular resection with a large (generally 36, 38, or 40 mm) annuloplasty ring prevents the development of SAM.[52] Additionally, this type of resection is less technically complex compared with Carpentier's sliding annuloplasty to correct posterior leaflet prolapse, thus possibly prompting more surgeons to repair rather than replace some valves.[53]

After correcting leaflet prolapse, attention is then turned to repair of the annulus. Following ventricular insufflation, a flexible annuloplasty ring that best approximates the entire surface of the valve is chosen. Interrupted sutures are placed to anchor the annuloplasty ring at the trigones of the valve, and a running suture is used to attach the ring within the intertrigonal portions of the annulus.[28]

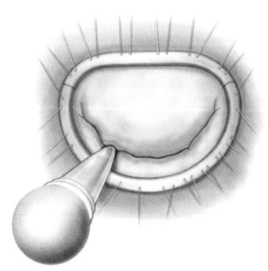

Fig. 16. Testing valve competency with a bulb syringe. (*From* Carpentier A, Adams DH, Filsoufi F. Techniques in type I dysfunction. In: Carpentier A, editor. Carpentier's reconstructive valve surgery: from valve analysis to valve reconstruction. Philadelphia: Elsevier Saunders; 2010. p. 78; with permission.)

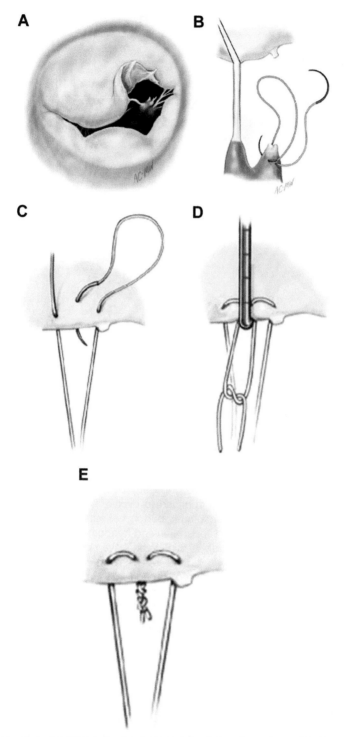

Fig. 17. Placement of artificial chordae to correct leaflet prolapse from chordal rupture. (*A*) Prolapsed anterior leaflet from ruptured chord. (*B*) A nonelongated chord is pulled taut for

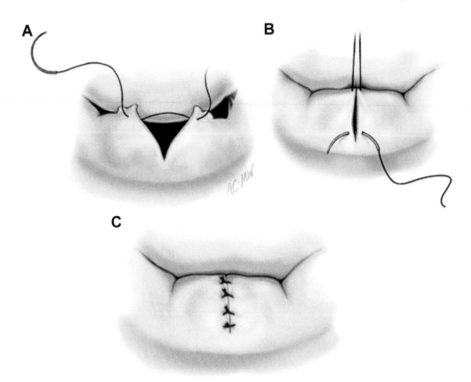

Fig. 18. Limited triangular resection of prolapsed posterior leaflet. (*A*) Triangular resection of prolapsed posterior leaflet. (*B*) Placement of interrupted sutures to reapproximate resected leaflet edges. (*C*) Completed triangular resection. (*From* Carpentier A, Adams DH, Filsoufi F. Techniques in type II posterior leaflet prolapse. In: Carpentier A, editor. Carpentier's reconstructive valve surgery: from valve analysis to valve reconstruction. Philadelphia: Elsevier Saunders; 2010. p. 116; with permission.)

This American correction has gained popularity over the past several years[54] as limited resection repair techniques continue to evolve.[55] Results demonstrate that these limited or nonresectional techniques perform at least as well as Carpentier's French correction. Freedom from reoperation and freedom from recurrent significant MR (as assessed by echocardiography) at 10 years have been reported at 90.1% and 93.9%, respectively. Additionally, studies have demonstrated almost no postoperative SAM when ventricular filling is optimized through adequate preload and afterload, there is atrioventricular synchrony, and hypercontractility is limited.[52] Although this limited or nonresectional technique has only been cultivated over the past decade, it seems to be a reasonable and durable approach to repair of the mitral valve.

reference, and a figure-of-eight suture is placed through the free papillary muscle head corresponding to the area of the ruptured chord. (*C*) The free ends of the suture are passed through to the ventricular side of the leaflet. (*D*) The first knot is tied while adjusting the length of the artificial chord to match that of the reference chord. (*E*) Completed artificial chordae. (*From* Carpentier A, Adams DH, Filsoufi F. Techniques in type II anterior leaflet prolapse. In: Carpentier A, editor. Carpentier's reconstructive valve surgery: from valve analysis to valve reconstruction. Philadelphia: Elsevier Saunders; 2010. p. 102; with permission.)

With the evidence supporting mitral valve repair over replacement for most degenerative mitral valve pathology, it is expected that these methods of valvular correction will continue to develop, given the wide variety of mitral valve pathology that exists. Carpentier was able to classify these various pathologies, thus providing a framework from which methods of mitral valve repair could develop in an organized and reproducible fashion. Relying on pathologic and autopsy specimens, the French correction aimed to restore normal valvular anatomy and has proven to be a durable method of repair. A purely anatomic correction, however, neglects the valve's functionality as an integral component of its competency. Furthermore, the technically demanding nature of Carpentier's techniques has remained an obstacle to widespread adoption of mitral valve repair techniques, leaving many patients who would have done well with a repaired mitral valve with a valve replacement.

With improved imaging capabilities and greater knowledge of the intricacies of mitral valve motion and function, the American correction was developed. This limited or nonresectional method of repair naturally follows the French correction as a consequence of innovation and reflects an evolution in the principles of mitral valve repair. Developed to first and foremost correct mitral valve function, these techniques may be somewhat technically less complex than Carpentier's methods, thus a greater number of surgeons will feel confident in repairing rather than replacing more mitral valves. These repair techniques will undoubtedly continue to evolve, ideally resulting in lower rates of recurrence and reoperation and better patient outcomes.

There are clearly many methods to repair a mitral valve, but the unifying principles include a comprehensive understanding of the valve pathology, correction of leaflet prolapse, and reduction of annular dilatation. Most importantly, one cannot leave the operating room with a leaky valve. If these essential principles are followed, a durable repair usually results.

REFERENCES

1. Goldstone AB, Woo YJ. Surgical treatment of the mitral valve in sabiston and spencer surgery of the chest. 9th edition. Philadelphia: Saunders; 2016.
2. Ling LH, Enriquez-Sarano M, Seward JB, et al. Clinical outcome of mitral regurgitation due to flail leaflet. N Engl J Med 1996;335(19):1417–23.
3. Enriquez-Sarano M, Avierinos JF, Messika-Zeitoun D, et al. Quantitative determinants of the outcome of asymptomatic mitral regurgitation. N Engl J Med 2005; 352(9):875–83.
4. Goldman ME, Mora F, Guarino T, et al. Mitral valvuloplasty is superior to valve replacement for preservation of left ventricular function: an intraoperative two-dimensional echocardiographic study. J Am Coll Cardiol 1987;10(3):568–75.
5. Gillinov AM, Blackstone EH, Nowicki ER, et al. Valve repair versus valve replacement for degenerative mitral valve disease. J Thorac Cardiovasc Surg 2008; 135(4):885–93, 893.e1-2.
6. Shuhaiber J, Anderson RJ. Meta-analysis of clinical outcomes following surgical mitral valve repair or replacement. Eur J Cardiothorac Surg 2007;31(2):267–75.
7. Vassileva CM, Mishkel G, McNeely C, et al. Long-term survival of patients undergoing mitral valve repair and replacement: a longitudinal analysis of Medicare fee-for-service beneficiaries. Circulation 2013;127(18):1870–6.
8. Zhou YX, Leobon B, Berthoumieu P, et al. Long-term outcomes following repair or replacement in degenerative mitral valve disease. Thorac Cardiovasc Surg 2010; 58(7):415–21.

9. Grossi EA, Goldberg JD, LaPietra A, et al. Ischemic mitral valve reconstruction and replacement: comparison of long-term survival and complications. J Thorac Cardiovasc Surg 2001;122(6):1107–24.

10. Zalaquett R, Scheu M, Campla C, et al. Long-term results of repair versus replacement for degenerative mitral valve regurgitation. Rev Med Chil 2005; 133(10):1139–46 [in Spanish].

11. Daneshmand MA, Milano CA, Rankin JS, et al. Mitral valve repair for degenerative disease: a 20-year experience. Ann Thorac Surg 2009;88(6):1828–37.

12. Gillinov AM, Wierup PN, Blackstone EH, et al. Is repair preferable to replacement for ischemic mitral regurgitation? J Thorac Cardiovasc Surg 2001;122(6): 1125–41.

13. Reece TB, Tribble CG, Ellman PI, et al. Mitral repair is superior to replacement when associated with coronary artery disease. Ann Surg 2004;239(5):671–5 [discussion: 675–7].

14. Magne J, Girerd N, Senechal M, et al. Mitral repair versus replacement for ischemic mitral regurgitation: comparison of short-term and long-term survival. Circulation 2009;120(11 Suppl):S104–11.

15. Al-Radi OO, Austin PC, Tu JV, et al. Mitral repair versus replacement for ischemic mitral regurgitation. Ann Thorac Surg 2005;79(4):1260–7 [discussion: 1260–7].

16. Nishimura RA, Otto CM, Bonow RO, et al. 2014 AHA/ACC guideline for the management of patients with valvular heart disease: executive summary: a report of the American College of Cardiology/American Heart Association Task Force on Practice Guidelines. J Am Coll Cardiol 2014;63(22):2438–88.

17. LaPar DJ, Kron IL. Should all ischemic mitral regurgitation be repaired? When should we replace? Curr Opin Cardiol 2011;26(2):113–7.

18. Davila JC, Glover RP. Circumferential suture of the mitral valve for the correction of regurgitation. Am J Cardiol 1958;2(3):267–75.

19. Lillehei CW, Gott VL, Dewall RA, et al. The surgical treatment of stenotic or regurgitant lesions of the mitral and aortic valves by direct vision utilizing a pump-oxygenator. J Thorac Surg 1958;35(2):154–91.

20. McGoon DC. Repair of mitral insufficiency due to ruptured chordae tendinae. J Thorac Cardiovasc Surg 1960;39:357–62.

21. Carpentier A. Reconstructive valvuloplasty. A new technique of mitral valvuloplasty. Presse Med 1969;77(7):251–3 [in French].

22. Carpentier A, Deloche A, Dauptain J, et al. A new reconstructive operation for correction of mitral and tricuspid insufficiency. J Thorac Cardiovasc Surg 1971; 61(1):1–13.

23. Carpentier A, Relland J, Deloche A, et al. Conservative management of the prolapsed mitral valve. Ann Thorac Surg 1978;26(4):294–302.

24. Carpentier A, Chauvaud S, Fabiani JN, et al. Reconstructive surgery of mitral valve incompetence: ten-year appraisal. J Thorac Cardiovasc Surg 1980;79(3): 338–48.

25. Carpentier A. Cardiac valve surgery: the "French correction". J Thorac Cardiovasc Surg 1983;86(3):323–37.

26. Lawrie GM, Earle EA, Earle NR. Feasibility and intermediate term outcome of repair of prolapsing anterior mitral leaflets with artificial chordal replacement in 152 patients. Ann Thorac Surg 2006;81(3):849–56 [discussion: 856].

27. Lawrie GM, Earle EA, Earle NR. Nonresectional repair of the Barlow mitral valve: importance of dynamic annular evaluation. Ann Thorac Surg 2009;88(4):1191–6.

28. Spratt JA. Non-resectional repair of myxomatous mitral valve disease: the "American Correction". J Heart Valve Dis 2011;20(4):407–14.

29. Lawrie GM. Structure, function, and dynamics of the mitral annulus: importance in mitral valve repair for myxamatous mitral valve disease. Methodist Debakey Cardiovasc J 2010;6(1):8–14.

30. Carpentier A, Adams DH, Filsoufi F. Surgical anatomy and physiology [of the mitral valve]. Philadelphia: Saunders Elsevier; 2010.

31. Jouan J. Mitral valve repair over five decades. Ann Cardiothorac Surg 2015;4(4): 322–34.

32. Carpentier AF, Lessana A, Relland JY, et al. The "physio-ring": an advanced concept in mitral valve annuloplasty. Ann Thorac Surg 1995;60(5):1177–85 [discussion: 1185–76].

33. Gallerstein PE, Berger M, Rubenstein S, et al. Systolic anterior motion of the mitral valve and outflow obstruction after mitral valve reconstruction. Chest 1983;83(5): 819–20.

34. Mihaileanu S, Marino JP, Chauvaud S, et al. Left ventricular outflow obstruction after mitral valve repair (Carpentier's technique). Proposed mechanisms of disease. Circulation 1988;78(3 Pt 2):I78–84.

35. Lee KS, Stewart WJ, Lever HM, et al. Mechanism of outflow tract obstruction causing failed mitral valve repair. Anterior displacement of leaflet coaptation. Circulation 1993;88(5 Pt 2):II24–9.

36. Carpentier A, Adams DH, Filsoufi F. Techniques in systolic anterior leaflet motion (SAM). Philadelphia: Elsevier; 2010.

37. Adams DH, Anyanwu AC, Rahmanian PB, et al. Large annuloplasty rings facilitate mitral valve repair in Barlow's disease. Ann Thorac Surg 2006;82(6):2096–100 [discussion: 2101].

38. Jebara VA, Mihaileanu S, Acar C, et al. Left ventricular outflow tract obstruction after mitral valve repair. Results of the sliding leaflet technique. Circulation 1993;88(5 Pt 2):II30–4.

39. David TE, Ivanov J, Armstrong S, et al. A comparison of outcomes of mitral valve repair for degenerative disease with posterior, anterior, and bileaflet prolapse. J Thorac Cardiovasc Surg 2005;130(5):1242–9.

40. Chang BC, Youn YN, Ha JW, et al. Long-term clinical results of mitral valvuloplasty using flexible and rigid rings: a prospective and randomized study. J Thorac Cardiovasc Surg 2007;133(4):995–1003.

41. Flameng W, Meuris B, Herijgers P, et al. Durability of mitral valve repair in Barlow disease versus fibroelastic deficiency. J Thorac Cardiovasc Surg 2008;135(2): 274–82.

42. Chung CH, Kim JB, Choo SJ, et al. Long-term outcomes after mitral ring annuloplasty for degenerative mitral regurgitation: Duran ring versus Carpentier-Edwards ring. J Heart Valve Dis 2007;16(5):536–44 [discussion: 544–5].

43. Itoh A, Ennis DB, Bothe W, et al. Mitral annular hinge motion contribution to changes in mitral septal-lateral dimension and annular area. J Thorac Cardiovasc Surg 2009;138(5):1090–9.

44. Lansac E, Lim KH, Shomura Y, et al. Dynamic balance of the aortomitral junction. J Thorac Cardiovasc Surg 2002;123(5):911–8.

45. Kaplan SR, Bashein G, Sheehan FH, et al. Three-dimensional echocardiographic assessment of annular shape changes in the normal and regurgitant mitral valve. Am Heart J 2000;139(3):378–87.

46. Pini R, Devereux RB, Greppi B, et al. Comparison of mitral valve dimensions and motion in mitral valve prolapse with severe mitral regurgitation to uncomplicated mitral valve prolapse and to mitral regurgitation without mitral valve prolapse. Am J Cardiol 1988;62(4):257–63.

47. Nazari S, Carli F, Salvi S, et al. Patterns of systolic stress distribution on mitral valve anterior leaflet chordal apparatus. A structural mechanical theoretical analysis. J Cardiovasc Surg (Torino) 2000;41(2):193–202.

48. Salgo IS, Gorman JH 3rd, Gorman RC, et al. Effect of annular shape on leaflet curvature in reducing mitral leaflet stress. Circulation 2002;106(6):711–7.

49. Kunzelman KS, Reimink MS, Cochran RP. Annular dilatation increases stress in the mitral valve and delays coaptation: a finite element computer model. Cardiovasc Surg 1997;5(4):427–34.

50. Gillinov AM, Cosgrove DM, Blackstone EH, et al. Durability of mitral valve repair for degenerative disease. J Thorac Cardiovasc Surg 1998;116(5):734–43.

51. Ben Zekry S, Lang RM, Sugeng L, et al. Mitral annulus dynamics early after valve repair: preliminary observations of the effect of resectional versus non-resectional approaches. J Am Soc Echocardiogr 2011;24(11):1233–42.

52. Gazoni LM, Fedoruk LM, Kern JA, et al. A simplified approach to degenerative disease: triangular resections of the mitral valve. Ann Thorac Surg 2007;83(5):1658–64 [discussion: 1664–5].

53. Suri RM, Orszulak TA. Triangular resection for repair of mitral regurgitation due to degenerative disease. Oper Tech Thorac Cardiovasc Surg 2005;10(3):194–9.

54. Kshettry VR, Aranki SF. Current trends in mitral valve repair techniques in North America. J Heart Valve Dis 2012;21(6):690–5.

55. Woo YJ, MacArthur JW Jr. Simplified nonresectional leaflet remodeling mitral valve repair for degenerative mitral regurgitation. J Thorac Cardiovasc Surg 2012;143(3):749–53.

Updates in Minimally Invasive Cardiac Surgery for General Surgeons

Muhammad Habib Zubair, MD[a], John Michael Smith, MD[b],*

KEYWORDS

- Minimally invasive cardiac surgery • Atrial septal defect
- Coronary artery bypass graft • Mitral valve • Robot

KEY POINTS

- Significant improvement and development have occurred in minimally invasive cardiac surgery over the past 20 years.
- Although most studies have consistently demonstrated equivalent or improved outcomes compared with conventional cardiac surgery, with significantly shorter recovery times, adoption continues to be limited.
- In addition, cost data have been inconsistent. Further ongoing trials are needed to help determine the exact roles for these innovative procedures.

HISTORY OF MINIMALLY INVASIVE CARDIAC SURGERY

The era of minimally invasive mitral valve (MV) surgery began in 1948 when Harken and Ellis[1] first described mitral valvulotomy through an intercostal approach. In 1994, Benetti and Ballester[2] from Argentina first described the left internal mammary artery (LIMA) to left anterior descending artery (LAD) anastomosis through a small left anterolateral thoracotomy; this was the first description of minimally invasive direct coronary artery bypass (MIDCAB) and was followed by Subramanian[3] in the United States in 1996. Cosgrove and Sabik[4] first described minimally invasive cardiac procedures in the United States in 1996 for the aortic valve (AV) followed by the MV.[5] Stevens and colleagues[6] invented the heart port platform in 1996, which opened the door to minimally invasive endoaortic cardiopulmonary bypass (CPB). Carpentier and colleagues[7] in 1996 did the first right minithoracotomy for a mitral valve replacement (MVR) followed shortly thereafter with the first robotic-assisted mitral valve procedure.

Conflicts of Interests: Consultant for Edwards Lifesciences, Intuitive Surgical, and AtriCure.
Funding: None.
[a] Division of General Surgery, Good Samaritan Hospital, TriHealth Heart Institute, Cincinnati, OH, USA; [b] Division of Cardiothoracic Surgery, Good Samaritan Hospital, TriHealth Heart Institute, 3219 Clifton Avenue, Cincinnati, OH 45220, USA
* Corresponding author.
E-mail address: jmichaelsmith62@gmail.com

Techniques involving a nonsternotomy or partial sternotomy incision with or without the use of CPB are included under the later section, Minimally invasive cardiac surgery.

HEARTPORT

The basic CPB requirements for robotic or minimally invasive cardiac surgery are achieved by a remote access system. One such system is the endoaortic balloon occlusion (EBO) system (Heartport, Redwood City, CA).[8] EBO is the only established system that enables port-only endoscopic cardiac surgery, without any cardioplegia cannula in the ascending aorta. A recent long-term follow-up by Kiessling and colleagues[9] showed no aortic degeneration or major complications over the course of 9 years. The ThruPort cannula (IntraClude, Edwards, Irvine, CA) is inserted into the common femoral artery. Then, under transthoracic echocardiography, a guide wire is advanced under transesophageal echocardiography into the ascending aorta. Then, the cannula is advanced. Venous drainage is provided by a single- or double-stage femoral venous cannula (Biomedicus 22–28 F, Edwards 24–28 F, or an ESTECH 23 or 25 F). After CPB initiation, the aortic occlusion balloon is inflated, and cardiac arrest is induced by injecting cardioplegia via the cardioplegia line. Bilateral radial artery pressure curves are used to avoid accidental occlusion of the innominate artery and to assist in monitoring balloon position. Major complications include aortic dissection, major vessel perforation, injury of intrapericardial structures, limb ischemia, myocardial infarction (MI), and neurologic events. Minor complications include minor vessel injury, groin bleeding, and lymphatic fistula. This platform allows most intracardiac procedures to be performed without sternotomy in a similar fashion to routine cardiac surgery (**Fig. 1**).

Minimally Invasive Direct Coronary Artery Bypass

Coronary artery bypass grafting (CABG) can be performed with CPB or without. CABG without CPB can be performed with or without open sternotomy or with minimally invasive anterior small thoracotomy; anterior small thoracotomy can include MIDCAB and minimally invasive cardiac surgery off-pump coronary artery bypass (MICS-OPCAB).

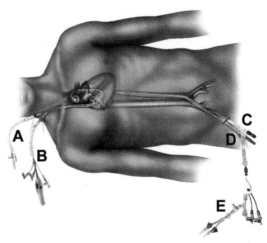

Fig. 1. (A) Endovent; (B) EndoPlege; (C) femoral venous cannula; (D) femoral arterial cannula; (E) Endoaortic balloon.

MIDCAB is also known as minimal or limited access CABG, defined as any nonster-notomy approach for CABG through a limited anterolateral thoracotomy. The LIMA is harvested through a left anterior thoracotomy or through a limited sternal split incision. The procedure can be performed with robotic assistance or without. The da Vinci system is the robotic system used and can be used for LIMA harvest. A stabilizer enables an anastomosis on the beating heart.[10]

Kettering[11] reported early and late mortalities of 1.3% and 3.2%, respectively. Conversion to sternotomy or CPB was 1.8%. At 6 months follow-up, 3.6% of the 445 grafts that were studied angiographically were occluded; 7.2% had significant stenosis. Better pulmonary function, quality of life, and pain management are reported in MID-CAB.[12–14] Excessive rib spreading for a LIMA harvest increases the incidence of wound complications, up to 9%.[15] To minimize this, thoracoscopic LIMA harvest was developed. A recent review by Dieberg and colleagues[16] showed decreased intensive care unit (ICU) length of stay and cost in MIDCAB compared with conventional surgery. This procedure is most suitable for coronary arteries on the anterior surface of the heart. For isolated LAD lesions, MIDCAB is associated with decreased requirements for revascularization and major adverse coronary events compared with percutaneous coronary intervention.[17]

Minimally Invasive Multivessel Coronary Artery Bypass Grafting

Introduced by Joseph McGinn and colleagues[18] in 2009, this procedure involves access to all myocardial territories via a 4- to 6-cm left fifth intercostal thoracotomy. An apical positioner and epicardial stabilizer are introduced into the chest through the subxiphoid and left seventh intercostal spaces, respectively. The left internal thoracic artery is used to graft the LAD artery, and radial artery or saphenous vein segments are used to graft the lateral and inferior myocardial territories. Proximal anastomoses are performed directly onto the aorta or from the left internal thoracic artery as a T-graft. In carefully selected patients, minimally invasive multivessel coronary artery bypass grafting (MICS CABG) has comparable mortality and outcomes to conventional CABG in the short term.[18] MICS CABG was found to be cost-effective in a small study.[19]

OFF-PUMP CORONARY ARTERY BYPASS GRAFTING

In 1967, Kolessov[20] first described a beating heart CABG via left anterolateral thoracotomy. Beating heart CABG via a left anterolater thoracotomy involves performing a CABG without the use of a CPB machine. Off-pump CABG requires excellent teamwork and devices to stabilize the heart and coronary blood vessels. A recent meta-analysis by Dieberg and colleagues[21] showed no difference in mortality, stroke, and MI for patients with OPCAB when compared with on-pump CABG, although the time on mechanical ventilation, time in ICU, and hospital stay were shorter in the OPCAB group compared with on-pump CABG.

PARTIAL STERNOTOMY VALVE REPAIR AND REPLACEMENT

Partial sternotomy can be used for aortic valve replacement (AVR) and MVR. For an aortic valve replacement through a partial sternotomy (defined as any sternal incision other than median sternotomy and/or smaller than median sternotomy) inverted "T" partial upper sternotomy, "J" upper partial sternotomy, "I" sternotomy performed between the second and fifth intercostal spaces, midline lower-half sternotomy, and a "C" mini-sternotomy, leaving the upper and lower ends of the sternum intact. Right parasternal approaches have also been described, with or without resection of costal cartilages. All of these techniques promote a regular CPB and cardioplegia with a routine AV replacement. As expected, this approach improves cosmesis, reduces the duration of mechanical ventilation and hospital stay, and decreases postoperative pain, facilitating an earlier return to normal activity.[10] Partial sternotomy was associated with a lower cost compared with anterolateral thoracotomy and intraoperative blood loss compared with a conventional AV replacement (**Fig. 2**).[22,23]

For minimally invasive mitral valve replacement (MIMVR), a parasternal incision, inverted J-type ministernotomy over the xiphoid, upper midline sternotomy, as well as a right minithoracotomy incision have been described. Chitwood and colleagues[24] proposed a classification system for minimally invasive approaches, whether the surgeon uses direct vision, thoracoscopic visualization, or robotics. Direct vision consists of surgery through a 5- to 7-cm right anterolateral minithoracotomy with or without video assistance. CPB is instituted through the femoral vessels; cardioplegia is administered, and the left ventricle is vented percutaneously. Compared with conventional MVR, MIMVR has a similar rate of reoperation, stroke, death, MV durability, shorter hospital and ICU stays, and fewer transfusions, although the incidence of complications from peripheral vascular cannulation and reexpansion pulmonary edema from a single lung ventilation are higher; furthermore, use of the parasternal approach has been abandoned because of sustained pain and chest wall instability (**Fig. 3**).[25,26]

HISTORY OF ROBOTIC CARDIAC SURGERY

Carpentier and colleagues[27] did the first robotic surgery in the world by repairing an atrial septal defect (ASD) followed by an MV repair in 1998. Nifong[28] did the first complete robotic MV repair in the United States in 2002. Mohr and colleagues[29] in 1998 did the first robot-assisted CABG followed by Loulmet and colleagues,[30] who did a totally endoscopic CABG. The first-in-human robot-assisted endoscopic AV replacement was reported by Folliquet and colleagues in 2005.[31] **Table 1** shows the milestones in robotic cardiac surgery.

ROBOTIC MITRAL VALVE SURGERY

Patients with asymptomatic MV disease and preserved LV function are ideal candidates for robotic MV repair. CPB is established through a femoral approach, and aortic

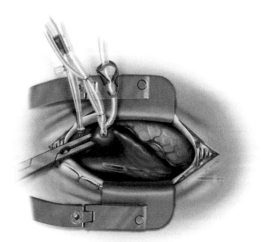

Fig. 2. Partial upper sternotomy.

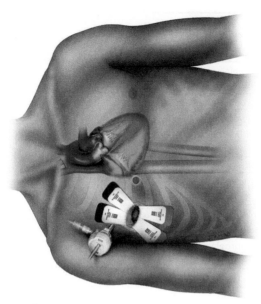

Fig. 3. Right chest port placement.

occlusion is performed with a Chitwood cross-clamp. Five ports are inserted in the right pleural cavity to repair the MV. In specialized centers, robotic MV repair has excellent outcomes, high survival, phenomenal durability, and minimal complications regardless of disease complexity.[32] Although there is a lack of proprioception or tactile feedback, robotic MV replacement enhances surgical dexterity and decreases intra-operative transfusions, hospital stay, time to return to work, and postoperative pain with outcomes comparable to that of conventional MV repair.[33] Although the experience is limited with MV replacement, it can be performed with low morbidity and mortality.[34] Compared with MIMVR, 30-day mortality for robotic MV repair is 2-fold lower.[35] A recent systematic review showed the cost of robotic MV surgery is slightly higher than conventional surgery (**Fig. 4**).[36]

Totally Endoscopic Coronary Artery Bypass

First described by Loulmet and colleagues in 1998,[30] LIMA is harvested endoscopically; a femorofemoral CPB is obtained, and the heart is arrested by occluding the ascending aorta with an endovascular balloon and infusing cardioplegic solution into the aortic root. Then, an LIMA-to-LAD anastomosis is performed using a total of 3 left-sided robotic ports. The totally endoscopic coronary artery bypass (TECAB) procedure is associated with comparable morbidity and mortality outcomes in carefully selected patients, although it is technically challenging, with longer operative times, and can be used for LAD disease only.[37–41] No death, stroke, or myocardial infarction occurred in the follow-up of 41.1 months in patients with LIMA-LAD anastomosis in a recent large series; LIMA patency over the course of 3 years was 97%.[42] The rate of major adverse cardiac event at 1 year was 7.0% in the TECAB group and 12.4% in the traditional CABG patients. The graft occlusion rate was also lower in the TECAB patients (1.8%) compared with 2.5% in the SYNTAX trial patients.[43] Cost of TECAB is higher than conventional CABG.[44]

Table 1
Milestones in robotic cardiac surgery

Surgery	Author, y
Robotic mitral valve repair	Carpentier et al, 1998
Robotic mammary harvesting	Mohr, 1998
Totally endoscopic coronary artery bypass with arrested heart	Loulmet et al, 1998
Totally endoscopic coronary artery bypass off pump	Falk, 2000
Use of BIMA in TECAB in arrested heart	Kappert, 2000
ASD closure	Torraca, 2000
Totally endoscopic mitral valve repair	Lange, 2002
LV lead implantation	DeRose, 2003
Use of BIMA in TECAB in beating heart	Farhat, 2004
Aortic valve replacement	Folliguet, 2004
Left atrial myxoma resection	Murphy et al, 2005
Aortic valve papillary fibroelastoma resection	Woo, 2005
Triple vessel TECAB	Bonatti & Srivastava, 2010
Combined mitral valve repair and CABG	Balkhy, 2013

Abbreviation: BIMA, bilateral internal mammary artery.
Data from Canale LS, BJ. Current state of robotically assisted coronary artery bypass surgery, in Coronary Graft Failure: State of the Art. 2016. p. 65–74.

ROBOTIC ATRIAL SEPTAL DEFECT REPAIR

Robotic ASD repair has excellent outcomes.[45–48] CPB is established through the femoral vessels. Five ports are used to access the right pleural cavity; aortic occlusion is performed with a Chitwood cross-clamp, and ASD is closed directly using 4-0

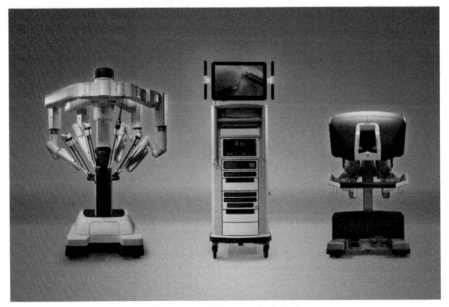

Fig. 4. The da Vinci Xi system. (©2017 Intuitive Surgical, Inc.)

Gore-Tex running suture or autologous pericardial patching, depending on the size and location of ASD. Non-CPB robotic ASD repair can be done but is associated with increased blood in the operative field and inability to perform large ASD repairs. There were no reoperations, conversion to sternotomy, or residual defect in a recent series from China (see Benjamin Wei and Robert J. Cerfolio's article, "Robotic Lobectomy and Segmentectomy: Technical Details and Results," in this issue). Ishikawa and colleagues[49] reported 2-port robotic cardiac surgery for ASD using the cross-arm technique, which only used 2 ports, further improving clinical and cosmetic outcomes. Cost of robotic ASD is greater than conventional ASD closure.[50]

ROBOTIC MYXOMA EXCISION

Murphy and colleagues[51] first reported the robotic excision in 2005. The largest series reported to date showed excellent outcomes for robotic atrial myxoma excision.[52] Compared with conventional surgery, robotic atrial myxoma excision is associated with better quality of life, pain control, earlier return to work, and decreased hospital length of stay.[53] The authors' group experienced similar outcomes.[54]

ROBOTIC SEPTAL MYECTOMY

Endoscopic septal myectomy was first described by Casselman and Vanermen[55] in 2002, followed by a robotic transmitral septal myectomy by Chitwood[56] in 2012. CPB is established through the femoral vessels. A 4.5-cm minithoracotomy is made in the right fourth intercostal space followed by insertion of 4 ports; then septal myectomy is done through a transmitral approach. Septal myectomy provides excellent exposure to the interventricular septum and has good outcomes.[57,58]

SUMMARY

Significant improvement and development have occurred in minimally invasive cardiac surgery over the past 20 years. Although most studies have consistently demonstrated equivalent or improved outcomes compared with conventional cardiac surgery, with significantly shorter recovery times, adoption continues to be limited. In addition, cost data have been inconsistent. Further ongoing trials are needed to help determine the exact roles for these innovative procedures.

REFERENCES

1. Harken DE, Ellis LB. The surgical treatment of mitral stenosis; valvuloplasty. N Engl J Med 1948;239(22):801–9.
2. Benetti FJ, Ballester C. Use of thoracoscopy and a minimal thoracotomy, in mammary-coronary bypass to left anterior descending artery, without extracorporeal circulation. Experience in 2 cases. J Cardiovasc Surg (Torino) 1995;36(2):159–61.
3. Subramanian VA. Clinical experience with minimally invasive reoperative coronary bypass surgery. Eur J Cardiothorac Surg 1996;10(12):1058–62.
4. Cosgrove DM 3rd, Sabik JF. Minimally invasive approach for aortic valve operations. Ann Thorac Surg 1996;62(2):596–7.
5. Navia JL, Cosgrove DM 3rd. Minimally invasive mitral valve operations. Ann Thorac Surg 1996;62(5):1542–4.
6. Stevens JH, Burdon TA, Peters WS, et al. Port-access coronary artery bypass grafting: a proposed surgical method. J Thorac Cardiovasc Surg 1996;111(3):567–73.

7. Carpentier A, Loulmet D, Carpentier A, et al. Open heart operation under video-surgery and minithoracotomy. First case (mitral valvuloplasty) operated with success. C R Acad Sci 1996;319(3):219–23 [in French].

8. Krapf C, Wohlrab P, Häußinger S, et al. Remote access perfusion for minimally invasive cardiac surgery: to clamp or to inflate? Eur J Cardiothorac Surg 2013; 44(5):898–904.

9. Kiessling AH, Kisker P, Miskovic A, et al. Long-term follow-up of minimally invasive cardiac surgery using an endoaortic occlusion system. Heart Surg Forum 2014;17(2):E93–7.

10. Kalavrouziotis D, Dagenais F. Minimally invasive cardiac surgery. In: Yuh DD, et al, editors. Johns Hopkins textbook of cardiothoracic surgery. New York: McGraw-Hill Education; 2014. p. 861.

11. Kettering K. Minimally invasive direct coronary artery bypass grafting: a meta-analysis. J Cardiovasc Surg (Torino) 2008;49(6):793–800.

12. d'Amato TA, Savage EB, Wiechmann RJ, et al. Reduced incidence of atrial fibrillation with minimally invasive direct coronary artery bypass. Ann Thorac Surg 2000;70(6):2013–6.

13. Lichtenberg A, Hagl C, Harringer W, et al. Effects of minimal invasive coronary artery bypass on pulmonary function and postoperative pain. Ann Thorac Surg 2000;70(2):461–5.

14. Wray J, Al-Ruzzeh S, Mazrani W, et al. Quality of life and coping following minimally invasive direct coronary artery bypass (MIDCAB) surgery. Qual Life Res 2004;13(5):915–24.

15. Ng PC, Chua AN, Swanson MS, et al. Anterior thoracotomy wound complications in minimally invasive direct coronary artery bypass. Ann Thorac Surg 2000;69(5): 1338–40 [discussion: 1340–1].

16. Dieberg G, Smart NA, King N. Minimally invasive cardiac surgery: a systematic review and meta-analysis. Int J Cardiol 2016;223:554–60.

17. Wang XW, Qu C, Huang C, et al. Minimally invasive direct coronary bypass compared with percutaneous coronary intervention for left anterior descending artery disease: a meta-analysis. J Cardiothorac Surg 2016;11(1):125.

18. McGinn JT Jr, Usman S, Lapierre H, et al. Minimally invasive coronary artery bypass grafting: dual-center experience in 450 consecutive patients. Circulation 2009;120(Suppl 11):S78–84.

19. King RC, Reece TB, Hurst JL, et al. Minimally invasive coronary artery bypass grafting decreases hospital stay and cost. Ann Surg 1997;225(6):805–9 [discussion: 809–11].

20. Kolessov VI. Mammary artery-coronary artery anastomosis as method of treatment for angina pectoris. J Thorac Cardiovasc Surg 1967;54(4):535–44.

21. Dieberg G, Smart NA, King N. On- vs. off-pump coronary artery bypass grafting: a systematic review and meta-analysis. Int J Cardiol 2016;223:201–11.

22. Hassan M, Miao Y, Maraey A, et al. Minimally invasive aortic valve replacement: cost-benefit analysis of ministernotomy versus minithoracotomy approach. J Heart Valve Dis 2015;24(5):531–9.

23. Bowdish ME, Hui DS, Cleveland JD, et al. A comparison of aortic valve replacement via an anterior right minithoracotomy with standard sternotomy: a propensity score analysis of 492 patients. Eur J Cardiothorac Surg 2016;49(2):456–63.

24. Chitwood WR, Rodriguez E. Minimally invasive and robotic mitral valve surgery. In: Cohn LH, editor. Cardiac surgery in the adult. New York: McGraw-Hill; 2008. p. 1079–100.

25. Downs EA, Johnston LE, LaPar DJ, et al. Minimally invasive mitral valve surgery provides excellent outcomes without increased cost: a multi-institutional analysis. Ann Thorac Surg 2016;102(1):14–21.

26. Sakaguchi T. Minimally invasive mitral valve surgery through a right mini-thoracotomy. Gen Thorac Cardiovasc Surg 2016;64(12):699–706.

27. Carpentier A, Loulmet D, Aupècle B, et al. Computer assisted open heart surgery. First case operated on with success. C R Acad Sci 1998;321(5):437–42 [in French].

28. Nifong LW, Chu VF, Bailey BM, et al. Robotic mitral valve repair: experience with the da Vinci system. Ann Thorac Surg 2003;75(2):438–42 [discussion: 443].

29. Mohr FW, Falk V, Diegeler A, et al. Computer-enhanced coronary artery bypass surgery. J Thorac Cardiovasc Surg 1999;117(6):1212–4.

30. Loulmet D, Carpentier A, d'Attellis N, et al. Endoscopic coronary artery bypass grafting with the aid of robotic assisted instruments. J Thorac Cardiovasc Surg 1999;118(1):4–10.

31. Folliguet TA, Vanhuyse F, Konstantinos Z, et al. Early experience with robotic aortic valve replacement. Eur J Cardiothorac Surg 2005;28(1):172–3.

32. Suri RM, Taggarse A, Burkhart HM, et al. Robotic mitral valve repair for simple and complex degenerative disease: midterm clinical and echocardiographic quality outcomes. Circulation 2015;132(21):1961–8.

33. Suri RM, Dearani JA, Mihaljevic T, et al. Mitral valve repair using robotic technology: safe, effective, and durable. J Thorac Cardiovasc Surg 2016;151(6):1450–4.

34. Changqing G, Ming Y. Robotic Mitral valve surgery. In: Changqing G, editor. Robotic Cardiac Surgery. New York: Springer; 2015. p. 105.

35. Hassan M, Miao Y, Lincoln J, et al. Cost-benefit analysis of robotic versus nonrobotic minimally invasive mitral valve surgery. Innovations (Phila) 2015;10(2):90–5.

36. Canale LS, Colafranceschi AS. Is robotic mitral valve surgery more expensive than its conventional counterpart? Interact Cardiovasc Thorac Surg 2015;20(6):844–7.

37. Halkos ME, Liberman HA, Devireddy C, et al. Early clinical and angiographic outcomes after robotic-assisted coronary artery bypass surgery. J Thorac Cardiovasc Surg 2014;147(1):179–85.

38. Kofler M, et al. 138 Robotic versus conventional coronary artery bypass graft: a propensity score-based comparison of perioperative and long-term results. Interact Cardiovasc Thorac Surg 2014;19(Suppl 1):S42.

39. Bonatti J, Lehr EJ, Schachner T, et al. Robotic total endoscopic double-vessel coronary artery bypass grafting–state of procedure development. J Thorac Cardiovasc Surg 2012;144(5):1061–6.

40. Cavallaro P, Rhee AJ, Chiang Y, et al. In-hospital mortality and morbidity after robotic coronary artery surgery. J Cardiothorac Vasc Anesth 2015;29(1):27–31.

41. Gao C, Yang M, Wu Y, et al. Early and midterm results of totally endoscopic coronary artery bypass grafting on the beating heart. J Thorac Cardiovasc Surg 2011;142(4):843–9.

42. Yang M, Wu Y, Wang G, et al. Robotic total arterial off-pump coronary artery bypass grafting: seven-year single-center experience and long-term follow-up of graft patency. Ann Thorac Surg 2015;100(4):1367–73.

43. Canale LS, Bonatti J. Current State of robotically assisted coronary artery bypass surgery. In: Tintoiu IC, Underwood MJ, Cook SP, et al, editors. Coronary graft failure. New York: Springer; 2016.

44. Yanagawa F, Perez M, Bell T, et al. Critical outcomes in nonrobotic vs robotic-assisted cardiac surgery. JAMA Surg 2015;150(8):771–7.

45. Argenziano M, Oz MC, DeRose JJ Jr, et al. Totally endoscopic atrial septal defect repair with robotic assistance. Heart Surg Forum 2002;5(3):294–300.

46. Bonaros N, Schachner T, Oehlinger A, et al. Robotically assisted totally endoscopic atrial septal defect repair: insights from operative times, learning curves, and clinical outcome. Ann Thorac Surg 2006;82(2):687–93.

47. Torracca L, Ismeno G, Alfieri O. Totally endoscopic computer-enhanced atrial septal defect closure in six patients. Ann Thorac Surg 2001;72(4):1354–7.

48. Wimmer-Greinecker G, Dogan S, Aybek T, et al. Totally endoscopic atrial septal repair in adults with computer-enhanced telemanipulation. J Thorac Cardiovasc Surg 2003;126(2):465–8.

49. Ishikawa N, Watanabe G, Tarui T, et al. Two-Port Robotic Cardiac Surgery (TROCS) for Atrial Septal Defect (ASD) using Cross-Arm Technique–TROCS ASD repair. Circ J 2015;79(10):2271–3.

50. Morgan JA, Thornton BA, Peacock JC, et al. Does robotic technology make minimally invasive cardiac surgery too expensive? A hospital cost analysis of robotic and conventional techniques. J Card Surg 2005;20(3):246–51.

51. Murphy DA, Miller JS, Langford DA. Robot-assisted endoscopic excision of left atrial myxomas. J Thorac Cardiovasc Surg 2005;130(2):596–7.

52. Gao C, Yang M, Wang G, et al. Excision of atrial myxoma using robotic technology. J Thorac Cardiovasc Surg 2010;139(5):1282–5.

53. Yang M, Yao M, Wang G, et al. Comparison of postoperative quality of life for patients who undergo atrial myxoma excision with robotically assisted versus conventional surgery. J Thorac Cardiovasc Surg 2015;150(1):152–7.

54. Schilling J, Hassan M, Engel A, et al. Robotic excision of atrial myxomas. J Card Surg 2012;27:423–6.

55. Casselman F, Vanermen H. Idiopathic hypertrophic subaortic stenosis can be treated endoscopically. J Thorac Cardiovasc Surg 2002;124(6):1248–9.

56. Chitwood WR. Idiopathic hypertrophic subaortic septal obstruction: robotic transatrial and transmitral ventricular septal resection. Oper Tech Thorac Cardiovasc Surg 2013;17(4):251–60.

57. Kim HR, Yoo JS, Lee JW. Minimally invasive trans-mitral septal myectomy to treat hypertrophic obstructive cardiomyopathy. Korean J Thorac Cardiovasc Surg 2015;48(6):419–21.

58. Khalpey Z, Korovin L, Chitwood WR Jr, et al. Robot-assisted septal myectomy for hypertrophic cardiomyopathy with left ventricular outflow tract obstruction. J Thorac Cardiovasc Surg 2014;147(5):1708–9.

Transcatheter Aortic Valve Replacement: A Review

John H. Braxton, MD, MBA[a],*, Kelly S. Rasmussen, MS, RN, NP-C, AACC[b],
Milind S. Shah, MD, FSCAI[c]

KEYWORDS

- Transcatheter aortic valve replacement • Surgical aortic valve replacement
- Aortic stenosis • Valvular heart disease • Catheter

KEY POINTS

- The treatment of aortic stenosis is changing and being treated more with catheter-based technology: inoperable, high risk, and intermediate risk are now approved.
- Gated multislice CT angiogram has emerged as the gold standard for assessment of valve anatomy and sizing of the transcatheter heart valve.
- Long-term results are needed before its use in lower risk categories.

Video content accompanies this article at http://www.surgical.theclinics.com/.

INTRODUCTION

With the recent approval of the intermediate-risk category for transcatheter aortic valve replacement (TAVR), medicine is undergoing a dramatic paradigm shift in the way aortic valve stenosis is treated. At this time, cardiac surgeons with their expertise in valve replacement remain the gatekeepers for TAVR; however, cardiac surgeons are no longer the sole providers for the advanced treatment of aortic stenosis (AS). The Centers for Medicare and Medicaid Services (CMS) in conjunction with the Food and Drug Administration (FDA) developed detailed criteria to ensure the best adoption of this new technology. A threshold of surgical experience and structural heart procedural experience was required to be a TAVR center.[1] Not only did CMS and the FDA selectively choose centers based on experience, they required a collaborative, multidisciplinary team approach to treatment decision making and participation in the

Disclosures: None.
[a] Structural Heart Services, Marshfield Clinic, Saint Joseph Hospital, 1000 North Oak Avenue, Section 2C2, Marshfield, WI 54449, USA; [b] Structural Heart Services, Department of Cardiology, Marshfield Clinic, Saint Joseph Hospital, 1000 North Oak Avenue, Section 2C2, Marshfield, WI 54449, USA; [c] Structural Heart Services, Section of Cardiology, Marshfield Clinic, Saint Joseph Hospital, 1000 North Oak Avenue, Section 2C2, Marshfield, WI 54449, USA
* Corresponding author.
E-mail address: braxton.john@marshfieldclinic.org

Surg Clin N Am 97 (2017) 899–921
http://dx.doi.org/10.1016/j.suc.2017.03.011
0039-6109/17/© 2017 Elsevier Inc. All rights reserved.

surgical.theclinics.com

Transcatheter Valve Therapy (TVT) Registry. This national registry was created in collaboration between the Society of Thoracic Surgery (STS) and American College of Cardiology (ACC), which mirrors the collaborative approach mandated by CMS and the FDA.

HISTORY

The paradigm shift in treatment of AS did not occur overnight but started in the laboratory with catheter-based concepts that transformed into catheter-based interventions and eventually translated into clinical trials. The first catheter-based therapy was performed in September 1977 in Switzerland by Andreas Gruentzig,[2,3] ushering in the era of interventional cardiology for the treatment of coronary disease. Within 10 years, the first balloon valvuloplasty was performed on a child for treatment of pulmonic stenosis.[4] In 1985, Cribier and coworkers[5] performed the first in-human balloon aortic valvuloplasty on an inoperable 77-year-old man. Cribier and coworkers[6,7] later went on to create the first percutaneous valve, which was subsequently acquired by Edwards Lifesciences (Irvine, CA). The Cribier-Edwards valve was further refined to become the Sapien, balloon expandable transcatheter heart valve (THV).

The Initial Registry of Endovascular Implantation of Valves in Europe[8] and the Registry of Endovascular Critical Aortic Stenosis Treatment were the first trial registries that evaluated feasibility of TAVR. The initial TAVR procedures were done on a compassionate basis. An antegrade approach with transseptal puncture was used for implantation. Although less than perfect, the results demonstrated that patients suffering from severe AS could be helped with a catheter-based procedure. The next several years were spent on refining the devices and implantation technique to produce a safer, more successful procedure.

THE HEART VALVE TEAM

The heart valve team approach has become the standard of care for the treatment of aortic valve stenosis, more specifically TAVR, in the United States.[9,10] CMS has mandated that a team of professionals have joint treatment decision making for these patients. This mandate by CMS clearly puts the patient at the center of the care model.

There are many stakeholders within the multidisciplinary heart valve team. A typical valve team consists of one or more each of the following physicians: cardiothoracic surgeon, interventional cardiologist, imaging specialist/radiologist, cardiac anesthesiologist, and noninvasive cardiologist. However, the most important stakeholder within the team is not one of these physicians but rather is the valve clinical coordinator. The coordinator is typically a registered nurse or advanced practice nurse that understands and oversees all processes within the valve clinic and aims to keep the patient at the center of care. This individual is responsible for overseeing the patient from the initial referral into the valve clinic through the entirety of the diagnostic process. The coordinator also oversees and coordinates the procedural process. He or she is available for coordination of hospital care and ensures all aspects of the follow-up care are arranged. The valve clinical coordinator is responsible for managing and collecting information for the TVT Registry.

The heart valve team should also include other ad hoc members for special, patient-specific circumstances, such as an oncologist for newly diagnosed malignancies, a gerontologist to help address complex medical issues, or a neuropsychologist for evaluation of cognitive impairment. Backup with additional cardiac and noncardiac services, such as a heart failure team, a vascular surgery team, and social services, is a force multiplier and only serves to strengthen the program.[11]

Once the TAVR work-up is completed (discussed next), all members of the multidisciplinary heart valve team meet to review and discuss all of the patient's diagnostic imaging and clinical evaluations. All unresolved issues or concerns are addressed and the team agrees on a treatment plan including THV selection, route of implantation, anesthesia method, and postoperative anticoagulation regimen. The decisions are disseminated to all team members. The decision is also communicated to the patient's other care providers including referring provider, primary care provider, and primary cardiologist.

The multidisciplinary heart valve team develops an expertise over time. With this expertise, the rhythm of patient care is perfected as the team dynamics change and strengthen. It is important that the heart valve team perform robust internal audits of their data and use this information to proactively change procedural and nonprocedural processes for the betterment of the program leading to improved patient outcomes.[12]

TRANSCATHETER AORTIC VALVE REPLACEMENT WORK-UP

The pre-TAVR work-up is best accomplished in a systematic fashion; however, it is well known and understood that the sequence of the diagnostic evaluations may not always be linear and follow the same path. Patients enter the valve clinic at different stages of evaluation. It is important to develop tools to help organize the evaluation process and ensure key diagnostics are not missed (**Fig. 1**).

There are certain key diagnostic procedures and clinical evaluations that every TAVR patient undergoes. There are some diagnostic procedures and clinical evaluations that are performed as needed on a patient-specific basis (**Table 1**).

Key Diagnostic Evaluations

Transthoracic echocardiogram
This is used to diagnose severe AS. Both aortic valve anatomy and aortic valve hemodynamics are assessed. The presence of concomitant mitral, tricuspid, and/or pulmonic valve disease is also determined. This examination is typically performed before referral into the valve clinic but may be repeated if the heart valve team determines the quality of the study is not satisfactory or specific diagnostic criterion are missing.

Coronary angiography
This is performed to determine the presence of coronary artery disease. If significant coronary artery disease is noted, this can add to the surgical risk if both coronary artery bypass grafting and aortic valve replacement are indicated. The team determines if percutaneous revascularization is necessary before TAVR.

Right and left heart catheterization
This is performed at the same time as coronary angiography. It confirms the presence of severe AS. It also serves as a baseline for invasive hemodynamics.

Gated multislice computed tomography angiography of the chest/abdomen/pelvis
This is considered the gold standard for aortic annulus measurements for preprocedural TAVR assessment. Specific acquisition protocols are performed and vary depending on scanner platform. It determines overall suitability for TAVR. It also determines access method and prosthesis size by using the following:

- Suitability of the peripheral access vessels (ileofemoral, subclavian, and aorta) including size, amount, and distribution of calcium and tortuosity
- Dimensions of the ascending aorta, aortic root, and aortic annulus
- Distribution of calcium within the aortic valve
- Annular plane for intraprocedural[11,13] fluoroscopy images

TAVR WORKUP CHECKLIST

Referring Provider: _____
Primary Cardiologist: _____

Key Clinical Evaluations	Name	Date
Interventional Cardiologist:	_____	_____
CV Surgeon #1:	_____	_____
CV Surgeon #2:	_____	_____

	Date	
VC Coordinator:	_____	
Education	_____	
Functional Assessment	_____	
TVT Registry	_____	
Patient Database	_____	
CTA Uploaded for Reconstruction	_____	
Reconstructions Received	_____	

Key Testing	Date	Sig Findings
TTE	_____	_____
Coronary/Heart Cath	_____	_____
CTA chest/abdomen/pelvis	_____	_____
Dental Clearance	_____	_____
Team Discussion	_____	_____

PRN Testing/Evaluation		
TEE	_____	_____
PFT	_____	_____
Carotid Duplex	_____	_____
DSE	_____	_____
Neuropsychology	_____	_____
Pulmonology	_____	_____
Gerontology	_____	_____
Other	_____	_____
Other	_____	_____

Fig. 1. Check list for TAVR work-up at Marshfield Clinic.

Table 1
Pre-TAVR evaluations

Key Evaluations	As Needed Evaluations
Transthoracic echocardiogram	Transesophageal echocardiogram
Coronary angiography	Pulmonary function tests
Right and left heart catheterization	Carotid duplex
Two cardiothoracic surgery evaluations	Dobutamine stress echo
Interventional cardiology evaluation	Neuropsychology
Valve clinical coordinator evaluation and education	Pulmonology
Computed tomography angiogram of chest/ abdomen/pelvis	Gerontology
Functional/frailty assessment	Other
Multidisciplinary team discussion	

Key Clinical Evaluations

Valve clinic interventional cardiologist

This team member is mandated by the CMS national coverage decision to be a stakeholder in the heart valve team. They review diagnostic evaluations, confirm the presence of symptomatic heart disease secondary to severe AS, and evaluate for contraindications to a TAVR procedure.[14]

Valve clinic cardiothoracic surgeon

It is mandated by the CMS national coverage decision that two cardiac surgeons independently examine the patient face-to-face and evaluate the patient's suitability for surgical aortic valve replacement (SAVR). They document risk category (low, intermediate, high, or prohibitive) and rationale in medical record, and provide to the entire heart valve team.[14]

Valve clinical coordinator

This member was initially seen in collaboration with the valve clinic interventional cardiologist and valve clinic cardiothoracic surgeon. They provide ongoing evaluation and discussion with patient and family as need arises, and pivotal patient and family education and coordination of care. They collaborate with all multidisciplinary providers involved in the patient's care.

Personal dentist or oral surgeon

Clinical guidelines recommended evaluation before surgical cardiac procedures to reduce the rates of infective endocarditis. There are no specific studies or guideline recommendations for TAVR. Whether dental procedures should delay the definitive cardiac treatment has been questioned and should be determined on a patient-specific basis.[15]

As-Needed Diagnostic Evaluations

Three-dimensional transesophageal echocardiogram

This may be completed before referral into the valve clinic and is used along with computed tomography (CT) to determine suitability for TAVR and aortic annulus measurements. In the presence of degenerated surgical aortic valve, it determines the cause of degeneration and hemodynamic abnormalities on transthoracic echocardiogram.

Pulmonary function tests

These are not routinely performed but consideration should be given to complete on all patients because many patients have some level of abnormality documented even when lung disease was not initially suspected. Consideration should be given to perform on all patients with documented pulmonary abnormalities on CT scan. Consideration should be given to perform in patients with known lung disease if not previously completely within 1 year.[16]

Carotid duplex

There has been no significant correlation between amount of carotid artery disease and periprocedural stroke documented. It is typically left to the surgeon's discretion. Higher consideration could be given in patients with suspected symptomatic disease.[17]

Dobutamine stress echocardiogram

This is performed when patients are diagnosed with stage D2 severe AS (symptomatic low-flow/low-gradient, severe AS with reduced left ventricular ejection fraction [LVEF]) to confirm presence of severe AS with a Vmax greater than 4.0 m/s or mean gradient greater than or equal to 40 mm Hg at any level of dobutamine infusion. Special attention should be paid to baseline hemodynamic numbers because baseline evaluation may confirm the presence of stage D1 or stage D3 severe AS.[9]

As-Needed Clinical Evaluations

Pulmonologist
Consideration for referral for preprocedural optimization should be given in patients with documented severe pulmonary disease. Consideration should be given for referral for patients with newly diagnosed moderate-severe pulmonary disease.

Gerontologist
Consideration should be given for referral in patients with multiple comorbid conditions to assist with determination of suitability for TAVR and for management of medical issues before the procedure.

Neuropsychologist
Consideration should be given for referral in patients with abnormal neurologic evaluation (montreal cognitive assessment or mini–mental state examination) to assist with determination of suitability for TAVR, of the patient's ability to understand the brevity of the medical situation, and of the patient's ability to participate in necessary care following procedure.

Other specialties
As the patients move through the pre-TAVR work-up, often abnormalities, either suspected or incidental, are noted. This may require consultation with other subspecialties for further evaluation and/or treatment.

METHODS OF IMPLANTATION

The valve implants are done with either retrograde or antegrade approach and the selection of the approach is based on the patient's vascular anatomy and diameters (**Tables 2 and 3**).

For the retrograde approach, most of the procedures are performed via percutaneous transfemoral (TF) approach. In the absence of femoral access, transaortic (TAo) or transsubclavian (TS) accesses are more common. Transcarotid and transcaval accesses can be considered but are significantly less common at the current time. Most of the TF procedures are performed under monitored anesthesia care or conscious sedation. All other types of retrograde and antegrade implant procedures are mini-surgical procedures and require general anesthesia. They are usually performed with transesophageal echocardiogram guidance.

All TAVR procedures (retrograde and antegrade) require a temporary pacemaker for rapid burst pacing (for Edwards Lifesciences) or rhythm override (for Medtronic, Dublin, Republic of Ireland). A pigtail catheter is also needed for aortic root injections to guide valve implantation. For Edwards Lifesciences, it is placed in the right cusp and for Medtronic it is placed in the noncoronary cusp. The pigtail catheter is inserted thru femoral, radial, or brachial arterial access. The temporary pacemaker is usually inserted via femoral or internal jugular venous access.

A core team is identified for the valve implant procedure. At our institution, this team includes a cardiovascular surgeon (first operator), an interventional cardiologist (second operator), hemodynamic technician (to operate the pacemaker), and an anesthesiologist. If a second interventional cardiologist is available, he or she acts as an assistant. For implantation of the Edwards Lifesciences THV, the first operator is responsible for the finer adjustment of the delivery system. The second operator is

Table 2
Current Edwards Lifesciences transcatheter heart valves

Valve		Valve Size (mm)	Annulus Size (mm²)	Access	Sheath Size (French catheter)
Sapien (first-generation)		23	18–22 mm (diameter)	TF TA	22 26
		26	21–25 mm (diameter)	TF TA	24 26
Sapien XT (second-generation)		23	338–430	TF TAo, TA	16 24
		26	430–546	TF TAo, TA	18 24
		29	540–683	TF TAo, TA	20 26
Sapien 3 (third-generation)		20	273–345	TF, TAo, TS	14
		23	338–430	TF, TAo, TS TA	14 18
		26	430–546	TF, TAo, TS TA	14 18
		29	540–683	TF, TAo, TS TA	16 21

Abbreviations: TA, transapical; TAo, transaortic; TF, transfemoral; TS, transsubclavian.

Table 3
Current Medtronic transcatheter heart valves

Valve		Valve Size (mm)	Annulus Size (Diameter)	Access	Sheath Size (French catheter)
CoreValve		26 29 31	20–23 23–27 26–29	TF, SC, TAo	18
CoreValve Evolut R		23 26 29	18–20 20–23 23–26	TF, SC, TAo	14
		34	26–30	TF, SC, TAo	16

Abbreviations: SC, subclavian, TAo, transaortic; TF, transfemoral.

in-charge of initiating the implant sequence and is responsible for aortography and inflating balloon to deploy the valve. For implantation of the Medtronic THV, the responsibilities remain the same; however, the second operator is also responsible to unsheath the valve. The valve team is constantly in sync with each other throughout the procedure. It is essential to check the orientation of the valve before inserting into the sheath. It is also important to standardize the valve implantation sequence with the team and practice it multiple times before the real procedure.

Anticoagulation is maintained with a target activated clotting time of 300 ± 25 seconds. Rapid burst pacing is kept to the minimum for patients with compromised left ventricular (LV) function. At our institution, we try to maintain systolic blood pressure of approximately 110 to 120 mm of Hg before the valve implantation sequence.

For TAo and transapical (TA) accesses, a shorter delivery system is used thru a larger 24F catheter sheath. Apart from the access site management, the valve deployment sequences remain the same. The only change in TA access is the orientation of the mounted valve, which is exactly opposite to the valve mounted for the retrograde access (**Figs. 2** and **3**, Videos 1–4).

EVOLUTION OF THE TRANSCATHETER HEART VALVE

Currently there are only two companies that offer commercially available THVs: Edwards Lifesciences and Medtronic.

EDWARDS LIFESCIENCES

Edwards Lifesciences was the first company to market with a commercial THV, in November 2011, the Sapien THV. The Edwards Sapien THV was comprised of a balloon-expandable, stainless steel frame, three bovine pericardial tissue leaflets and a polyethylene terephthalate (PET) fabric skirt. The PET fabric skirt was sewn on the inner portion of the bottom of the stent frame to help seal the aortic annulus

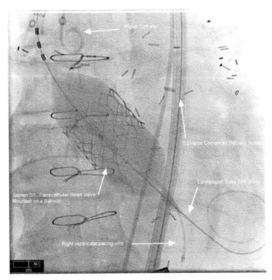

Fig. 2. Annotated TF Sapien S3 valve.

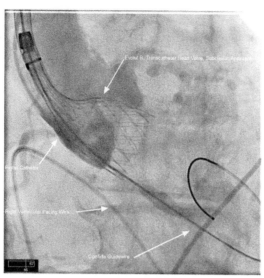

Fig. 3. Annotated TS: Evolut R, valve, aortogram.

and reduce the amount of paravalvular leak (PVL). The leaflets were treated according to the Carpentier-Edwards ThermaFix process, which is intended to reduce the buildup of calcium overtime. The Sapien THV is currently no longer available for implantation but was available in two sizes, 23 mm and 26 mm. The 23-mm valve was delivered through a 22F catheter sheath if placed using TF access or a 26F catheter sheath if delivered using TA access. The 26-mm valve was delivered through a 24F catheter sheath if placed using TF access or 26F catheter is placed using TA access.

In March of 2010 Sapien XT, Edwards Lifesciences second-generation THV, received CE mark for approval. The Sapien XT THV also consists of a balloon-expandable frame; however, the frame is constructed using cobalt-chromium instead of stainless steel. Three bovine pericardial leaflets treated with the Carpentier-Edwards ThermaFix process and an inner PET fabric skirt were also used. The improvements seen in the Sapien XT THV allows for expanded annular size coverage, smaller sheath sizes, and expanded access routes to include TAo. Four sizes of Sapien XT THV are available: 20 mm, 23 mm, 26 mm, and 29 mm. When delivered using TF access, a sheath size of either 16F, 18F, or 20F catheter is used. When delivered using TAo or TA access, a 24F catheter sheath for the 23-mm or 26-mm valve is used and a 26F catheter sheath for the 29-mm valve is used.

In June 2015, Edwards Lifesciences received FDA approval for their third-generation THV: Sapien 3. This valve also consists of a balloon-expandable cobalt chromium frame; however, the frame's geometry was altered to allow for lower delivery height and reduction in delivery profile. There are still three bovine pericardial leaflets, which are also treated with the Carpentier-Edwards ThermaFix process. A PET fabric outer skirt was added in addition to the PET fabric inner skirt to further seal the aortic annulus and further reduce the amount of PVL. The Sapien 3 THV has been approved for TF, TA, TAo, or TS. When delivered using TF, TAo, or TS access, a 14F catheter sheath is used for the placement of a 23-mm or 26-mm valve and a 16F catheter sheath is used for the placement of a 29-mm valve. When delivered using TA access, an 18F catheter sheath is used for the 23-mm or 26-mm valve and a 21F catheter sheath for the 29-mm valve (see **Table 2**).

MEDTRONIC

In January of 2014, Medtronic announced FDA approval of its CoreValve THV, making it the second commercially available system on the market. The second-generation Medtronic THV, CoreValve Evolut R, was approved by the FDA in June of 2015. Both the CoreValve and CoreValve Evolut R THV systems are comprised of three porcine leaflets and an inner porcine skirt sutured to a self-expanding nitinol frame. Both the CoreValve and CoreValve Evolut R have "three distinct segments: the base portion which exerts a high radial force that expands and pushes aside the calcified leaflets [of the native valve]; the central portion which carries the valve; and the top portion which flares to fixate and stabilize the valve in the ascending aorta".[18] The Evolut R features an improved design to the nitinol frame with a lower delivery height, reduced delivery profile, and expanded sealing skirt to further reduce the amount of PVL. The other significant improvement in the CoreValve Evolut R is the ability to recapture the THV once partially deployed allowing for repositioning within the annulus. The CoreValve THV is available in three sizes: 26 mm, 29 mm, and 31 mm fitting annular dimensions ranging from 20 mm to 30 mm using an 18F catheter sheath. The CoreValve Evolut R THV is available in four sizes: 23 mm, 26 mm, 29 mm, and 34 mm fitting annular dimension ranging from 18 mm to 30 mm using a 14F catheter sheath for the 23 mm, 26 mm, or 29 mm and a 16F catheter sheath for the 34 mm. Both the CoreValve and CoreValve Evolut R THV are delivered using TF, TAo, or TS access (see **Table 3**).

CURRENT INDICATIONS FOR TRANSCATHETER AORTIC VALVE REPLACEMENT

TAVR using all commercially available THV has an indication for use in patients with symptomatic heart disease caused by severe, calcific native, or prosthetic AS who meet an indication for SAVR but are considered to have at least intermediate surgical risk for implantation of the Edwards Lifesciences S3 or Sapien XT THVs or high to prohibitive surgical risk for the Medtronic CoreValve and CoreValve Evolut R THVs.

DEFINITION OF SEVERE AORTIC STENOSIS

According to the American Heart Association (AHA)/ACC Guidelines for the Management of Patients with Valvular Heart Disease,[9] which was updated most recently in 2014, severe AS is broken down into three stages: D1, D2, and D3. Patients must qualify for one of these three stages to be considered for TAVR.

Stage D1 Severe Aortic Stenosis

Stage D1 AS is defined as "severe symptomatic severe high-gradient AS."[9] Echocardiographic valve anatomy findings reveal leaflet calcification with reduced leaflet motion. Hemodynamic findings of the aortic valve typically reveal an aortic valve area of less than or equal to 1.0 cm^2 (may be larger with mixed AS/aortic regurgitation), an aortic Vmax of greater than 4.0 m/s, or a mean gradient greater than or equal to 40 mm Hg.

Stage D2 Severe Aortic Stenosis

Stage D2 AS is defined as "symptomatic severe low-flow/low-gradient AS with reduced LVEF less than 50%."[9] Echocardiographic valve anatomy findings reveal leaflet calcification with reduced leaflet motion. Hemodynamic findings of the aortic valve typically show an aortic valve area of less than or equal to 1.0 cm^2 with a resting aortic Vmax less than 4.0 m/s or mean gradient less than 40 mm Hg. Dobutamine stress echocardiogram shows aortic valve area less than or equal to 1.0 cm^2 and an aortic Vmax greater than or equal to 4.0 m/s or a mean gradient greater than or equal to 40 mm Hg at any flow rate of dobutamine.

Stage D3 Severe Aortic Stenosis

Stage D3 AS is defined as "symptomatic severe low-gradient AS with normal LVEF $\geq$50%."[9] Echocardiographic valve anatomy findings reveal leaflet calcification with reduced leaflet motion. Hemodynamic findings of the aortic valve show an aortic valve area of less than or equal to 1.0 cm^2 with an aortic Vmax less than or equal to 4 m/s or mean gradient less than or equal to 40 mm Hg and an indexed stroke volume of less than 35 mL/m^2 (**Table 4**).

SURGICAL RISK EVALUATION

Initially, when TAVR was first approved by the FDA, it was indicated only for patients with prohibitive/high surgical risk. Since that time, the level of surgical risk needed for TAVR indication has decreased. Operative mortality is typically calculated using a scoring system or tool. Two of the most common cardiovascular surgical risk estimators are the euroSCORE II and the STS Risk Score. The STS risk model is the more widely used of the two and is referred to in the AHA/ACC Guidelines for the Management of Patients with Valvular Heart Disease and was also used to determine risk in all of the major TAVR clinical trials. The STS offers a free online STS risk calculator tool.[19] The STS predicted risk of operative mortality (PROM) correlates to surgical risk category as follows: high risk = STS PROM greater than 8%, intermediate risk = STS PROM 4% to 8%, and low risk = STS PROM less than 4%.

Using only the STS Risk Score has limitations because it does not take into consideration other patient-specific factors, such as frailty, comorbid conditions with major organ system compromise, or surgical procedure barriers (**Table 5**). These factors should also be considered when determining risk.

According to the ACC/AHA Guidelines,[9] the following are examples of major organ system compromise:

- Cardiac: LV systolic dysfunction, LV diastolic dysfunction, right ventricular (RV) dysfunction, or pulmonary hypertension
- Renal: chronic kidney disease stage 3 or more
- Pulmonary: moderate or greater restrictive or constrictive lung disease based on pulmonary function test analysis
- Neurologic: dementia of any type, significant cognitive dysfunction, Parkinson disease, stroke with persistent deficit
- Gastrointestinal: Crohn's disease, ulcerative colitis, nutritional impairment with serum albumin less than 3
- Gastrointestinal (liver specific): cirrhosis, variceal bleeding
- Oncologic: active malignancy

Some of the surgical procedure barriers that could be encountered that would increase risk of surgical AVR are presence of tracheostomy, calcification in the ascending aorta (porcelain aorta), radiation damage, chest structure malformation, coronary anatomy/grafts adherent to the chest wall, or coronary bypass grafts crossing midline.[9]

Frailty is a state of vulnerability to poor resolution of homoeostasis after a stressor event and is a consequence of cumulative decline in many physiologic systems during a lifetime. This cumulative decline depletes homoeostatic reserves until minor stressor

Table 4
Stage of symptomatic severe aortic stenosis

		D: Symptomatic Severe AS		
D1	Symptomatic severe high-gradient AS	• Severe leaflet calcification or congenital stenosis with severely reduced leaflet opening	• Aortic Vmax ≥4 m/s or mean ΔP ≥40 mm Hg • AVA typically ≤1.0 cm² (or AVAi ≤0.6 cm²/m²) but may be larger with mixed AS/AR	• LV diastolic dysfunction • LV hypertrophy • Pulmonary hypertension may be present	• Dyspnea or decreased exercise tolerance • Angina • Syncope/presyncope
D2	Symptomatic severe low-flow/low-gradient AS with reduced LVEF	• Severe leaflet calcification with severely reduced leaflet motion	• AVA ≤1.0 cm² with resting aortic Vmax <4 m/s or mean ΔP <40 mm Hg • Dobutamine stress echocardiography shows AVA ≤1.0 cm² with Vmax ≥4 m/s at any flow rate	• LV diastolic dysfunction • LV hypertrophy • LVEF <50%	• HF • Angina • Syncope/presyncope
D3	Symptomatic severe low-gradient AS with normal LVEF or paradoxic low-flow severe AS	• Severe leaflet calcification with severely reduced leaflet motion	• AVA ≤1.0 cm² with aortic Vmax <4 m/s or mean ΔP <40 mm Hg • Indexed AVA ≤0.6 cm²/m² and Stroke volume index <35 mL/m² • Measured when patient is normotensive (systolic BP <140 mm Hg)	• Increased LV relative wall thickness • Small LV chamber with low stroke volume • Restrictive diastolic filling • LVEF ≥50%	• HF • Angina • Syncope/presyncope

Abbreviations: AR, aortic regurgitation; AVA, aortic valve area; AVAi, aortic valve area indexed to body surface area; BP, blood pressure; HF, heart failure; Vmax, maximum aortic velocity; ΔP, pressure gradient.

From Nishimura RA, Otto CM, Bonow RO, et al. 2014 AHA/ACC guideline for the management of patients with valvular heart disease: a report of the American College of Cardiology/American Heart Association task force on practice guidelines. J Thorac Cardiovasc Surg 2014;148(1):e17–8; with permission.

Table 5
Risk assessment combining STS risk estimate, frailty, major organ system dysfunction, and procedure-specific impediments

	Low Risk (Must Meet ALL Criteria in This Column)	Intermediate Risk (Any One Criterion in This Column)	High Risk (Any One Criterion in This Column)	Prohibitive Risk (Any One Criterion in This Column)
STS PROM[a] Frailty[b]	<4% AND None AND	4%–8% OR 1 index (mild) OR	>8% OR ≥2 indices (moderate to severe) OR	Predicted risk with surgery of death or major morbidity (all-cause) >50% at 1 y OR
Major organ system compromise not to be improved postoperatively[c]	None AND	1 organ system OR	No more than 2 organ systems OR	≥3 Organ systems OR
Procedure-specific impediment[d]	None	Possible procedure-specific impediment	Possible procedure-specific impediment	Severe procedure-specific impediment

Abbreviations: CKD, chronic kidney disease; CNS, central nervous system; CVA, stroke; $DLCO_2$, diffusion capacity for carbon dioxide; FEV_1, forced expiratory volume in 1 s; GI, gastrointestinal; INR, international normalized ratio; RV, right ventricular; VKA, vitamin K antagonist.

[a] Use of the STS PROM to predict risk in a given institution with reasonable reliability is appropriate only if institutional outcomes are within one standard deviation of STS average observed/expected ratio for the procedure in question.

[b] Seven frailty indices: Katz Activities of Daily Living (independence in feeding, bathing, dressing, transferring, toileting, and urinary continence) and independence in ambulation (no walking aid or assist required or 5-m walk in <6 s). Other scoring systems can be applied to calculate no, mild-, or moderate-to-severe frailty.

[c] Examples of major organ system compromise: cardiac—severe LV systolic or diastolic dysfunction or RV dysfunction, fixed pulmonary hypertension; CKD stage 3 or worse; pulmonary dysfunction with FEV_1 less than 50% or $DLCO_2$ less than 50% of predicted; CNS dysfunction—dementia, Alzheimer disease, Parkinson disease, CVA with persistent physical limitation; GI dysfunction—Crohn's disease, ulcerative colitis, nutritional impairment, or serum albumin less than 3.0; cancer—active malignancy; and liver—any history of cirrhosis, variceal bleeding, or elevated INR in the absence of VKA therapy.

[d] Examples: tracheostomy present, heavily calcified ascending aorta, chest malformation, arterial coronary graft adherent to posterior chest wall, or radiation damage.

From Nishimura RA, Otto CM, Bonow RO, et al. 2014 AHA/ACC guideline for the management of patients with valvular heart disease: a report of the American College of Cardiology/American Heart Association task force on practice guidelines. J Thorac Cardiovasc Surg 2014;148(1):e14; with permission.

events trigger disproportionate changes in health status.[20] Frailty is an important factor as surgical risk prediction and is classified as either mild (one abnormal index), moderate (two abnormal indices), or severe (three or more abnormal indices).[9]

At our facility frailty assessment is initiated with the initial evaluation in the valve clinic and is documented on a frailty/functional assessment form (**Fig. 4**). This form is placed in the electronic medical record and is immediately available to all members of the valve team for review. The following indices are measured:

- Grip strength. A functional measurement to determine muscle strength. Muscle weakness has been shown to increase the risk of 1-month functional decline and need for new social help.[21]
- 5-m gait speed. An average gait speed greater than or equal to 6 seconds is considered slow and is an indication of frailty. The test is performed with any patient able to walk 5 m. The following guidelines should be used. (1) Accompany the patient to the designated area that has been marked at 0 and 5 m. (2) Position the patient with his/her feet behind and just touching the 0-m start line. (3) Instruct

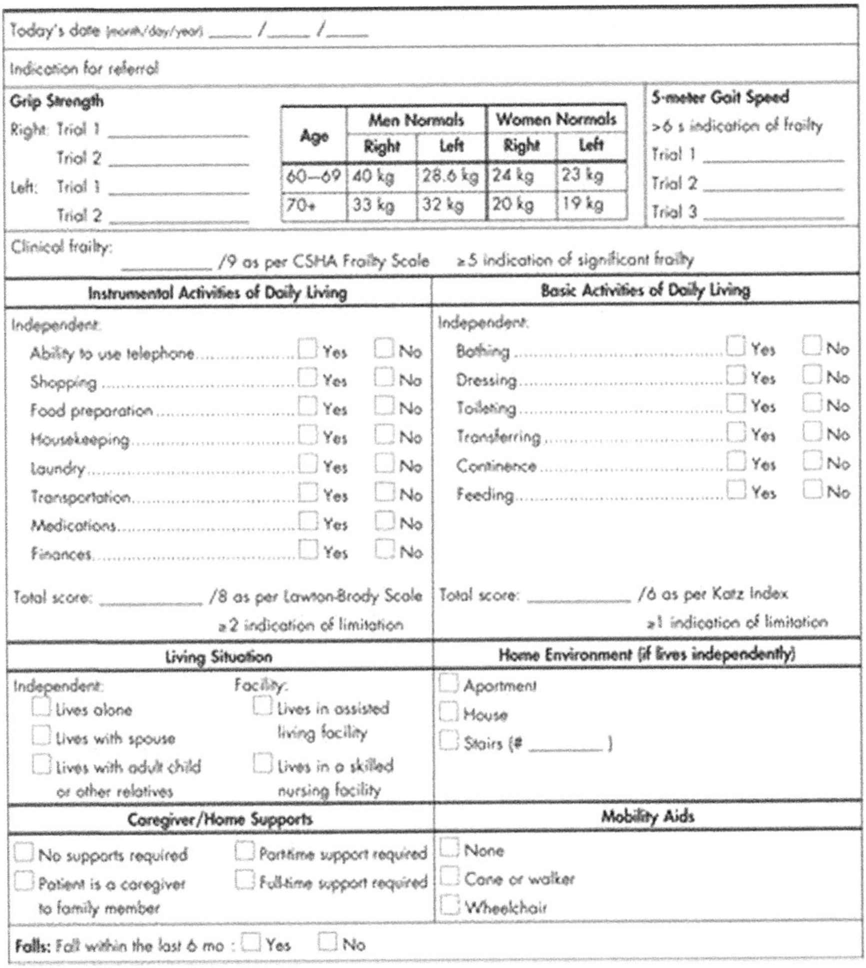

Today's date (month/day/year) ____ / ____ / ____

Indication for referral

Grip Strength

Right: Trial 1 _____
      Trial 2 _____
Left: Trial 1 _____
      Trial 2 _____

Age	Men Normals		Women Normals	
	Right	Left	Right	Left
60–69	40 kg	28.6 kg	24 kg	23 kg
70+	33 kg	32 kg	20 kg	19 kg

5-meter Gait Speed

>6 s indication of frailty

Trial 1 _____
Trial 2 _____
Trial 3 _____

Clinical frailty: _____ /9 as per CSHA Frailty Scale   ≥5 indication of significant frailty

Instrumental Activities of Daily Living	Basic Activities of Daily Living
Independent:	Independent:
Ability to use telephone........ ☐ Yes ☐ No	Bathing........ ☐ Yes ☐ No
Shopping........ ☐ Yes ☐ No	Dressing........ ☐ Yes ☐ No
Food preparation........ ☐ Yes ☐ No	Toileting........ ☐ Yes ☐ No
Housekeeping........ ☐ Yes ☐ No	Transferring........ ☐ Yes ☐ No
Laundry........ ☐ Yes ☐ No	Continence........ ☐ Yes ☐ No
Transportation........ ☐ Yes ☐ No	Feeding........ ☐ Yes ☐ No
Medications........ ☐ Yes ☐ No	
Finances........ ☐ Yes ☐ No	
Total score: _____ /8 as per Lawton-Brody Scale	Total score: _____ /6 as per Katz Index
≥2 indication of limitation	≥1 indication of limitation

Living Situation	Home Environment (if lives independently)
Independent:	☐ Apartment
☐ Lives alone	☐ House
☐ Lives with spouse	☐ Stairs (# _____)
☐ Lives with adult child	
or other relatives	
Facility:	
☐ Lives in assisted living facility	
☐ Lives in a skilled nursing facility	

Caregiver/Home Supports	Mobility Aids
☐ No supports required	☐ Part-time support required	☐ None
☐ Patient is a caregiver to family member	☐ Full-time support required	☐ Cane or walker
		☐ Wheelchair

Falls: Fall within the last 6 mo : ☐ Yes   ☐ No

Fig. 4. Frailty tool at Marshfield Clinic.

the patient to "Walk at your comfortable pace" until a few steps past the 5-m mark (the patient should not start to slow down before the 5-m mark). (4) Begin each trial on the word "Go." (5) Start the timer with the first step after the 0-m line. (6) Stop the timer with the first step after the 5-m line. (7) Repeat three times, allowing sufficient time for recuperation between trials. (8) Record the times in seconds on the data collection form. The patient may use a walking aid (cane, walker). If the patient is receiving an intravenous drip, he/she should perform the test without the intravenous drip if possible.[22]

- Canadian Study of Health and Aging frailty scale. The Clinical Frailty Scale has been shown to be an effective measure of frailty and can provide predictive information similar to that of other established tools.[23]
- Lawton-Brody Instrumental Activities of Daily Living Scale. This is an instrument used to assess independent living.[24] The instrument is most useful for identifying how a person is functioning at the present time. Requiring assistance in more than one functional domain represents limitation.
- Katz Index of Independence in Activities of Daily Living. This is an instrument used to identify a patient's ability to perform basic activities of daily living. Requiring assistance in any one or more functional domain represents limitation.[25]
- Montreal Cognitive Assessment. "Poorer Montreal Cognitive Assessment scores were significantly correlated with the higher likelihood of being frail, independent of age, sex, education, drinking, smoking, living alone, Independence in Activities of Daily Living and a history of comorbidities."[26]
- Psoas muscle area. Sarcopenia has been defined as progressive loss of skeletal muscle mass, strength, and power, and is regarded as a key component of frailty.[27] A reduced psoas muscle area is one way to determine presence of sarcopenia.[28] This is easily calculated and is determined with images available from the gated multislice CT scan already performed.

RANDOMIZED TRIALS

In 2010 the PARTNER investigators reported on the treatment of TAVR in high-risk patients with AS not believed to be candidates for conventional surgery.[29] Cohort B was the first multicenter trial that randomized 385 patients with critical AS to either a new balloon expandable transcatheter aortic valve versus the best in medical therapy, which also included balloon aortic valvuloplasty. The results from this trial lead the FDA to approve and CMS to pay for a commercially available THV for the treatment of symptomatic, severe AS in patients believed to have prohibitive risk for surgical treatment.

At 1 year, the rate of death from any cause (Kaplan-Meier analysis) was 50.7% with standard therapy and 30.7% with TAVR ($P<.001$). The rate of the composite end point of death from any cause or repeat hospitalization was 42.5% with TAVR as compared with 71.6% with standard therapy (hazard ratio, 0.46; 95% confidence interval, 0.35–0.59; $P<.001$). Among survivors at 1 year, the rate of cardiac symptoms (New York Heart Association class III or IV) was lower among patients who had undergone TAVR than among those who had received standard therapy (25.2% vs 58.0%; $P<.001$). At 30 days, TAVR, as compared with standard therapy, was associated with a higher incidence of major strokes (5.0% vs 1.1%; $P = .06$) and major vascular complications (16.2% vs 1.1%; $P<.001$). In the year after TAVR, there was no deterioration in the functioning of the bioprosthetic valve, as assessed by evidence of stenosis or regurgitation on an echocardiogram. The Sapien valve was found to be superior to medical management in cohort B.

A year later, the same PARTNER investigators reported on Cohort A, which randomized 699 high-risk patients with AS to either TAVR or SAVR.[30] TAVR was found not to be inferior to standard SAVR in patients with advanced symptomatic AS who were at high risk for surgical therapy. Each group had statistically the same mortality at 1 year with TAVR and SAVR each demonstrating equivalent 1-year mortality (TAVR, 24.2%; SAVR, 26.8%) and equivalent relief of symptoms at 1 year.

In 2014, US CoreValve clinical investigators reported on 795 patients that were randomized to high-risk surgical procedure versus the first self-expanding THV. This pivotal trial demonstrated a higher rate of survival with the CoreValve at 1 year than SAVR. In this as-treated analysis, the rate of death from any cause at 1 year was significantly lower in the TAVR group than in the surgical group (14.2% vs 19.1%), with an absolute reduction in risk of 4.9% points (upper boundary of the 95% confidence interval, −0.4; $P<.001$) for noninferiority ($P = .04$ for superiority).[31]

In April 2016, PARTNER 2 investigators published their result on patients with intermediate-risk TAVR. Intermediate risk was defined as an STS score 4% to 8%. In this trial, they randomized 2032 patients to SAVR versus TAVR either TF or TAo. At 2 years, the investigators found that TAVR and SAVR had similar results for mortality and disabling stroke. TAVR in essence was found to be noninferior to standard aortic valve surgery.[32] Of note is that the THV used in this study was Edwards Lifesciences' second-generation Sapien XT THV. In a separate propensity-matched observational trial Thourani and colleagues[33] suggested that TAVR might be the preferred treatment alternative in intermediate-risk patients; however, this trial used Edwards Lifesciences' newest THV Sapien 3 not the Sapien XT THV. The Sapien 3 THV system included several design changes believed to improve the procedural technique, safety, and success.

The 5-year results of PARNTER 1 were recently published and demonstrated that high-risk TAVR and SAVR seem to have equivalent overall outcomes.[34] There were no differences in overall mortality, stroke, and readmission to the hospital. There was no valve deterioration in either group and the hemodynamics for each group seemed to be the same with sustained low mean gradient across the valve along with LV mass regression. The slightly higher stroke rate demonstrated in the TAVR group was no longer demonstrated at 5 years. However, the higher PVL rate in the TAVR group still played a major role in a predictor of late mortality. Inherent to the early studies were the limitations of the early technology including the rudimentary understanding of valve sizing and the limited TAVR valve sizes of 23 mm and 26 mm for all patients.

DATABASE AND OBSERVATIONAL STUDIES

Although not randomized data, observational database reviews can reveal and demonstrate real world experiences and how devices and procedures behave in all comers. CE certification occurred many years before FDA approval and real world outcome experience may be informed from these databases. The German Aortic Valve Registry has done just that.[35] Unlike other registries, the German Aortic Valve Registry also includes patients that undergo SAVR along with coronary artery bypass graft. The first study that was published from this group demonstrated two things. First, excellent outcomes are possible on a national level. Second, the total number of aortic valve interventions in Germany increased more than 7% suggesting that more patients were receiving treatment of AS.[35] In addition, patients with intermediate- and low-risk TAVR were reviewed and found to have comparable outcomes to surgical patients. This registry identified patient-specific predictors of early mortality from PVL, such as higher baseline pulmonary artery pressure and the presence of 2+ mitral regurgitation.

The United Kingdom implantation TAVR registry demonstrated favorable survival rates at 3 and 5 years of 61.2% and 45.5%, respectively. Stroke within 30 days was the only procedural predictor of mortality. In addition, the authors believed there were specific underlying disease characteristics that were major factors in determining outcome, such as atrial fibrillation, respiratory dysfunction, ventricular dysfunction, and renal dysfunction.[36] Neither device type nor PVL were seen as a predictor of long-term outcome.

The STS/TVT database recently reported its finding on 26,414 patients with TAVR with procedure dates from 2011 through December 2014. The patients were grouped into two time periods: 2011 through 2012, and 2013 through December of 2014. There were a total of 346 centers that participated. This study provided an overview of current US TVT practice and trends. They compared the first time period (2011–2012) with the second time period (2013–December 2014). First, the data sets noted that these patients were elderly with a mean age 82 and this did not change between the two study periods. Second, patients in the later time period experienced an overall drop in the mean STS score, perhaps reflecting lower risk applications for TAVR. During the second time period, with the evolution of technology and changes in procedural characteristics the data sets noted the following:

- Increase in use of moderate sedation from 1.6% to 5.1%
- Increase in use of percutaneous techniques up to 66.8% in 2014
- Decrease in vascular complications from 5.6% to 4.2%
- Decrease in bleeding complication rates, reflected of lower profile devices

Despite the evolution in technology the stroke rates remained stable at 2.2% during both time periods.[37]

COMPLICATIONS OF TRANSCATHETER AORTIC VALVE REPLACEMENT

Complications associated with TAVR are categorized as early/procedural or late/postprocedural and typically are related to mechanical factors, such as design/type of THV or implantation technique, and independent patient factors, such as age, presence of Peripheral artery disease (PAD), or end-stage renal disease (ESRD).

Common early/procedural complications include the following:

- Bleeding. Mostly related to mechanical factors, such as sheath delivery size leading to vascular complications. Also can be related to the inability to maintain hemostasis at the vascular access points. These bleeds are confounded by the use of anticoagulation or antiplatelet medications.
- Low cardiac output/hypotension. Usually treatable with medications. Rarely needs to be treated with cardiopulmonary bypass. Could consider treatment with intra-aortic balloon pump or Impella device (Abiomed Danvers, MA, USA).[38]
- Coronary obstruction. More common with low ostia heights (<10 mm), small sinuses of Valsalva, and bulky leaflet calcification. Can be treated at the time of TAVR with emergent percutaneous coronary intervention.
- Stroke. Commonly related to manipulation of catheters in diseased vessels. Less commonly related to prolonged episodes of hypotension (hypoperfusion).
- Annular rupture. Rare, but life-threatening. More common with smaller annular size, smaller sinotublar junction size, bulky calcification at the annulus and LV outflow tract (LVOT), implantation of a balloon-expandable device. Can be treated aggressively with conversion to open procedure or with comfort measures. This contingency plan is determined before procedure with patient involvement.

- Vascular complications. More common with larger delivery sheath size and in patients with PAD.
- Heart block. Occurs in one out of six patients and is believed to be related to inflammation, swelling, or compression of the pacemaker tissue.[39] More common with pre-existing right bundle branch block or left anterior fascicular block, smaller LVOT diameter, and higher ratio of annulus diameter to LVOT diameter. More common with lower delivery height of the THV and in use of self-expanding devices.[40] If a patient at any point following TAVR develops type 2 atrioventricular block or complete Heart block, electrophysiology should be consulted for consideration of permanent pacemaker implantation.[41]
- Aortic regurgitation (paravalvular and central). Often caused by malpositioning of the THV, either too high or too low. Can also be caused by undersizing of the THV.
- Pericardial effusion/tamponade. Can occur from RV perforation from temporary transvenous pacemaker or LV perforation from wires/catheters. Typically treated with pericardiocentesis but may require open procedure.

Common late/postprocedural complications include the following:

- Bleeding. Although less common in this time period, the frequent types of late bleeds are gastrointestinal, neurologic, or traumatic fall-related. These bleeds are confounded by the use of anticoagulation or antiplatelet medications.
- Valve leaflet thrombosis. A more recently documented phenomenon, subclinical valve thrombosis that may lead to a rising AV gradient. Valves placed by TAVR and SAVR have been discovered to contain subclinical thrombus. Four-dimensional CT scan is the best way to document this problem and a trial of anticoagulation should be considered.[42]
- Heart block. In patients who develop a new left branch bundle block or type 1 heart block, close monitoring with an event monitor at the time of discharge may be considered to allow for closer monitoring of potential late atrioventricular block.
- Aortic regurgitation (paravalvular and central). May not be discovered until after the patient has left the procedure room. If PVL is greater than moderate, this is associated with a poorer long-term prognosis at 2 years.[31,32] It is important that all members of the heart care team communicate in the same language and quantify the amount of PVL in a consistent and concise manner. The Valve Academic Research Consortium (VARC) has settled on common language and criteria that should be used.[33,34] If significant by VARC 2 criteria, the implanting physicians should consider a second procedure to "plug" the leak, postdilate the implanted THV, or implant a second THV if believed to be related to malpositioning.
- Patient prosthetic mismatch. Although patient prosthetic mismatch occurs more with SAVR, it is still noted with TAVR. In some patients with patient prosthetic mismatch, symptoms never resolve or worsen. There may not be the typical LV mass regression.[43]
- Prosthetic valve endocarditis. Occurs in 1.13% to 2.3% of patients in large TAVR cohorts. Diagnosed by transthoracic echocardiogram or transesophageal echocardiogram. The bacteria are usually *Staphylococcus*, *Streptococcus*, and *Enterococci*. The onset of endocarditis is early or late. Overall the diagnosis carries a poor prognosis given the inherent population.[44,45]

SPECIAL CIRCUMSTANCES

As the indications for TAVR expand, more patients will be served with this treatment modality leading to use of TAVR in patient populations that may not have been specifically studied initially. These special circumstances should be evaluated on a case by case basis until more research is available and long-term durability is documented.

End-Stage Renal Disease

Patients with ESRD were excluded from the PARTNER trials but were included in the CoreValve US Expanded Use Study. There has been at least one database/observation study using TVT Registry data that reviewed all patients with renal-replacement therapy. Mack and coworkers[46] reported that patients on renal-replacement therapy were compared with nondialysis patients undergoing TAVR. They found that patient on renal-replacement therapy had higher mean STS PROM scores (13.8% vs 6.8%; $P<.0001$), a higher incidence of bleeding complications (7.7% vs 3.3%; $P<.001$), a higher major vascular complication rate (9.5% vs 6.1%; $P = .006$), and a higher in-hospital mortality (9.7% vs 5.3%; $P = .0002$). The risk of stroke seemed to be the same for both groups. Of note was a lower than expected observed mortality for patients with TAVR and ESRD.

Patients with ESRD in the CoreValve US Expanded Use Study were found to have a higher risk for mortality and complications.[47] Stroke and major vascular injury were infrequent and valve durability was maintained at 1 year.[48]

In summary, TAVR in patients with ESRD carries a higher risk than seen in the general pool of patients undergoing the procedure, but still is offered with caution.[49]

Pregnancy

Women represent close to 50% of all patients undergoing TAVR.[50] Although extremely rare, there have been case reports of pregnant patients undergoing TAVR with successful outcomes.[51] Pre-TAVR work-up may need to be altered to reduce the amount of radiation and contrast exposure to the patient and the baby. The procedural steps should remain as close to routine as possible to help ensure optimal THV placement and patient outcomes.

Incidental Pulmonary Nodules

Single pulmonary nodules (<5 mm in size) are a common finding in elderly patients with AS. With the gated multislice CT angiography performed on all patients during pre-TAVR work-up, incidental findings are bound to be found[52] and may be noted in up to 18% of patients screened.[53] Often these incidental findings include pulmonary nodules. Unless advanced thoracic malignancy is obvious, the reduction of morbidity and mortality by TAVR outweighs potentially harmful delays regarding further diagnostics. Standard, guideline-approved evaluation of single pulmonary nodules is safely performed after TAVR.[54]

THE FUTURE

TAVR and other transcatheter valve therapies are here to stay. Currently in the United States there are only two THVs available for commercial implantation; however, in Europe there are eight THVs for commercial implantations. Some of the valves commercially available in Europe are currently under study in the United States. After the recent approval for TAVR in the intermediate-risk group (PROM 4%–8%), the only group left to be treated with SAVR is the low-risk group (PROM <4%). As new THVs become available and TAVR indications expand, the future of advanced treatment of AS is predicted to shift even further from SAVR to TAVR.

A recent study reported by the Northern New England Cardiovascular Disease Study Group confirmed the longevity of SAVR noting that patients younger than 80 had a median survivorship of 11.5 years, patients between the ages of 80 and 84 had a median survivorship of 6.8 years, and those older than age 85 had a median survivorship of 6.2 years. Knowing the median survival with SAVR, to rationally approve TAVR in the low-risk group, long-term data on valve durability need to be evaluated[55,56] with documentation of freedom from structural valve deterioration that approaches 80% at 20 years for one biologic valve.[57]

History does not repeat itself, but is an important gauge into the future. It is not hard to recall the initial celebration within the surgical community with the results of the first-generation biologic valves at 5 years, only to be met with the sobering results of the 10-year durability data. Many unanswered questions remain about TAVR, such as the effect of PVL on long-term outcomes, the effect of permanent pacemaker implant in this subset of patients on mortality, and of course the 10- or 20-year THV durability data. However, it is important that the modern cardiac surgeon take a page from vascular surgery colleagues and continue to acquire endovascular skills. For the modern cardiac surgeon with the appropriate skill sets,[58] the future is bright.

SUPPLEMENTARY DATA

Supplementary data related to this article can be found at http://dx.doi.org/10.1016/j.suc.2017.03.011.

REFERENCES

1. Tommaso CL, Bolman RM 3rd, Feldman T, et al. Multisociety (AATS, ACCF, SCAI, and STS) expert consensus statement: operator and institutional requirements for transcatheter valve repair and replacement, part 1: transcatheter aortic valve replacement. J Am Coll Cardiol 2012;59(22):2028–42.
2. Meier B. The first patient to undergo coronary angioplasty — 23-year follow-up. N Engl J Med 2001;344(2):144–5.
3. Gruentzig A. Results from coronary angioplasty and implications for the future. Am Heart J 1982;103(4 Pt 2):779–83.
4. Kan JS, White RI Jr, Mitchell SE, et al. Percutaneous balloon valvuloplasty: a new method for treating congenital pulmonary-valve stenosis. N Engl J Med 1982; 307(9):540–2.
5. Cribier A, Remadi F, Koning R, et al. Emergency balloon valvuloplasty as initial treatment of patients with aortic stenosis and cardiogenic shock. N Engl J Med 1992;326(9):646.
6. Cribier A, Eltchaninoff H, Tron C. First human transcatheter implantation of an aortic valve prosthesis in a case of severe calcific aortic stenosis. Ann Cardiol Angeiol (Paris) 2003;52(3):173–5 [in French].
7. Cribier A, Eltchaninoff H, Bash A, et al. Percutaneous transcatheter implantation of an aortic valve prosthesis for calcific aortic stenosis: first human case description. Circulation 2002;106(24):3006–8.
8. Cribier A, Eltchaninoff H, Tron C, et al. Treatment of calcific aortic stenosis with the percutaneous heart valve: mid-term follow-up from the initial feasibility studies: the French experience. J Am Coll Cardiol 2006;47(6):1214–23.
9. Nishimura RA, Otto CM, Bonow RO, et al. 2014 AHA/ACC guideline for the management of patients with valvular heart disease a report of the American College

of Cardiology/American Heart Association task force on practice guidelines. J Am Coll Cardiol 2014;63(22):e57–185.

10. Vahanian A, Alfieri O, Andreotti F, et al. Guidelines on the management of valvular heart disease (version 2012): the joint task force on the management of valvular heart disease of the European Society of Cardiology (ESC) and the European Association for Cardio-Thoracic Surgery (EACTS). Eur J Cardiothorac Surg 2012;42(4):S1–44.

11. Achenbach S, Delgado V, Hausleiter J, et al. SCCT expert consensus document on computed tomography imaging before transcatheter aortic valve implantation (TAVI)/transcatheter aortic valve replacement (TAVR). J Cardiovasc Comput Tomogr 2012;6(6):366–80.

12. Chambers J, Ray S, Prendergast B, et al. Standards for heart valve surgery in a 'heart valve centre of excellence'. Open Heart 2015;2(1):e000216.

13. Litmanovich DE, Ghersin E, Burke DA, et al. Imaging in transcatheter aortic valve replacement (TAVR): role of the radiologist. Insights Imaging 2014;5(1):123–45.

14. CMS, NCD decision memo. Available at: https://www.cms.gov/medicare-coverage-database/details/nca-decision-memo.aspx?NCAId=257&ver=4&NcaName=Transcatheter+Aortic+Valve+Replacement+(TAVR)&bc=ACAAAAAAIAAA&. Accessed January 7, 2017.

15. Smith MM, Barbara DW, Mauermann WJ, et al. Morbidity and mortality associated with dental extraction before cardiac operation. Ann Thorac Surg 2014;97(3): 838–44.

16. Henn MC, Zajarias A, Lindman BR, et al. Preoperative pulmonary function tests predict mortality after surgical or transcatheter aortic valve replacement. J Thorac Cardiovasc Surg 2016;151(2):578–85, 586.e1-2.

17. Condado JF, Jensen HA, Maini A, et al. Should we perform carotid Doppler screening before surgical or transcatheter aortic valve replacement? Ann Thorac Surg 2017;103(3):787–94.

18. Available at: http://www.openaccessjournals.com/articles/evolution-in-transcatheter-aortic-valve-replacement-the-corevalve-selfexpanding-prosthetic-aortic-valve.pdf.

19. Available at: http://riskcalc.sts.org. Accessed January 7, 2017.

20. Clegg A, Young J, Iliffe S, et al. Frailty in elderly people. Lancet 2013;381(9868): 752–62.

21. Vidan MT, Blaya-Novakova V, Sánchez E, et al. Prevalence and prognostic impact of frailty and its components in non-dependent elderly patients with heart failure. Eur J Heart Fail 2016;18(7):869–75.

22. STS. Using gate speed as a measure of frailty. Available at: http://www.sts.org/news/using-gait-speed-measure-frailty. Accessed January 7, 2017.

23. Rockwood K, Song X, MacKnight C, et al. A global clinical measure of fitness and frailty in elderly people. CMAJ 2005;173(5):489–95.

24. Graf C. The Lawton instrumental activities of daily living (IADL) Scale. Medsurg Nurs 2009;18(5):315–6.

25. Wallace M, Shelkey M. Katz index of independence in activities of daily living (ADL). Urol Nurs 2007;27(1):93–4.

26. Nasreddine ZS, Phillips NA, Bédirian V, et al. The Montreal Cognitive Assessment, MoCA: a brief screening tool for mild cognitive impairment. J Am Geriatr Soc 2005;53(4):695–9.

27. Morrell GR, Ikizler TA, Chen X, et al. Psoas muscle cross-sectional area as a measure of whole-body lean muscle mass in maintenance hemodialysis patients. J Ren Nutr 2016;26(4):258–64.

28. Paknikar R, Friedman J, Cron D, et al. Psoas muscle size as a frailty measure for open and transcatheter aortic valve replacement. J Thorac Cardiovasc Surg 2016;151(3):745–50.

29. Leon MB, Smith CR, Mack M, et al. Transcatheter aortic-valve implantation for aortic stenosis in patients who cannot undergo surgery. N Engl J Med 2010; 363(17):1597–607.

30. Smith CR, Leon MB, Mack MJ, et al. Transcatheter versus surgical aortic-valve replacement in high-risk patients. N Engl J Med 2011;364(23):2187–98.

31. Adams DH, Popma JJ, Reardon MJ. Transcatheter aortic-valve replacement with a self-expanding prosthesis. N Engl J Med 2014;371(10):967–8.

32. Leon MB, Smith CR, Mack MJ, et al. Transcatheter or surgical aortic-valve replacement in intermediate-risk patients. N Engl J Med 2016;374(17):1609–20.

33. Thourani VH, Kodali S, Makkar RR, et al. Transcatheter aortic valve replacement versus surgical valve replacement in intermediate-risk patients: a propensity score analysis. Lancet 2016;387(10034):2218–25.

34. Mack MJ, Leon MB, Smith CR, et al. 5-year outcomes of transcatheter aortic valve replacement or surgical aortic valve replacement for high surgical risk patients with aortic stenosis (PARTNER 1): a randomised controlled trial. Lancet 2015; 385(9986):2477–84.

35. Hamm CW, Möllmann H, Holzhey D, et al. The German aortic valve registry (GARY): in-hospital outcome. Eur Heart J 2014;35(24):1588–98.

36. Duncan A, Ludman P, Banya W, et al. Long-term outcomes after transcatheter aortic valve replacement in high-risk patients with severe aortic stenosis: the U.K. transcatheter aortic valve implantation registry. JACC Cardiovasc Interv 2015;8(5):645–53.

37. Holmes DR Jr, Nishimura RA, Grover FL, et al. Annual outcomes with transcatheter valve therapy from the STS/ACC TVT registry. J Am Coll Cardiol 2015;66(25):2813–23.

38. Singh V, Yarkoni A, O'Neill WW. Emergent use of Impella CP during transcatheter aortic valve replacement: transaortic access. Catheter Cardiovasc Interv 2015; 86(1):160–3.

39. Young Lee M, Chilakamarri Yeshwant S, Chava S, et al. Mechanisms of heart block after transcatheter aortic valve replacement: cardiac anatomy, clinical predictors and mechanical factors that contribute to permanent pacemaker implantation. Arrhythm Electrophysiol Rev 2015;4(2):81–5.

40. Siontis GC, Jüni P, Pilgrim T, et al. Predictors of permanent pacemaker implantation in patients with severe aortic stenosis undergoing TAVR: a meta-analysis. J Am Coll Cardiol 2014;64(2):129–40.

41. Kalathiya R, Upadhyay GA. Available at: http://www.acc.org/latest-in-cardiology/articles/2016/04/26/15/22/risk-stratification-for-pacemaker-placement-after-tavr. Accessed January 7, 2017.

42. Mack MJ, Douglas PS, Holmes DR. Shedding more light on valve thrombosis after transcatheter aortic valve replacement. J Am Coll Cardiol 2016;67(6):656–8.

43. Pibarot P, Weissman NJ, Stewart WJ, et al. Incidence and sequelae of prosthesis-patient mismatch in transcatheter versus surgical valve replacement in high-risk patients with severe aortic stenosis: a partner trial cohort analysis. J Am Coll Cardiol 2014;64(13):1323–34.

44. Latib A, Naim C, De Bonis M, et al. TAVR-associated prosthetic valve infective endocarditis results of a large, multicenter registry. J Am Coll Cardiol 2014;64(20): 2176–8.

45. Eisen A, Shapira Y, Sagie A, et al. Infective endocarditis in the transcatheter aortic valve replacement era: comprehensive review of a rare complication. Clin Cardiol 2012;35(11):E1–5.

46. Mack MJ, Brennan JW, Peterson E, et al. The Outcomes of Transcatheter Aortic Valve Replacement in Patients with End-stage Renal Disease: A Report from the STS/ACC TVT Registry. J Am Coll Cardiol 2014;63(12).

47. O'Hair D, Petrossian GA, Bajwa T, et al. TCT-100 transcatheter aortic valve replacement in patients with end-stage renal disease: one year outcomes from the Corevalve US expanded use study. J Am Coll Cardiol 2015;66(15_S).

48. Petrossian GA, Robinson N, Yakubov S, et al. Transcatheter aortic valve replacement in patients with end-stage renal disease: early outcomes from the Corevalve US expanded use study. J Am Coll Cardiol 2015;65(10_S).

49. Szerlip M, Kim RJ, Adeniyi T, et al. The outcomes of transcatheter aortic valve replacement in a cohort of patients with end-stage renal disease. Catheter Cardiovasc Interv 2016;87(7):1314–21.

50. Chieffo A, Petronio AS, Mehilli J, et al. Acute and 30-day outcomes in women after TAVR: results from the WIN-TAVI (Women's INternational Transcatheter Aortic Valve Implantation) real-world registry. JACC Cardiovasc Interv 2016;9(15): 1589–600.

51. Gandhi S, Ganame J, Whitlock R, et al. Double trouble: a case of valvular disease in pregnancy. Circulation 2016;133(22):2206–11.

52. Budoff MJ, Fischer H, Gopal A. Incidental findings with cardiac CT evaluation: should we read beyond the heart? Catheter Cardiovasc Interv 2006;68(6):965–73.

53. Stachon P, Kaier K, Milde S, et al. Two-year survival of patients screened for transcatheter aortic valve replacement with potentially malignant incidental findings in initial body computed tomography. Eur Heart J Cardiovasc Imaging 2015;16(7):731–7.

54. Schmidt LH, Vietmeier B, Kaleschke G, et al. Thoracic malignancies and pulmonary nodules in patients under evaluation for transcatheter aortic valve implantation (TAVI): incidence, follow up and possible impact on treatment decision. PLoS One 2016;11(5):e0155398.

55. Kron IL, Ailawadi G. Low risk TAVR: the long view. Ann Thorac Surg 2016;102(2):357.

56. Mack MJ. Does transcatheter aortic valve implantation mean the end of surgical aortic valve replacement? Tex Heart Inst J 2010;37(6):658–9.

57. Dellgren G, David TE, Raanani E, et al. Late hemodynamic and clinical outcomes of aortic valve replacement with the Carpentier-Edwards Perimount pericardial bioprosthesis. J Thorac Cardiovasc Surg 2002;124(1):146–54.

58. Lazar HL. What is the best method for cardiac surgeons to acquire catheter-based interventional skills? Can J Cardiol 2016;32(3):289–90.

Surgical Treatment of Heart Failure

Robert S.D. Higgins, MD, MSHA[a],*, Ahmet Kilic, MD[b], Daniel G. Tang, MD[c]

KEYWORDS

- Surgical treatment of heart failure • Coronary revascularization
- End-stage myocardial dysfunction

KEY POINTS

- Coronary revascularization is the mainstay of surgical treatment of heart failure in patients with left ventricular ejection fraction less than 35% based on demonstration of viable or hibernating myocardium.
- Patients with end-stage myocardial dysfunction refractory to revascularization may require mechanical circulatory support as a bridge to transplantation or destination therapy.
- Mechanical circulatory support using left ventricular assist devices has developed as an effective means of circulatory support and end-organ perfusion; however, complications of left ventricular assist devices are common, including driveline infection, pump thrombosis, allosensitization, and gastrointestinal bleeding.
- Heart transplantation is the gold standard of biological replacement for end-stage congestive heart failure; however its long-term success and growth is limited by donor availability, perioperative infections, and cellular rejection as complications of chronic immunosuppression, as well as the development of malignancies and transplant allograft vasculopathy.

INTRODUCTION: EVOLVING BURDEN OF DISEASE

Cardiac surgery, as it is applied to patients with advanced heart failure, has evolved significantly in the past 50 years. From the time when anatomic replacement of the heart was conceived and executed by Lower, Shumway, and Barnard as the best definitive way to treat heart failure, advances in surgical technique, myocardial

Disclosure: The authors have nothing to disclose.
[a] Department of Surgery, Johns Hopkins Medicine, 720 Rutland Avenue, Room 759, Baltimore, MD 21205, USA; [b] Heart Transplantation and Mechanical Circulatory Support, Advanced Heart Failure Program, Clinical and Academic Affairs, Division of Cardiac Surgery, The Ohio State University Wexner Medical Center, Columbus, OH, USA; [c] Division of Cardiothoracic Surgery, Virginia Commonwealth University, MCV Campus, West Hospital, 7th Floor, South Wing, 1200 East Broad Street, PO Box 980068, Richmond, VA 23298-0068, USA
* Corresponding author.
E-mail address: Robert.Higgins@jhmi.edu

Surg Clin N Am 97 (2017) 923–946
http://dx.doi.org/10.1016/j.suc.2017.04.003
0039-6109/17/© 2017 Elsevier Inc. All rights reserved.

surgical.theclinics.com

protection during cardiopulmonary bypass, and evolution of mechanical circulatory support (MCS) have revolutionized the field. Along the way, several innovative approaches to ventricular restoration, myocardial revascularization by direct coronary and percutaneous interventions as hybrid procedures, and stem cell therapies have been attempted to mitigate the impact and pathophysiology of ischemic cardiomyopathy as a primary cause of heart failure. Landmark clinical trials, such as the Surgical Treatment for Ischemic Heart Failure (STICH) trial, document the challenges with managing these complex patients and the intense efforts necessary to study the natural history of the heart failure patients before, during, and after interventions designed to treat the growing heart failure patient population.

More than 5 million Americans suffer from heart failure and more than 250,000 die annually. Heart failure has been called the cardiovascular epidemic of the twenty-first century.[1] The diagnosis of heart failure carries an ominous prognosis, with a nearly 40% annual mortality despite optimal treatment with medications. Renin-angiotensin system inhibition with angiotensin-converting enzyme (ACE) inhibitors or angiotensin receptor blockers in conjunction with beta blockers and aldosterone antagonists remain the cornerstone of optimal medical management.

ACE inhibitors, beta blockers, and other medical therapies have evolved to reduce the progression of heart failure and subsequent morbidity and mortality. The pharmacologic armamentarium has recently expanded with the introduction of angiotensin receptor and neprilysin inhibitors (valsartan-sacubitril) and sinoatrial node modulators (ivabradine).Other nonsurgical modalities in the treatment of heart failure include cardiac resynchronization therapy or implantable defibrillators and catheter-based interventions for the treatment of valvular heart disease. The rapid expansion and evolution in heart failure therapy underscores the need for integrated multidisciplinary treatment teams.

Current therapeutic interventions are focused on the appropriate assessment of myocardial dysfunction as a means to select the right patient for the appropriate procedure using state of the art myocardial viability testing and metabolic testing to determine if patients with advanced heart failure are candidates for conventional interventions, mechanical devices, or transplant. This is particularly germane in the era of aggressive percutaneous coronary interventions, multivessel percutaneous coronary intervention, left main stenting, and invasive valve procedures. Patients with nonischemic cardiomyopathy secondary to viral or congenital disease serve as a compelling group of patients with limited surgical options who present with advanced heart failure refractory to conventional medical therapies.

Advances in MCS with more efficient and less morbid ventricular assist devises, including potential enhancements in biventricular failure treatment using the total artificial heart (TAH) as a bridge to transplant (BTT), offer the potential to change the trajectory of this growing epidemiologic dilemma. The ultimate goal of creating a biologically compatible replacement for advanced heart failure is still the holy grail of surgical treatment and involves a combination of strategies, which are enumerated in this article.

HISTORICAL PERSPECTIVE

The introduction of the heart-lung machine and the ability to support vital end-organ and neurologic functions has enabled the surgical treatment of patients with heart failure.[2] In 1953, John Gibbon performed the first open heart procedure using the heart-lung machine. Evolution of this seminal work at the University of Minnesota using a bubble oxygenator enhanced safety and visibility for procedures.[3] Coronary revascularization became a standard approach to improve myocardial perfusion in patients with critical atherosclerotic disease leading to myocardial dysfunction and advanced heart failure.

Based on techniques developed by Lower and Shumway[4] in the laboratory, the modern era of cardiac transplantation captured the collective imagination in 1967 when Barnard[5] reported the first successful human-to-human cardiac transplant. Ironically, the donation occurred after withdrawal of medical care (donation after cardiac death). Dr Adrian Kantrowitz performed the first pediatric transplant on Dec 6, 1967, in New York. He also laid the foundation for formulating the brain death criteria, which later came out of the Ad Hoc Committee of the Harvard Medical School.

Although technical success was demonstrated by many surgeons after this success, immunologic consequences of rejection presented an almost insurmountable challenge until the introduction of cyclosporine in the 1970s. This powerful interleukin cytokine inhibitor revolutionized transplantation for thousands of transplant recipients. Organ availability continues to be a limited resource; approximately 2000 cardiac transplants are performed in the United States each year. This chronic shortage of donors has provoked the development of MCS as a BTT or even as a permanent solution. In 1969, Cooley performed the first TAH procedure as a BTT.[6] Continuous axial or centrifugal flow pumps have replaced pulsatile displacement pumps as the most effective long-term support devices in the current era.[7]

ABANDONED INTERVENTIONS

Many patients with congestive heart failure have significant left ventricular (LV) dilatation, which was thought to be amenable to volume reduction techniques as an alternative to transplantation or mechanical assist devices. Ventricular dilatation in progressive stages of congestive heart failure serves as a compensatory mechanism to maintain stroke volume because the ventricle becomes more globular and less ellipsoid. Changes in ventricular geometry without ventricular muscle hypertrophy leads to further deterioration in systolic function and progressive heart failure (**Fig. 1**).[8]

Volume reduction procedures excising nonfunctional or infarcted muscle using the Dor or Batista procedure were intended to restore the LV cavity to a more normal geometry (**Fig. 2**).[9]

Reductions in end-systolic and end-diastolic volume theoretically reduce wall stress. Unfortunately, these procedures did not demonstrate a significant reduction in morbidity or mortality and many have been abandoned.[10]

The Batista procedure specifically involved excision of the LV free wall between the papillary muscles.[8] Despite some early improvements in LV function and functional status, excess morbidity and mortality limited the application and adoption of these procedures.

The Surgical Anterior Ventricular Endocardial Restoration procedure was evaluated as part of the STICH trial, a prospective, randomized study specifically evaluating LV reconstruction in subjects with ischemic cardiomyopathy randomly assigned to high-risk coronary artery bypass grafting (CABG) alone or CABG with LV reconstruction.[11] Preliminary results demonstrated significantly reduced end-systolic volumes; however, there was no significant difference in mortality.

CURRENT OPTIONS
High-Risk Coronary Artery Bypass Grafting

Coronary revascularization has been the cornerstone of surgical treatments for patients with significant atherosclerotic heart disease since the 1970s. An important

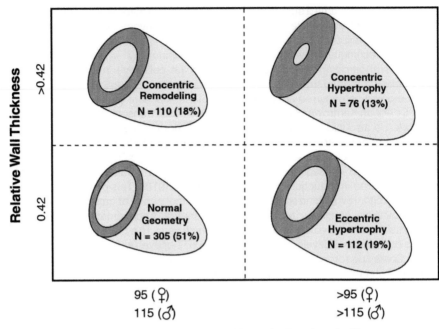

Fig. 1. Patterns of remodeling. The echocardiographic substudy of the VALsartan In Acute myocardial iNfarcTion (VALIANT) trial defined 3 patterns of LV remodeling in patients with heart failure and/or LV ejection fraction equal to or less than 35%, based on measurement of LV mass index (LVMi) and relative wall thickness (RWT): concentric remodeling (normal LVMi and increased RWT), eccentric hypertrophy (increased LVMi and normal RWT), and concentric hypertrophy (increased LVMi and increased RWT). (*From* Konstam MA, Kramer DG, Patel AR, et al. Left ventricular remodeling in heart failure: current concepts in clinical significance and assessment. JACC Cardiovasc Imaging 2011;4(1):101; with permission.)

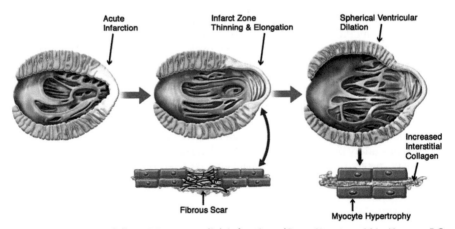

Fig. 2. Post-MI remodeling. MI, myocardial infarction. (*From* Konstam MA, Kramer DG, Patel AR, et al. Left ventricular remodeling in heart failure: current concepts in clinical significance and assessment. JACC Cardiovasc Imaging 2011;4(1):101; with permission.)

subgroup that was excluded from many of these studies has been the patient population with LV dysfunction secondary to ischemic cardiomyopathy. Classically, ejection fractions less than 35% have been observed in these patients.

To evaluate the role of cardiac surgery and, in particular, coronary revascularization in the treatment of patients with CAD and LV dysfunction, the STICH trial was initiated as a multicenter, randomized study at 127 clinical sites.[10]

Between 2002 and 2007, a total of 1212 subjects with ejection fraction of 35% or less and coronary artery disease (CAD) amenable to CABG were randomly assigned to medical therapy alone (602) or medical therapy plus CABG (610). In this randomized trial, there was no significant difference between medical therapy alone and medical therapy plus CABG, with respect to death from any cause. Subjects assigned to CABG, as compared with those assigned to medical care alone, and had lower rates of death from cardiovascular causes (**Fig. 3**).

In the STICH trial, which looked at long-term effects of CABG in subjects with ischemic cardiomyopathy, the rates of death from cardiovascular causes were significantly lower (by 16%) over 10 years among the subjects who underwent CABG in addition to receiving medical therapy compared with medical therapy alone (**Fig. 4**).[12]

Patients with ischemic cardiomyopathy have significant abnormalities in hemodynamics and myocardial energetics that may lead to significant abnormalities in metabolism. Decisions regarding who would be the most appropriate candidate for revascularization often depend on appropriate assessments of myocardial viability. Predicting whether a patient with ischemic cardiomyopathy will ultimately improve or have survival benefit from CABG and recovery of myocardial function depends on the presence of viable myocardium (hibernating or stunned myocardium).[13]

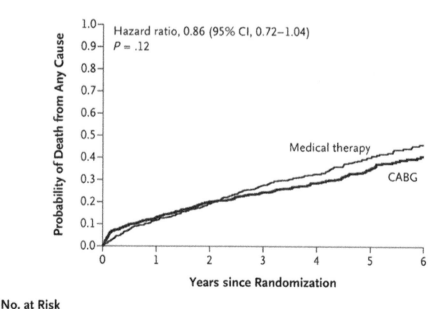

Fig. 3. Kaplan-Meier curves for the probability of death from any cause. (*From* Jones R, Velasquez E, Michler R, et al. Coronary bypass with or without surgical ventricular reconstruction. N Engl J Med 2009;360:1705; with permission.)

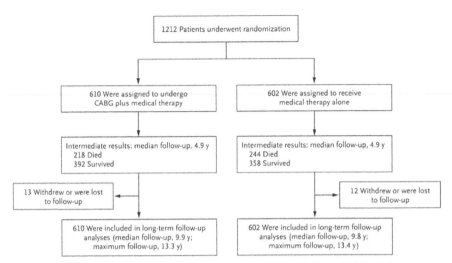

Fig. 4. Randomization and follow-up. (*From* Velazquez EJ, Lee KL, Jones RH, et al. Coronary-Artery Bypass Surgery in Patients with Ischemic Cardiomyopathy. N Engl J Med 2016;374(16):1516; with permission.)

Assessment of myocardial viability

Myocardial perfusion imaging using SPECT has been validated in several studies as a useful screening tool for CAD in patients with risk factors and for the detection of extent and degree of myocardial ischemia.[14] Glucose metabolism substitutes free fatty acid metabolism as the main energy source in ischemic but viable myocardium. F-fluorodeoxyglucose (F-FDG), a glucose analogue combined with a tracer (rubidium-82) is used to evaluate the glucose metabolism in the myocyte. Following the detection of a fixed perfusion defect on perfusion imaging, preservation of F-FDG uptake in that region by a PET scan is suggestive of hibernating myocardium and indicates the beneficial effect of revascularization in patients with ventricular dysfunction.[14]

Kim and colleagues[15] observed that contrast MRI in combination with cine MRI could identify acute myocardial infarction (hyperenhanced with contractile dysfunction), injured but viable myocardium (not hyperenhanced but with contractile dysfunction), and normal myocardium (not hyperenhanced and with normal function). Subsequently, the same group investigated the use of contrast-enhanced MRI to predict improvements following revascularization in regions of abnormal ventricular contraction. Gadolinium-enhanced MRI was performed in 50 subjects with ventricular dysfunction before either surgical or percutaneous revascularization to assess the transmural extent of the hyperenhanced myocardium postulated to represent nonviable myocardium. In addition, cine MRI was performed to assess the regional contractility at the same locations before and after revascularization. Following analysis of the data, the investigators demonstrated that the likelihood of improvement in regional contractility after revascularization decreased progressively as the transmural extent of the hyperenhancement before revascularization increased. The amount of LV mass that was dysfunctional and not hyperenhanced before revascularization strongly related to the degree of improvement in the wall motion score and ejection fraction after revascularization. The investigators clearly demonstrated that reversible myocardial dysfunction can be identified by contrast-enhanced MRI before coronary revascularization. Further confirmatory studies established the value of delayed enhancement MRI as a powerful predictor of myocardial viability after surgery.[12]

Mitral Valve Repair

Many patients with dilated cardiomyopathy develop or manifest mitral valve incompetence either secondary to ischemia or annular dilatation. The mechanism of ischemic mitral regurgitation (MR) is complex and must be understood as an ultimate manifestation of a decompensating ventricle, not an intrinsic disease of the valve. Ischemic MR is a consequence of adverse LV remodeling with distortion of the ventricle and mitral annulus, along with apical and lateral migration of the papillary muscles (**Fig. 5**).[16] This remodeling creates a tethering force that distorts the papillary muscles and surrounding myocardium and, therefore, pulls the valve leaflets away from the annulus during systole, preventing valve coaptation and leading to regurgitation.[17] Ischemic MR may be addressed at the time of coronary revascularization leading to improvements in ventricular perfusion or as a complementary mitral valve repair and annuloplasty.[18] By reducing LV volume demands, volume loads, and myocardial oxygen demands, LV function can be improved with or without a ring. If repair is to be performed, many surgeons favor partial or less rigid, autologous pericardial strips to augment the posterior annulus. Current evidence now demonstrates that CABG candidates with moderate MR will not benefit from simultaneous mitral valve repair in the short run, and every patient with severe symptomatic ischemic MR should not undergo attempt at valve repair.[19] In patients with moderate ischemic MR, the addition of mitral valve repair to CABG did not result in a higher degree of LV reverse remodeling. Mitral valve repair was associated with a reduced prevalence of moderate or severe MR but an increased number of untoward events. Thus, at 1 year, this trial did not show a clinically meaningful advantage of adding mitral valve repair to CABG.

Ventricular Assist Device

MCS has been used for advanced heart failure since the 1990s when volume displacement pumps (LV assist devices [LVADs]) were approved by the US Food and Drug

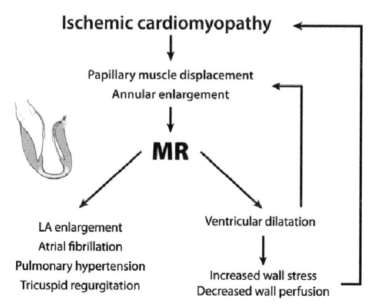

Fig. 5. Ischemic cardiomyopathy mechanism. (*From* Anyanwu A, Rahmanian P, Filoufi F, et al. The pathophysiology of ischemic mitral regurgitation: implications for surgical and percutaneous intervention. J Interv Cardiol 2006;19:S80; with permission.)

Administration (FDA). Two general indications to support the failing heart have evolved: as a BTT and as a destination therapy to support cardiac function for the remainder of the patient's life.[20] Some patients may require support until their general medical condition improves or until they become a better candidate eligible for transplantation (bridge to decision or eligibility).[21] Other patients, in a rare circumstance, may have improvements or recovery of myocardial function (ie, myocarditis) so that their native heart recovers and the LVAD can be explanted.

Continuous-flow pumps have emerged as the preferred MCS for patients with LV failure awaiting heart transplantation or as destination therapy. LVADs restore cardiac output and tissue perfusion, therefore improving end-organ function. The 2 currently approved LVADs have inlet and outflow ports with a single rotary element that rotates to propel blood to the aorta, leading to increased arterial blood pressure and flow. Blood is drawn into the pump impeller from the LV apex and delivered to the aorta. There are 2 LVAD blood flow configurations: axial and centrifugal flow pumps. In the centrifugal pump, blood is captured between the blades, which spin at right angles to the outflow. In the axial flow pump, the rotating impeller operates like a propeller in a tube. The 2 commercially approved LVADs are the HeartMate II (Thoratec/St Jude Corp, Pleasanton, CA, USA) and the Heart Ware HVAD (Heart Ware/Medtronic Inc, Framingham, MA, USA) (**Fig. 6**A,[22] B[23]).

Pump outflow is determined by the revolutions per minute (RPMs) generating forward flow. Device flows are proportional to rotor speed and inversely related to the difference in pressure in the inflow and the outflow cannulas. Patient physiology and loading conditions that affect flow rates include right ventricular (RV) function, intravascular volume, afterload conditions, external kinking of the outflow graft, or tamponade. LVAD pump power is measured by the current and voltage delivered to the motor and varies with pump speed and flow. When flows are decreased, secondary to thrombus formation on the rotor, power may be increased. Pulsatility index correlates with the magnitude of flow pulse measured through the pump. It fluctuates with changes in the patient's volume status, and the heart's contractility. It increases with increased preload and contractility and decreases when blood volume and afterload is

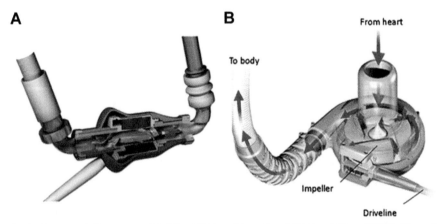

Fig. 6. Commercially approved LVADs: (*A*) HeartMate II and (*B*) Heart Ware HVAD. (*From* [*A*] St. Jude Medical. Available at: http://media.sjm.com/newsroom/media-kits/heart-failure-hypertension/international/default.aspx. Accessed June 16, 2017; with permission; and [*B*] Aaronson KD, Slaughter MS, Miller LW, et al. Use of an intrapericardial, continuous-flow, centrifugal pump in patients awaiting heart transplantation. Circulation 2012;125: 3192; with permission).

decreased. The HeartMate II has 2 modes of operation: fixed rate and auto mode, in which the LVAD can respond to the patient's activity and volume status. Both pumps require systemic anticoagulation.

The Interagency Registry for Mechanically Assisted Circulatory Support (INTER-MACS) is a collaborative database sponsored by the National Heart, Lung, and Blood Institute that collects outcomes data on FDA-approved durable (capable of patient discharged to home) MCS devices (MCSDs) implanted in the United States. Initiated in June 2006, more than 14,000 patients were entered into the INTERMACS database through January 2015. INTERMACS collects detailed demographics and outcomes data for implant and postimplant from event-driven episodes of care and at specific follow-up intervals. Between April 2008 and June 30, 2014, a total of 11,123 HeartMate II devices were implanted and recorded in the INTERMACS database.

Through documentation and reporting in clinical databases like INTERMACS and the International Society for Heart and Lung Transplantation (ISHLT) registry, both LVADs have demonstrated effective performance profiles and improved systemic perfusion and enhance outcomes. These databases also document that complications of MCSDs are common. The most common complications include driveline infections, cannula obstruction, gastrointestinal bleeding, and device thrombosis. RV dysfunction and postimplant failure occurs in approximately 10% to 20% of implants historically and a number predictive indices have been developed to predict and avoid RV failure in the perioperative period.[24] Echocardiographic assessments of RV function have been demonstrated to be effective parameters to evaluate and monitor in the perioperative period. Frequently identified risk factors include increased age, increased filling pressures (central venous pressure [CVP], CVP/pulmonary capillary wedge pressure), poor RV function (decreased right ventricular stroke work index, low right ventricular ejection fracture, increased RV dimension, severe tricuspid regurgitation), and increased illness severity (inotropes, intubation, intra-aortic balloon pump [IABP], renal dysfunction, hepatic dysfunction). Typical interventions to manage and improve RV function include inotropes, afterload reduction using phosphodiesterase inhibitors or pulmonary vasodilators, and carefully monitored filling pressures and pump flows to maintain the RV-LV septum in its normal position.[25]

Among the most challenging complications to identify and manage is device thrombosis (**Fig. 7**).[26] Device thrombosis can lead to inflow or outflow obstruction and subsequent device power surges. Predisposing factors include shear stresses in blood flow, cannula malposition, disturbances in von Willebrand factor levels (deficiency), and heparin-induced thrombocytopenia. Starling and colleagues[27] reported an increase in the rate of device thrombosis in patients with HeartMate II in 2014. Based on data from 3 institutions with experience in 837 patients, a total of 72 pump thromboses were confirmed in 66 patients. They reported that elevated lactate dehydrogenase (LDH) levels presaged thrombosis. Most patients underwent pump replacement and 11 patients underwent urgent transplantation.

These findings were confirmed in a report from INTERMACS in 2015. INTERMACS identified 9808 adult patients from 144 institutions receiving a primary HeartMate II implant between April 2008 and June 30, 2014 (**Fig. 8**). Risk factors for pump thrombosis included younger age, higher body mass index, history of noncompliance, severe right heart failure, later date of implant, and elevated LDH during the first month postimplant. Subsequent pump thrombosis was more likely if the initial pump exchange indication was pump thrombosis. Identification of marked elevation of LDH during the first month offers an opportunity for early intervention strategies.

Several pump and patient characteristics can contribute to the development of thrombosis. Based on these characteristics, an algorithm for the diagnosis and

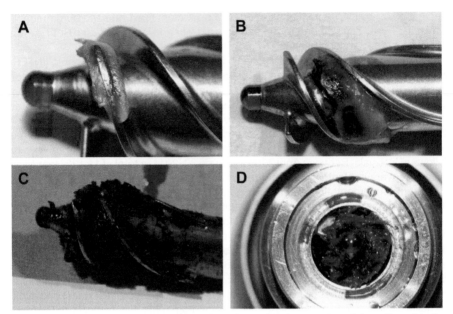

Fig. 7. Examples of HeartMate II device thrombosis. (*A–C*) HeartMate II impeller with the ruby bearing and different types of clots in the same location. (*A*) Fibrin-only clot. (*B*) Fibrin and blood clot. (*C*) Blood-only clot. (*D*) Cross-section of the HeartMate II motor with significant combined fibrin and blood clot. (*From* Uriel N, Han J, Morrison KA, et al. Device thrombosis in HeartMate II continuous-flow left ventricular assist devices: a multifactorial phenomenon. J Heart Lung Transplant 2014;33(1):53; with permission.)

management of suspected thrombus has been developed and validated as the standard of care in the field (**Fig. 9**). Based on expert opinion, this stepwise approach has been used to manage and assist in early detection. Recent emphasis on serial monitoring of LDH or signs of hemolysis (hemoglobinuria with tea-colored urine) has improved the management of these problems. Changes inpatient management, including strict adherence to an international normalized ratio of 2 to 3, early initiation of aspirin therapy (81–325 mg), and use of perioperative heparin, have been reported to decrease the rate of device exchange secondary to pump thrombosis by 450%.[28] The PREVENtion of HeartMate II Pump Thrombosis through Clinical Management (PREVENT) study was designed to evaluate the rates of thrombosis when these management practices were adopted.[29] Full adherence to implant techniques, heparin bridging, and pump speeds greater than 9000 RPMs resulted in a significantly lower risk of pump thrombosis (1.9% vs 8.9%; po 0.01) and lower composite risk of suspected thrombosis, hemolysis, and ischemic stroke (5.7% vs 17.7%; po 0.01) at 6 months.

LVADs can stimulate the development of alloreactive antibodies.[30] Panel reactive antibody (PRA) screening is done in all heart transplant candidates, and further evaluation is needed if PRA levels are elevated above 10% to 20%. The factors involved leading to sensitization are homograft use in congenital surgery, female sex, prior pregnancies, black race, ventricular assist device (VAD) surface exposure, retransplantation, perioperative blood products usage, and infections. Acute antibody-mediated rejection occurs in about 10%, usually due to antibodies driven by T cells to donor vascular antigens. This leads to B-cell activation and production of plasma cells. It is difficult to diagnose but usually associated with detection of

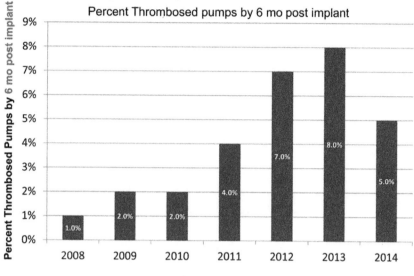

INTERMACS: HMII Pump Investigation
Implants: April 2008 – June 2014, n = 9808
Follow-up: Thru September 2014

Percent Thrombosed pumps by 6 mo post implant

Implant Year

Fig. 8. Pump thrombosis in the Thoratec HeartMate II device: an update analysis of the IN-TERMACS Registry. (*From* Kirklin JK, Naftel DC, Pagani FD, et al. Pump thrombosis in the Thoratec HeartMate II device: an update analysis of the INTERMACS registry. J Heart Lung Transplant 2015;34(12):1521; with permission.)

immunoglobulins, complement fragments, CD68 positive cells, and de novo anti-human leukocyte antigen (HLA) antibodies.

PRA levels greater than 10% are treated, and aggressive desensitization with plasmapheresis, intravenous immunoglobulin (IVIG), and rituximab is associated with significantly improved survival. IVIG is used to neutralize preformed antibodies before and after transplantation. The effectiveness is variable. Plasmapheresis is fast, short-lived, and can be done immediately before transplantation. Rituximab (anti-CD20) is frequently used and is effective in the long term. Immunoabsorption and splenectomy are rarely used.[31] The rate of infection is very high with these therapies.

As MCS evolves, the interface between patient physiology, potential allosensitization, selection for durable devices, psychosocial suitability, and support and device variables will continue to be the critical success factors for long-term complication-free survival. The ability to screen appropriate candidates who have advanced heart failure physiology but lack the social supports or physical wherewithal to benefit from LVAD insertion will be pivotal to the success of this technology to enhance outcomes and save lives. Increasingly, concepts like frailty, which is the aggregate of subclinical impairments that decrease patients reserve and vulnerability to stress, may be the critical measures of potential success in the future.[32]

Heart Transplantation

Heart transplantation has been and continues to be the ultimate surgical intervention for patients with advanced heart failure refractory to medical therapies. Several critical

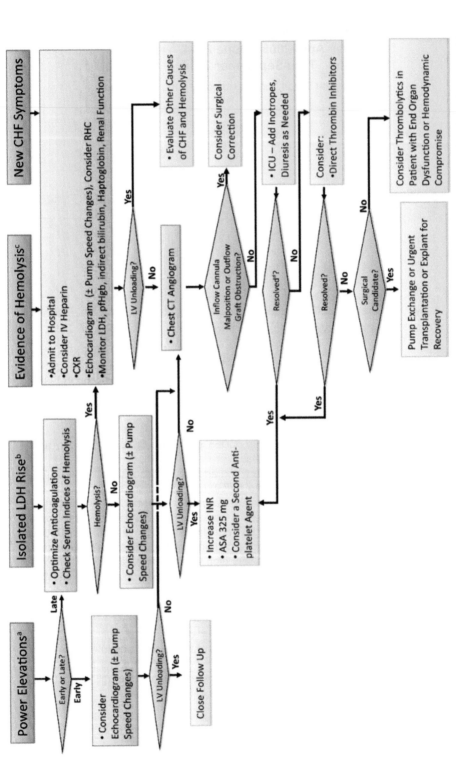

Fig. 9. Algorithm for the diagnosis and management of suspected pump thrombus. Definitions: [a] Power Elevations: Sustained (>24 hours) Power >10 W; or Sustained (>24 hours) Power increase >2 W from Baseline; [b] Isolated LDH Rise: LDH >3× Upper Limit of Normal (ULN); [c] Hemolysis: Clinical Diagnosis;

technical and management advancements over the past 50 years have helped to overcome inherent obstacles imposed by the body's immunologic response to biological replacement by a foreign organ. The original technique described by Lower and Shumway[4] and perfected in the laboratory confirmed that the denervated heart could function to support the circulation in the transplant recipient. The development of a technique to perform transvenous endomyocardial biopsies for immunologic surveillance was also a breakthrough milestone that provided tissue to characterize the nature of acute cellular rejection and enabled early detection and treatment with augmented immunosuppression. However, among the most influential advances in the modern transplant era was the development and application of cyclosporine, the powerful immunosuppressant used as part of a triple immunosuppression protocol in solid organ transplant programs around the world.

Cyclosporine reduces the activity of the immune system by interfering with the activity and growth of T cells. Its immunosuppressant activity is manifest by binding to the cytosolic protein cyclophilin (immunophilin) of lymphocytes. This complex of cyclosporin and cyclophilin inhibits calcineurin that, under normal circumstances, is responsible for activating the transcription of interleukin 2. The success of cyclosporin in preventing organ rejection was shown in kidney transplants by Calne and colleagues[33] at the University of Cambridge and in liver transplants performed by Thomas Starzl[34] at the University of Pittsburgh Hospital. Cyclosporin was subsequently approved for use in 1983.

Current indications for heart transplantation are well described in guidelines developed by professional organizations well versed in the care of patients with advanced heart failure.[35,36] Cardiopulmonary stress testing is the most reliable and objective criteria to determine the extent of critical, advanced heart failure and it has predictive value as to the morbidity and mortality associated with class IV congestive heart failure. Peak oxygen consumption per unit time (V_{O_2}) less than 10 mL/kg/min with respiratory exchange ratio greater than 1.05 is predictive of poor outcome and this value has been used as criteria for transplant waiting list selection.[30] Additional listing criteria supportive of placement on the heart transplant waiting list include a history of repeated hospitalizations for heart failure, progressive increases in heart failure medications, and the need for MCS (ie, IABP, LVAD).

The major physiologic problem that can prevent a patient from being eligible for cardiac transplantation is irreversible pulmonary hypertension. Patients with irreversible pulmonary hypertension have an increased risk of RV failure in the immediate postoperative period. Pulmonary hypertension can often be improved by using nitroprusside, nesiritide, dobutamine, milrinone, prostaglandin E1, prostacyclin, and inhaled nitric oxide. Milrinone therapy is highly effective and is often used to determine if pulmonary hypertension is reversible and or treatable. If pulmonary hypertension is controlled, a patient may be considered for transplantation. Diabetes and/or end-organ complications of diabetes, renal failure, previous malignancy within 5 years of transplant consideration, hepatic insufficiency, psychosocial noncompliance, active substance abuse (ie, smoking or illicit drug abuse), and lack of sufficient social support can all limit consideration for transplantation.

---

or LDH >3× ULN and pfHgb > 40; [d] Resolved: Normal Powers, Normal LDHs, Sufficient LV Unloading, and No Clinical Evidence of Hemolysis. CXR, Chest X ray; LDH, Lactate Dehydrogenase; LV, Left Ventricle; pfHgb, Plasma-free Hemoglobin; RHC, Right Heart Cath. (*From* Goldstein DJ, John R, Salerno C, et al. Algorithm for the diagnosis and management of suspected pump thrombus. J Heart Lung Transplant 2013;32(7):668; with permission.)

Multidisciplinary selection criteria for heart transplantation have helped to identify the patients with the highest mortality and greatest risk of mortality on the waiting list. US heart allocation policy has evolved considerably since the inception of the National Organ Transplant Act in 1984. An urgency-based system with concentric geographic zones was first adopted in 1988, with 2 priority statuses: status 1, for all MCS patients and those with inotropic dependency, and status 2 for everyone else. Further modifications occurred in 1998 with the introduction of a 3-tiered system, with status 1A, the most urgent, intended for patients supported with MCS, mechanical ventilation, and inotropic dependency with continuous hemodynamic monitoring; status 1B for stable patients on VADs or inotrope infusions; and status 2 for all others.

The current system, which was last modified in 2006, allows greater regional sharing of organs according to clinical urgency; thus, organs are now offered only to status 1A or 1B candidates locally (organ procurement area), then in the nearest concentric zone (500 mile radius) before being offered to status 2 locally.

Candidates are considered adults if they are registered on the waiting list at age 18 years or older. Candidates qualify for status 1A if

- They require continuous infusion of a single high-dose intravenous inotrope or multiple intravenous inotropes and continuous hemodynamic monitoring
- They are supported by a TAH, an IABP, extracorporeal mechanical oxygenation (ECMO), mechanical ventilation, or a VAD (for a 30-day discretionary period)
- They are implanted with an MCSD and are experiencing a device-related complication
- They have an approved exception.[37]

Since the last significant revision to the adult heart allocation system in 2006, there has been an overall decline in waiting list mortality rates among adult heart transplant candidates intended to benefit from the policy changes. Even with these changes, there remains regional variation in waiting times and number of transplants performed on higher urgency candidates.[38]

The current system has identified 4 major limitations: there are too many status 1A candidates, too many exception requests required, increased use of mechanical support not accommodated by current system, and the geographic sharing scheme is not equitable. The Organ Procurement and Transplant Network/United Network for Organ Sharing (OPTN/UNOS) Thoracic Organ Transplantation Committee proposes modifications to the adult heart allocation system to better stratify the most medically urgent heart transplant candidates, reflect the increased use of MCSDs and prevalence of MCSD complications, and address geographic disparities in access to donors among heart transplant candidates. This may evolve as a heart allocation score similar to the Lung Allocation Score and the Model for End-Stage Liver Disease scores used for lung and liver transplantation.

The technique of orthotopic heart transplantation has historically used a biatrial technique with the benefit of ease of implantation, shorter clamp times, and reduced ischemic times. Since 1997, the use of a bicaval anastomosis has been associated with theoretic improvements in atrial function (**Figs. 10** and **11**). Recent literature has reported improved long-term survival and freedom from permanent pacemaker implantation.[39] In addition, short-term benefits, including decreased length of stay (likely related to reductions in the need for pacemakers before discharge), have also been clearly demonstrated.

Organ rejection can manifest as hyperacute, acute cellular, or acute antibody-mediated rejection. Hyperacute rejection occurs within minutes to hours due to binding of preformed antibodies to donor antigens leading to complement fixation in vessels and tissue death. The traditional immunosuppressive regimen after orthotopic heart

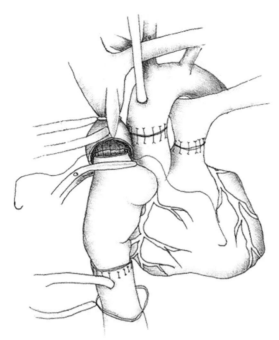

Fig. 10. Bicaval anastomotic technique. (*From* Tsilimingas, Nikolaos B. Modification of bicaval anastomosis: an alternative technique for orthotopic cardiac transplantation. The Annals of Thoracic Surgery 2003; 75(4);1333–4; with permission.)

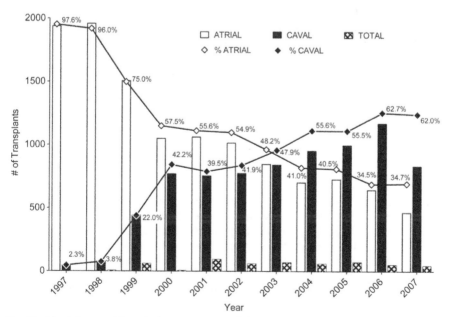

Fig. 11. Biatrial versus bicaval anastomosis in orthotopic transplantation. (*From* Steinman T, Becker B, Frost A, et al. Guidelines for the referral and management of patients eligible for solid organ transplantation. Transplantation 2001;71:1189; with permission.)

transplant has consisted of calcineurin inhibitors (CNIs), such as cyclosporine or tacrolimus, combined with mycophenolate mofetil or azathioprine and glucocorticoids. The introduction of cyclosporine microemulsion, sirolimus, rapamycin protein inhibitors, new-generation monoclonal antibodies (anti-interleukin-2 receptor antagonists, daclizumab, basiliximab, alemtuzumab), OKT3, and the depleting polyclonal biologic thymoglobulin has significantly increased the ability of physicians to fight rejection.[40]

Complications after transplantation are most commonly related to the level or adequacy of immunosuppression. Acute cellular rejection is more common in the first 6 months, occurring in 20% to 40% of recipients secondary to T-cell–mediated activity against the donor's HLA. Acute antibody-mediated rejection occurs in about 10% of patients, usually due to antibodies driven by T cells to donor vascular antigens.[41] This leads to B-cell activation and production of plasma cells. It is difficult to diagnose but usually associated with detection of immunoglobulins, complement fragments, CD68 positive cells, and de novo anti-HLA antibodies.[35] Surveillance endomyocardial biopsies are essential in the first year to detect rejection at the subclinical level before the development of cardiac dysfunction. Infants and children have lower rejection rates, whereas adolescents have higher rates.

Within the first 30 days after transplantation, the patient is at greatest risk for infections associated with health care, often due to antibiotic-resistant organisms. Immunosuppressive agents target either single or multiple sites in the immune system. Therefore, these drugs represent a double-edged sword, potentially predisposing heart transplant recipients to all categories of pathogens by impairing host defenses. Immunosuppressive drug–induced antiproliferative activity can lead to mucosal erosions, transient cytopenias, uremia, hyperglycemia, and malnutrition; and, with the use of invasive mechanical devices (leading to drive-line colonization and infection), abnormalities in tissue perfusion (vascular or surgery-related causes), abscesses, cytomegalovirus (CMV) infection, Epstein-Barr virus (EBV) infection, and human immunodeficiency virus infection.

Cyclosporine administration increases the risk of post-transplant lymphoproliferative disorder, an EBV-associated condition. An important difference between cyclosporine and tacrolimus is that the latter is far more potent than cyclosporine. During the 1 to 6 months after transplantation, infections occur based on the presence or absence of pathogens, whether or not there are ongoing prophylactic antibiotics against *Pneumocystis* or viruses such as CMV or hepatitis B; or herpesviruses, such as herpes simplex virus, varicella-zoster virus, and EBV.

Transplant CAD (TCAD; accelerated atherosclerosis of the transplant heart) is a thought to be a manifestation of chronic rejection driven by an inflammatory milieu consisting of multiple cell types that contribute to fibromuscular and smooth muscle cell proliferation with subsequent coronary obstruction (**Fig. 12**). The prevalence and prognosis of cardiac allograft vasculopathy (CAV) after cardiac transplantation vary considerably depending on how vasculopathy is defined and which method is used to detect it.[42] Some studies have defined CAV as coronary artery stenosis ranging from 30% to 70% by coronary angiography (**Fig. 13**). Other studies have diagnosed CAV using the much more sensitive technique of intravascular ultrasound.[43–45]

The heart is denervated at the time of transplant and reinnervation is generally incomplete. As a result, vasculopathy (TCAD) generally progresses silently and, in some cases, rapidly. Because of afferent denervation, affected patients seldom present with classic symptoms of angina. Silent myocardial infarction, sudden death, and progressive heart failure are common presentations.

Current treatments for TCAD include pharmacotherapy, percutaneous coronary intervention, and repeat transplantation. Although percutaneous coronary intervention

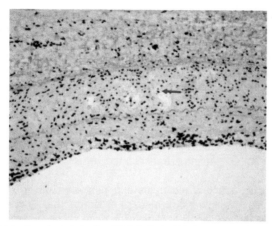

Fig. 12. Immunohistochemical stain for CD4 Cells in TCAD. Immunohistochemical stain for CD4 cells in an epicardial coronary artery of a patient with TCAD demonstrating subendothelial accumulation of T lymphocytes (*arrow*) characteristic of endotheliitis, which is a manifestation of chronic rejection. (*From* Zimmer RJ, Lee MS. Transplant coronary artery disease. JACC Cardiovasc Interv 2010;3(4):368; with permission.)

has generally demonstrated high procedural success rates, it has been plagued by a high incidence of in-stent restenosis. Drug-eluting stents reduce in-stent restenosis compared with bare metal stents.

Proliferation signal inhibitors (sirolimus and its derivative everolimus) are increasingly playing an important role in the treatment and prevention of TCAD. Sirolimus has been used as a substitute for CNIs as a way of averting nephrotoxicity.

The results of heart transplantation have markedly improved with the use of modern immunosuppression agents (calcineurin inhibitors cyclosporine and tacrolimus), better selection criteria, enhancements in donor management and selection, and vigilant

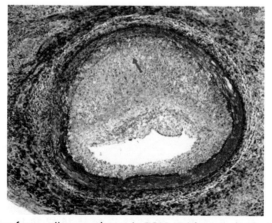

Fig. 13. Lipid-Laden foam cell macrophages in TCAD. Trichrome elastic stain of a coronary artery demonstrating progressive arterial occlusion with lipid-laden foam cell macrophages (*arrow*) in a patient with TCAD. (*From* Zimmer RJ, Lee MS. Transplant coronary artery disease. JACC Cardiovasc Interv 2010;3(4):370; with permission.)

post-transplant surveillance.[46] In 2016, the most recent report of the ISHLT registry reported on 118,788 heart transplants in recipients from 457 heart transplant centers. A total of 4157 adult transplants were performed in 2014. For the pediatric and adult patient transplants performed in 1982 to June 2015, survival was better for pediatric patients and younger adult recipients. Post-transplant survival decreased with increasing recipient and donor age (**Fig. 14**). Survival was not adversely affected by pretransplant MCS except for patients supported by extracorporeal membrane oxygenation (**Fig. 15**). The leading causes of death after transplant were primary graft failure, non-CMV infection, and multiorgan failure. The overall 1-year survival is now approximately 90% with 3-year survival of greater than 75%. More than 405 of patients awaiting transplant are now transplanted as BTT recipients requiring LVAD explant (**Fig. 16**).

Long-term cardiac transplant recipients experience increased risk for cutaneous malignancies and lymphoproliferative disease or lymphoma.[47] Multivariable analysis showed older age and earlier transplant year were highly significant risk factors. Aggregate malignancy incidence in the modern era (2001–2008) did not differ significantly from the normal population, which seemed to be attributable to a lower rate of malignancies other than lung cancer, lymphoma, and melanoma. From 2001 to 2008, rates were significantly higher for lung cancer and lymphoma than in the normal population. The highest risk for lymphoma was in younger adults who received transplants at ages 18 to 35 years. The highest risk for lung cancer was in patients who underwent transplantation at ages 55 to 65 years. Once diagnosed with malignancy, subsequent survival at 5 years was 21% for lung cancer and 32% for lymphoma.

FUTURE INTERVENTIONS
Stem Cells

Given the existing challenges in donor organ identification and availability, heart transplantation may be an inadequate solution to the existing clinical epidemic of heart failure.[48] Promising experimental work in stem cell biology has offered theoretic solutions to myocardial dysfunction and been supported by work in animal models.[40] Of critical

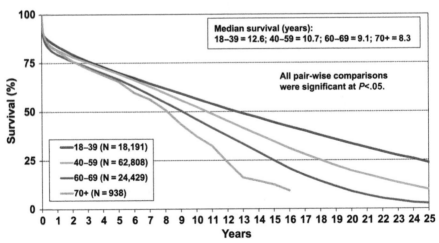

Fig. 14. Kaplan-Meier survival by recipient age. (*From* Zimmer RJ, Lee MS. Transplant coronary artery disease. JACC Cardiovasc Interv 2010;3(4):370; with permission.)

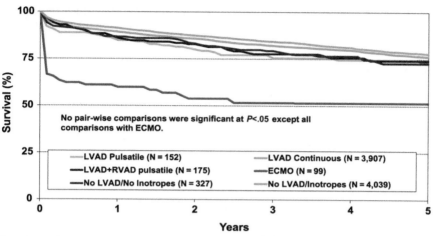

Fig. 15. Kaplan-Meier survival by pretransplant MCS. RVAD, right ventricular assist device. (*From* Lund LH, Edwards LB, Dipchand AI, et al. The registry of the International Society for Heart and Lung Transplantation: thirty-third adult heart transplantation report-2016. J Heart Lung Transplant 2016;35(10):1158–69; with permission.)

importance is the type of cells to be used, the effectiveness of cell type and delivery methods, the timing and dose of therapies, and overall clinical effectiveness and impact. Bone marrow derived stem cells delivered by direct injection have demonstrated very modest improvements in cardiac function. In the future, autologous cell regeneration may show promise for more effective regeneration based on refinements in isolation and expansion of these cells for clinical use.[49] Different cell types, including bone marrow–derived mesenchymal stem cells, mobilized CD34+ cells, and recently

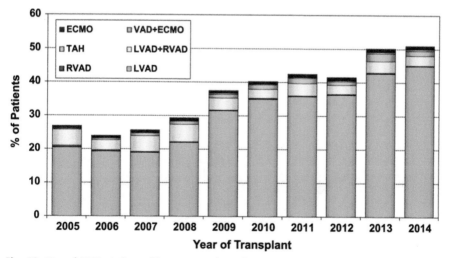

Fig. 16. Use of MCS at time of heart transplant. (*From* Lund LH, Edwards LB, Dipchand AI, et al. The registry of the International Society for Heart and Lung Transplantation: thirty-third adult heart transplantation report-2016. J Heart Lung Transplant 2016;35(10): 1158–69; with permission.)

cardiac-derived C-kit+ stem cells and cardiosphere-derived cells may be used to reduce cardiac scar size and to improve cardiac function in patients with ischemic cardiomyopathy.[50]

Total Artificial Heart

Although the almost all patients with advanced heart failure are adequately treated with isolated LV support, there is a small subset of patients that requires biventricular support or even biventricular replacement. Patients with advance late-stage biventricular failure represent a particularly ill cohort and often present with cardiogenic shock and multisystem organ dysfunction. As previously noted, evaluating risk for RV failure after LVAD can be difficult. Temporary support options (ECMO, Centrimag [Thoratec Corporation, Pleasanton, CA, USA], Impella [Abiomed Inc, Danvers, MA, USA], Tandem [CardiacAssist Technologies, Pittsburgh, PA, USA], IABP) can be used as a bridge to a bridge. Although this allows simultaneous resuscitation and evaluation, it potentially introduces the added morbidity of additional procedures.

Durable mechanical RV support options are limited. Early-generation pulsatile devices were limited by thromboembolism and limited dischargeability. There is growing experience with continuous flow LVADs adapted for RV support but this remains an off-label investigational use.

Biventricular replacement with the TAH offers several advantages over assist devices (**Fig. 17**). The larger and shorter blood flow pathway can generate higher cardiac outputs with lower inotropic requirements and thus facilitate resuscitation. Orthotopic excision and replacement can be an effective, albeit extreme, treatment of disease that is not well treated by LVADs or would otherwise require extensive repair. This includes postinfarction ventricular septal defect, aortic root aneurysm or dissection, cardiac allograft failure, massive ventricular thrombus, refractory malignant arrhythmias, hypertrophic or restrictive cardiomyopathy, and complex congenital heart disease.

The Syncardia (SynCardia Systems, Tucson, AZ, USA) device is currently the only FDA-approved device in clinical use. Its design has changed little since it was first introduced as the Jarvik 7 in 1982. Early adaptation was quickly tempered by the development of major complications common to all MCSDs. Subsequent refinement in patient selection and management led to markedly improved outcomes and FDA approval as a

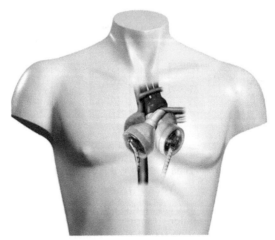

Fig. 17. SynCardia TAH. (*Courtesy of* SynCardia Systems, LLC, Tucson, AZ; with permission.)

BTT.[51] Although they share many of the same challenges seen with LVADs, TAH patients face increased risks with regard to anemia and renal failure. The Syncardia pneumatic design with 4 single-leaflet mechanical disks creates a greater hemolytic stress and accompanying anemia compared with continuous flow LVADs. Although the incidence of renal failure in TAH patients compared with continuous flow LVADs is confounded by underlying illness severity, biventricular excision is associated with an abrupt drop in natriuretic peptide that seems to contribute. Perioperative natriuretic peptide supplementation seems to have protective effects. The introduction of the 14 lb Freedom Driver has enabled Syncardia TAH patients to be discharged from the hospital and even return to work. However, unlike LVAD patients, TAH patients do not have the native myopathic heart as a backup should the device fail.

Since the 1980s when the TAH became a clinical reality, MCS for patients with biventricular failure has evolved to be an important consideration in the armamentarium of surgeons around the world. Theoretic advantages of TAH over LVADs include the ability to overcome significant pulmonary hypertension that would otherwise lead to RV failure after LVAD placement (see **Fig. 14**).

Despite promising experiences in many proficient centers, the medical management of anticoagulation, end-organ dysfunction, and poor outcomes challenge even the best centers. Arabia and colleagues[52] recently evaluated experience over 3 eras to ascertain the impact of implanting center experience an outcomes. Between 2006 and 2015, 359 patients received 362 TAH (3 patients received second device) implants as a BTT in 44 hospitals in the INTERMACS registry. The mean age of patients was 50 years old and 85% were male patients. The most common primary diagnoses were dilated cardiomyopathy (34%), ischemic cardiomyopathy (30%), and other (26%). There were 210 patients who were successfully transplanted and 114 patients who died while on the device. In their analysis, centers performing greater than 11 implants experienced 88% survival at 6-months postimplant. Hazard function analysis revealed that older age, elevated bilirubin, lower albumin, prior history of cancer, and valve surgery were risk factors for death. Implanting centers with the most experience had the best outcomes, probably secondary to better experience in patient selection, timing of intervention, and management. DePasquale and colleagues[53] reviewed post-transplant outcomes after biventricular mechanical support using UNOS national registration data. In 682 patients BTT with either TAH (120) or PVADs (562), 498 underwent successful heart transplant. Although overall short-term survival was comparable between groups, there was a trend toward worse survival with the TAH group.

In the future, the development of TAHs will require significant advancements in bioengineering with close collaborations between surgeons, cardiologists, physicians, biomedical engineers, vascular biologists, pharmacists, and material and tissue engineers. These collaborative teams will investigate specific flow dynamics that lead to alterations in sheer stresses in formed blood elements, deficiencies in von Willebrand factors, thrombosis, and hemolysis. Durable power sources that use percutaneous energy transfer without cables prone to infection or even implantable energy sources with high-energy isotopes are a possibility. Use of inducible pluripotent stem cells to create biocompatible tissue constructs that are resistant to thrombosis may be the next generation of MCS for the failing heart.

REFERENCES

1. Mozzafarian D, Benjamin EJ, Go AS, et al, on behalf of the American Heart Association Statistics Committee, Stroke Statistics Subcommittee. Heart disease and

stroke statistics—2016 update: a report from the American Heart Association. Circulation 2016;133:e38–360.

2. Gibbon JH. The development of the heart lung apparatus. Am J Surg 1978; 135(5):608–19.

3. Dewall R, Gott V, Lillehei C, et al. A simple expendable artificial oxygenator for open heart surgery. Surg Clin North Am 1956;1025–34.

4. Lower RR, Shumway NE. Studies on orthotopic homotransplantation of the canine heart. Surg Forum 1960;11:18–9.

5. Barnard CN. The operation: a human cardiac transplant: an interim report of a successful operation performed at Groote Schuur Hospital, Cape Town. S Afr Med J 1967;41(48):1271–4.

6. DeVries W, Anderson J, Joyce L, et al. Clinical use of the total artificial heart. N Engl J Med 1984;310(5):273–8.

7. Slaughter MS, Rogers JG, Milano CA, et al. Advanced heart failure treated with continuous-flow left ventricular assist device. N Engl J Med 2009;361(23): 2241–51.

8. Konstam M, Kramer D, Patel A, et al. Left ventricular remodeling in heart failure. JACC Cardiovasc Imaging 2011;4:98–108.

9. Batista R, Santos J, Takesshita N, et al. Partial left ventriculotomy to improve left ventricular function in end stage heart disease. J Card Surg 1996;11:96.

10. Etoch S, Koenig SC, Laureano MA, et al. Results after partial left ventriculotomy versus heart transplantation for idiopathic cardiomyopathy. J Thorac Cardiovasc Surg 1999;117:952.

11. Jones R, Velasquez E, Michler R, et al. Coronary bypass with or without surgical ventricular reconstruction. N Engl J Med 2009;360:1705.

12. Kim RJ, Wu E, Rafael A, et al. The use of contrast-enhanced magnetic resonance imaging to identify reversible myocardial dysfunction. N Engl J Med 2000; 343(20):1445–53 (Permission to be obtained.).

13. Hausmann H, Topp H, Sinlawski H, et al. Decision making in end stage coronary artery disease: revascularization or heart transplantation. Ann Thorac Surg 1997; 64:1296–301.

14. Selvanayagam J, Kardos A, Francis J, et al. Value of delayed-enhancement cardiovascular magnetic resonance imaging in predicting myocardial viability after surgical revascularization. Circulation 2004;110(12):1535–41.

15. Kim RJ, Fieno DS, Parrish TB, et al. Relationship of MRI delayed contrast enhancement to irreversible injury, infarct age, and contractile function. Circulation 1999;100(19):1992–2002.

16. Anyanwu A, Rahmanian P, Filoufi F, et al. The pathophysiology of ischemic mitral regurgitation: implications for surgical and percutaneous intervention. J Interv Cardiol 2006;19:S78–86.

17. Kumanohoso T, Otsuji Y, Yoshifuku S, et al. Mechanism of high incidence of ischemic mitral regurgitation in patients with inferior myocardial infarction: quantitative analysis of left ventricular and mitral valve geometry in 103 patients with prior myocardial infarction. J Thorac Cardiovasc Surg 2003;125:135–43.

18. Smith PK, Puskas JD, Ascheim DD, et al. Surgical treatment of moderate ischemic mitral regurgitation. N Engl J Med 2014;371:2178–88.

19. Smith P, Puskas J, Aschein D, et al. Surgical treatment of moderate mitral ischemic mitral regurgitation. N Engl J Med 2014;37(23):2178–88.

20. Miller L, Pagani F, Russell S, et al. Use of continuous flow device in patients awaiting heart transplantation. N Engl J Med 2007;357:885–97.

21. Pagani F, Miller L, Russell S, et al. Extended mechanical support with continuous flow rotary left ventricular assist device. J Am Coll Cardiol 2009;54:312–21.

22. St. Jude Medical. Available at: http://media.sjm.com/newsroom/media-kits/heart-failure-hypertension/international/default.aspx. Accessed April, 2017.

23. Aaronson KD, Slaughter MS, Miller LW, et al. Use of an Intrapericardial, Continuous-Flow, Centrifugal Pump in Patients Awaiting Heart Transplantation. Circulation 2012;125:3191–200.

24. Mathews J, Koelling T, Pagani F, et al. The right ventricular failure risk score a pre-operative tool for assessing the risk of right ventricular failure in left ventricular assist device candidates. J Am Coll Cardiol 2008;51:2163–72.

25. Dang N, Topkara V, Mercando M, et al. Right heart failure after left ventricular assist device implantation in patients with chronic congestive heart failure. J Heart Lung Transplant 2006;25:1–6.

26. Kirklin JK, Naftel DC, Kormos RL, et al. Interagency Registry for Mechanically Assisted Circulatory Support (INTERMACS) analysis of pump thrombosis in the HeartMate II left ventricular assist device. J Heart Lung Transplant 2014;33(1): 12–22.

27. Starling R, Moazami N, Silvestry S, et al. Unexpected abrupt increase in left ventricular assist device thrombosis. N Engl J Med 2014;370:1466–7.

28. Stulak JM, Maltais S. A different perspective on thrombosis and the HeartMate II. N Engl J Med 2014;370:1467–8.

29. Maltais S, Kilic A, Nathan S, et al. PREVENTion of HeartMate II Pump Thrombosis Through Clinical Management: The PREVENT multi-center Study. J Heart Lung Transplant 2016;36(1):1–12.

30. Alba AC, Tinckam K, Foroutan F, et al. Factors associated with anti-human leukocyte antigen antibodies in patients supported with continuous-flow devices and effect on probability of transplant and post transplant outcomes. J Heart Lung Transplant 2015;34:685–92.

31. Schaffer JM, Singh S, Reitz B, et al. Heart transplant survival is improved after a reduction in panel reactive antibody activity. J Thorac Cardiovasc Surg 2013;145: 555–65.

32. Flint K, Matlock D, Lindenfeld J, et al. Frailty and the selection of patients for Destination Therapy Left Ventricular Assist Device. Circ Heart Fail 2012;5(2): 286–93.

33. Calne RY, White DJG, Thiru S, et al. Cyclosporin A in patients receiving renal allografts from cadaver donors. Lancet 1978;II:1323–7.

34. Starzl TE, Klintmalm GB, Porter KA, et al. Liver transplantation with use of cyclosporin a and prednisone. N Engl J Med 1981;305(5):266–9.

35. Steinman T, Becker B, Frost A, et al. Guidelines for the referral and management of patients eligible for solid organ transplantation. Transplantation 2001;71:1189.

36. Mehra M, Canter C, Hannan M, et al. The 2016 International Society of Heart Lung Transplantation listing criteria for heart transplantation: a 10-year update. J Heart Lung Transplant 2016;35(1):1–23.

37. OPTN Final Rule §121.8(a)(8). Available at: http://www.ecfr.gov/cgi-bin/text-idx?tpl=/ecfrbrowse/Title42/42cfr121_main_02.tpl.

38. Schulze PC, Clerkin K, Kitada S, et al. Regional differences in recipient waitlist time and pre-and post-transplant mortality following the 2006 UNOS Policy Changes in the Donor Heart Allocation Algorithm. JACC Heart Fail 2014;2(2): 166–77.

39. Davies RR, Russo MJ, Morgan JA, et al. Standard versus bicaval techniques for orthotopic heart transplantation: an analysis of the United Network for Organ Sharing database. J Thorac Cardiovasc Surg 2010;140(3):700–8.

40. Vincenti F. Immunosuppression minimization: current and future trends in transplant immunosuppression. J Am Soc Nephrol 2003;14:1940–8.

41. Tait BD, Susal C, Gabel HM, et al. Consensus guidelines on the testing and clinical management issues associated with HLA and non-HLA antibodies in transplantation. Transplantation 2013;95:19–47.

42. Lund LH, Edwards LB, Kucheryavaya AY, et al. The registry of the International Society for Heart and Lung Transplantation: thirty-first official adult heart transplant report–2014; focus theme: retransplantation. J Heart Lung Transplant 2014;33:996.

43. Mehra MR, Crespo-Leiro MG, Dipchand A, et al. International Society for Heart and Lung Transplantation working formulation of a standardized nomenclature for cardiac allograft vasculopathy-2010. J Heart Lung Transplant 2010;29:717.

44. Costanzo MR, Naftel DC, Pritzker MR, et al. Heart transplant coronary artery disease detected by coronary angiography: a multiinstitutional study of preoperative donor and recipient risk factors. Cardiac Transplant Research Database. J Heart Lung Transplant 1998;17:744.

45. Tuzcu EM, Kapadia SR, Sachar R, et al. Intravascular ultrasound evidence of angiographically silent progression in coronary atherosclerosis predicts long-term morbidity and mortality after cardiac transplantation. J Am Coll Cardiol 2005; 45:1538.

46. Lund L, Edwards L, Dipchand A, et al. The registry of the International Society for Heart and Lung Transplantation: Thirty-third Adult Heart Transplantation Report-2016. J Heart Lung Transplant 2006;35(10):1158–69.

47. Higgins R, Brown R, Chang P, et al. A multi-institutional study of malignancies after heart transplantation and a comparison with the general United States population. J Heart Lung Transplant 2014;33:478–85.

48. Jakob P, Landmesser U. Current status of cell-based therapy for heart failure. Curr Heart Fail Rep 2013 Jun;10(2):165–76.

49. D'Alessandro DA, Michler RE. Current and future status of stem cell therapy in heart failure. Curr Treat Options Cardiovasc Med 2010;12(6):614–27.

50. Weisse AB. Cardiac surgery: a century of progress. Tex Heart Inst J 2011;38(5): 486–90.

51. Copeland JG, Smith RG, Arabia FA, et al. Cardiac replacement with a total artificial heart as a bridge to transplantation. N Engl J Med 2004;351:859–67.

52. Arabia F, Gregoric I, Kasirajan V, et al. Total Artificial Heart (TAH): survival outcomes, risk factors, adverse events in intermacs. J Heart Lung Transplant 2016;35:595.

53. DePasquale E, Salimbangon A, Howell E, et al. Biventricular Bridge to Transplant: Total Artificial Heart (TAH) vs Thoratec Paracorporeal VADs (PVADs) Outcomes Post Heart Transplant (HT). J Heart Lung Transplant 2016;35:594.

Printed and bound by CPI Group (UK) Ltd, Croydon, CR0 4YY

03/10/2024

01040398-0007